Neurological Disorders and Imaging Physics, Volume 4

Application to attention deficit hyperactivity disorder

Neurological Disorders and Imaging Physics, Volume 4

Application to attention deficit hyperactivity disorder

Edited by
Ayman El-Baz
University of Louisville, Louisville, KY, USA

Jasjit S Suri
AtheroPoint, Roseville, CA, USA

IOP Publishing, Bristol, UK

ISBN 978-0-7503-1822-8 (ebook)
ISBN 978-0-7503-1799-3 (print)
ISBN 978-0-7503-1805-1 (myPrint)
ISBN 978-0-7503-1825-9 (mobi)

DOI 10.1088/978-0-7503-1822-8

Version: 20201201

IOP ebooks

British Library Cataloguing-in-Publication Data: A catalogue record for this book is available from the British Library.

Published by IOP Publishing, wholly owned by The Institute of Physics, London

IOP Publishing, Temple Circus, Temple Way, Bristol, BS1 6HG, UK

US Office: IOP Publishing, Inc., 190 North Independence Mall West, Suite 601, Philadelphia, PA 19106, USA

With love and affection to my mother and father, whose loving spirit sustains me still

— Ayman El-Baz

To my late loving parents, immediate family, and children

— Jasjit S Suri

Contents

Preface

The book covers state-of-the-art approaches for automated and early diagnosis of attention deficit hyperactivity disorder (ADHD). ADHD is a common disorder that impacts focus, self-control and other skills important in daily life. It is caused by differences in brain anatomy and wiring, and often runs in families. It can be considered as one of the most common conditions in childhood. Moreover, it impacts how kids function in school and in everyday life. Recent advances in neuroimaging techniques have enabled imaging of different brain structures and correlating the results to clinical findings, which can help in the early diagnosis of this neurological disorder. This will be covered in the book. Among the topics discussed in the book are diagnostic models for ADHD based on neuroimaging methods, application of machine learning algorithms to diagnose ADHD, classification of ADHD by using statistical features of MR images, resting-state functional magnetic resonance imaging as a potential tool for ADHD early diagnosis, brain networks, criminal behavior, supporting academic activities of children with developmental disorders and application of augmented reality in education of children with ADHD.

In summary, the main aim of this book is to help advance scientific research within the broad field of early detection of ADHD. The book focuses on major trends and challenges in this area, and it presents work aimed to identify new techniques and their use in biomedical analysis.

Ayman El-Baz
Jasjit S Suri

Acknowledgements

The completion of this book could not have been possible without the participation and assistance of so many people whose names may not all be enumerated. Their contributions are sincerely appreciated and gratefully acknowledged. However, the editors would like to express their deep appreciation and indebtedness particularly to Dr Ali H Mahmoud and Ahmed Sleman for their endless support.

Ayman El-Baz
Jasjit S Suri

Editor biographies

Ayman El-Baz

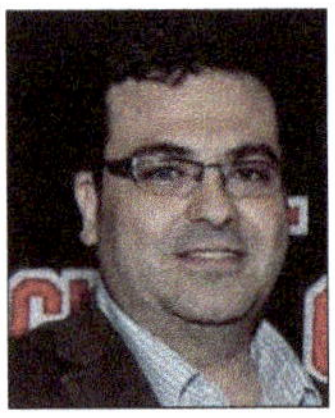

Ayman El-Baz is a Distinguished Professor, University Scholar, and Chair of the Bioengineering Department at the University of Louisville, Kentucky. He earned his BSc and MSc degrees in electrical engineering in 1997 and 2001, respectively. He earned his PhD in electrical engineering from the University of Louisville in 2006. He was named as a Fellow for Coulter, AIMBE and NAI for his contributions to the field of biomedical translational research. He has almost two decades of hands-on experience in the fields of bio-imaging modeling and non-invasive computer-assisted diagnosis systems. He has authored or coauthored more than 500 technical articles (151 journals, 29 books, 80 book chapters, 255 refereed-conference papers, 173 abstracts, and 35 US patents and Disclosures).

Jasjit S Suri

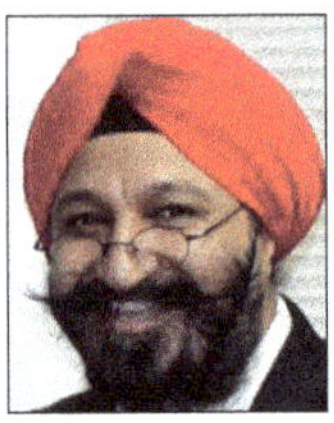

Jasjit S Suri is an innovator, scientist, visionary, industrialist and an internationally known world leader in biomedical engineering. He has spent over 25 years in the field of biomedical engineering/devices and its management. He received his PhD from the University of Washington, Seattle, and his Business Management Sciences degree from Weatherhead, Case Western Reserve University, Cleveland, Ohio. He was crowned with President's Gold medal in 1980 and made Fellow of the American Institute of Medical and Biological Engineering for his outstanding contributions. In 2018, he was awarded the Marquis Life Time Achievement Award for his outstanding contributions and dedication to medical imaging and its management

List of contributors

Dr Kamarulzaman Ab Aziz
Faculty of Management, Multimedia University, Selangor, Malaysia

Dr Nor Azlina Ab Aziz
Faculty of Engineering & Technology, Multimedia University, Melaka, Malaysia

Professor Aydin Akan
Department of Electrical and Electronics Engineering, Izmir University of Economics, Izmir, Turkey

Dr/Professor Emeritus L Eugene Arnold
Nisonger Center Clinical Trials Program/The Ohio State University, Columbus, OH, USA

Dr Alessandro O Caffò
Department of Educational Sciences, Psychology, Communication, University 'Aldo Mori' of Bari, Bari, Italy

Dr Tindara Caprì
Department of Clinical and Experimental Medicine, University of Messina, Messina, Italy

Research Assistant Gulay Cicek
Department of Software Engineering, Istanbul University-CerrahPasa, Istanbul, Turkey

Dr Pilar de Castro-Manglano
Departamento de Psiquiatria y Psicologia Medica, Clinica Universidad de Navarra, Madrid, Spain

Professor Rosa Angela Fabio
Department of Clinical and Experimental Medicine, University of Messina, Messina, Italy

Assistant Professor Saeed Farzi
K N Toosi University of Technology, Seyed khandan, Shariati Street, Tehran, Iran

Principal Researcher Won-Seok Kang
Division of Intelligent Robot/Convergence Research Center for Olfaction, DGIST, Daegu, Korea

Professor Lihua Li Li
Hangzhou Dianzi University, Xiasha, Hangzhou, Zhejiang, China

Dr Victor Pereria-Sanchez
NYU Grossman School of Medicine, New York, USA

Mr Marc Ruffinengo
Boise State University, Boise, ID, USA

Dr/Teaching assistant professor Yunhee Shin
Department of Behaviour Therapy, Daegu Cyber University, Gyeongsangbuk-do, Korea

Professor Fabrizio Stasolla
Giustino Fortunato University, Benevento, Italy

Miss Saedeh Tahery
K N Toosi University of Technology, Seyed khandan, Shariati Street, Tehran, Iran

Dr/Assistant Professor Pankhuree Vandana
Nationwide Children Hospital, Westerville, OH, USA

Dr/Assistant Professor Shikha Verma
Rogers Behavioral Health/ Rosalind Franklin University of Medicine and Science, Gurnee, IL, USA

Dr Anthony Walsh
Boise State University, Boise, ID, USA

Dr Xun-Heng Wang
Hangzhou Dianzi University, Xiasha, Hangzhou, Zhejiang, China

IOP Publishing

Neurological Disorders and Imaging Physics, Volume 4
Application to attention deficit hyperactivity disorder
Ayman El-Baz and Jasjit S Suri

Chapter 1

Diagnostic models for attention-deficit hyperactivity disorder based on neuroimaging methods

Xunheng Wang and Lihua Li

1.1 Introduction

Attention-deficit hyperactivity disorder (ADHD) is a highly prevalent brain disorder in the world. Compared to healthy normal controls, patients with ADHD exhibit inattention, hyperactivity as well as impulsivity, which are inappropriate to their age. ADHD is an ordinary disorder that is usually seen in school-age children. ADHD emerges in childhood and could persist into adulthood. According to a survey in 2005, ADHD affects nearly 5%–10% of children, and impacts about 4% of adults [1]. Although the clinical symptoms of some ADHD patients disappear with normal aging, a few adults still suffer from ADHD throughout their lives. Moreover, ADHD exhibits gender differences. Many patients are school-age boys. According to a statistical study in 2002, the rate of boy patients versus girl patients is 10:1 based on clinical investigations. However, the rate of boy patients versus girl patients is 3:1 based on community investigations [1]. Therefore, we should pay more attention to girl patients. In particular, considering the twice-exceptionality of ADHD [2], some patients exhibit high intellectual quotient (IQ) or giftedness [3]. Students with twice-exceptionality exhibit excellent performance in IQ tests, the arts and related fields, but have significant psychological or behavioral disorders, such as autism or ADHD. Previous evidence found that ADHD patients with high IQs had low risk for substance abuse and anti-social behaviors [3]. Thus, it is beneficial to investigate the brain mechanisms of ADHD and discover the twice-exceptionality for individuals, and their related families and society. However, the pathophysiology of ADHD remains unclear to the scientific community. There were several studies to investigate the neural basis of ADHD. The anterior cingulate cortex (ACC) of ADHD patients exhibited characteristic resting-state functional connectivity [4]. Altered amplitude of low-frequency fluctuations (ALFFs) of the

doi:10.1088/978-0-7503-1822-8ch1

right ACC, as well as the right inferior frontal cortex were reported in children with ADHD [5]. In addition to resting state fMRI-based studies, anatomical T1-weighted MRI has also been applied to detect the abnormal brain regions in ADHD. The cortical thickness of patients was decreased in the attention and executive brain regions [6]. The volumes of the basal ganglia were reduced in boys with ADHD [7]. Hence, it is feasible to explore the brain mechanisms for ADHD based on neuroimaging methods.

Machine learning methods are beneficial to the field of neuroscience through building the predictive models and mining the disease-related patterns. Patients with ADHD could be classified from normal controls using feature extraction and support vector machines (SVMs) [8, 9]. In order to discover the brain mechanisms of ADHD, the functional 1000 connectome projects released a datasets of patients and normal controls collected at the Medical Center of New York University, USA, in 2009. The population of these datasets were adults with ADHD and healthy individuals. The datasets contained T1-weighted structural MRI and resting state fMRI of 25 patients and age and gender matched typical developed individuals. Several studies have been published based on these datasets. In 2011, directed by Professor Michael Milham, the international neuroscience society released the ADHD-200 Consortium, which collected children with ADHD from eight medical centers around the world. In March 2011, ADHD-200 released 285 patients with ADHD and 491 typical developed individuals, which could be taken as the training samples for diagnostic models of ADHD. In July 2011, ADHD-200 released 197 individuals, which could be taken as testing samples for the diagnostic models. The goals of ADHD-200 were twofold: developing novel algorithms for discriminative analysis of ADHD based on structural MRI and resting state fMRI and developing novel methods to discover the biomarkers and the regularities of ADHD [10]. Overall, ADHD-200 Consortium provided the big data of neuroimaging for discovering the neural mechanisms of ADHD and building diagnostic models for ADHD. Based on the ADHD-200 Consortium [10], a great amount of machine learning methods were applied to diagnosis of ADHD, most of which were based on resting state fMRI techniques [11–13]. Although patients with ADHD could be identified using resting state fMRI, the functional measures were related to head motion and physiological confounds, which could bring challenges in feature extraction after data preprocessing. Notably, surface-based morphological patterns were reliable morphological measures, which exhibited excellent signal-to-noise ratio and were independent of the physiological artifacts. The regional surface-based morphological features could identify ADHD patients from healthy controls through extreme learning machines (ELMs) [14–16]. However, to the best of our knowledge, surface-based morphological features were local measures, which could not represent the brain topology of an individual with ADHD. The brain network could denote high-level cortical information than local features. Thus, building inter-regional morphological relationships from regional features is beneficial for a diagnostic model of ADHD.

The morphological connections between pairs of brain regions for a single subject remain unclear, due to the few features of the pairwise brain regions in individual anatomical MRI. So far, few studies focused on estimating the individual inter-regional morphological connectivity. Anatomical networks based on a hierarchical region of interest has been proposed to classify subjects with mild cognitive impairment (MCI) [17]. Recently, a similarity matrix using local density distribution function was applied to indicate the morphological connectivity between the two brain regions [18]. Moreover, the morphological connectivity is correlated to brain developments [19] and its test–retest reliability was excellent [20]. However, the aforementioned studies were based on voxel-based morphology (VBM) rather than surface-based morphology (SBM). Of note, cortical thickness-based inter-regional morphological features have been applied to diagnose autism spectrum disorder (ASD) [21], as well as Alzheimer's disease and MCI [22]. However, the inter-regional morphological measures based on complex regional morphological features remain unexplored to date.

In this chapter, we assumed that patients with ADHD could be classified using the inter-regional surface-based morphological features, and the predictive patterns of morphological connectivity could be revealed by machine learning methods. To test this hypothesis, a cohort of adults with and without ADHD was obtained from the publicly available functional 1000 connectome database. In the Methods section, the regional morphological features (i.e., cortical thickness, cortical curvature, brain volume, surface area, and folding index) are derived from surface-based analysis. Then, the Mahalanobis distance is used as an inter-regional surface-based morphological feature. The features of similarity matrix based on Mahalanobis distance are taken as inputs for the predictive model. The SVMs are applied to build the predictive model, which is validated by leave-one-out cross-validation (LOOCV). In addition, the diagnostic models based on functional connectivity are also investigated for comparison. In the Results section, the performance of the predictive model is evaluated by accuracy, sensitivity and specificity. In addition, the predictive weights of the features are reported by the weights of linear SVMs. In the Discussion section, we discuss the performance of the discriminative model, and explore the relationships between the discriminative patterns of morphological connectivity and clinical symptoms. In addition, the advantages and limitations are discussed for this study.

1.2 Methods

1.2.1 Study population

The subjects for this study were adults with ADHD and normal controls. The participants were recruited at the Medical Center of New York University (NYU). A cohort of 23 participants with ADHD (18 males; mean age 35.14 ± 9.75) and a cohort of 23 healthy participants (18 males; mean age 32.04 ± 9.23) were obtained from the functional 1000 connectome project. The participants were age and gender matched for this study. All patients met the criteria for combined type of ADHD in their lifetime. All participants provided signed informed consent which was approved by the institutional review boards of NYU School of Medicine. The demographics information is presented in table 1.1. The ADHD rating scale

Table 1.1. Subjects' demographic information.

	ADHD	TD	*p*-Value
Number of subjects	23	23	—
Gender (male:female)	18:5	18:5	1
Age (year)	35.14 ± 9.75	32.04 ± 9.23	0.28
Inattentive scores	17 ± 4.97	—	—
Impulsive scores	13 ± 5.28	—	—

(ADHD-RS) evaluations were only performed on the patient group, thus the ADHD-RS scores could not be obtained for the normal group.

1.2.2 MRI protocol

Anatomical and functional MRI images were obtained from the 1000 Functional Connectomes Project (http://www.nitrc.org/projects/fcon_1000/). The data-release is unrestricted for researchers to publish with any part of the dataset. Anatomical MRI and resting-state fMRI data were acquired on a Siemens Allegra 3.0 Tesla MRI scanner. A high-resolution T1-weighted three-dimensional image was scanned for each subject-based magnetization prepared gradient echo sequence with the following parameters: repetition time (TR) = 2500 ms; echo time (TE) = 4.35 ms; inversion time (T1) = 900 ms; flip angle = 8; 176 slices; field of view (FOV) = 256 mm. Resting-state fMRI images scan was scanned for each subject using the EPI sequence with the following parameters: TR = 2000 ms; TE = 25 ms; flip angle = 90; 39 slices; matrix = 64 × 64; FOV = 192 mm; acquisition voxel size = 3 mm × 3 mm × 3 mm; 192 continuous volumes.

1.2.3 Data preprocessing

1.2.3.1 Preprocessing of anatomical MRI

The anatomical MRI images were preprocessed using Freesurfer version 5.2 (http://surfer.nmr.mgh.harvard.edu). The processing procedure contained the following steps: motion correction to remove the effect of head motion; intensity normalization to remove the effect of imaging; skull strip to remove non-brain tissues; linear and nonlinear volumetric registration to normalize into standard brain space; volumetric labeling to segment the brain into sub-regions; white matter segmentation to obtain the boundaries of the cortex; surface inflation to transform into freesurfer space; spherical mapping and registration to normalize in the spherical space; cortical parcellation to segment the brain into sub-regions in the spherical space; cortical parcellation statistics to calculate the regional measures. After data processing, five features were obtained for each brain region: the mean cortical thickness, mean cortical curvature, folding index, surface area, and volume size. Of note, cortical thickness indicates the thickness of cortical ribbon between the brain skull and the whiter matter; cortical curvature and folding index represent the complex patterns of cortical folding; surface area indicates the size of cortical surface in the two-dimensional space; volume measures the size of the brain region in the three-dimensional space.

1.2.3.2 Preprocessing of resting state MRI

To obtain the normalized functional images, anatomical and resting state fMRI datasets were preprocessed using the following procedures. For each subject, the anatomical image was first skull stripped to remove non-brain tissues. Then, the anatomical image was segmented into white matter, gray matter and cerebral spinal fluid. Finally, the segmented brain volumes were nonlinearly normalized into standard MNI brain space. For each subject, the resting state fMRI datasets were preprocessed using the following steps: (1) discarding the first five functional volume to make sure the left functional volumes were in resting state; (2) slice timing to remove the effect of slice order; (3) motion correction to remove the effect of head motion; (4) skull stripping to remove non-brain tissues; (5) detrending to remove linear and nonlinear trends; (6) regressing out Friston-24 head motion parameters as well as global signals of white matter and cerebral spinal fluid; (7) temporally band-pass filtering to remove high frequency and low frequency noises; (8) nonlinearly normalizing into standard MNI space with spatial resolution of 3 mm × 3 mm × 3 mm. The above preprocessing procedures were carried out using AFNI (afni.nimh.nih.gov) and FSL (https://fsl.fmrib.ox.ac.uk/fsl/fslwiki). The batch preprocessing scripts could be found at the website of functional 1000 connectome project (http://fcon_1000.projects.nitrc.org/).

1.2.4 Feature extraction

1.2.4.1 Inter-regional morphological connectivity

For each individual, the inter-regional morphological connectivity was calculated from a pair of vectors that were composed of regional features. Here, the inter-regional morphological connectivity was calculated by the feature similarity using the Mahalanobis distance. The morphological connectivity matrix was derived from the sample covariance of the regional feature matrix. The morphological connectivity between pairwise regional measures is presented by the following formula:

$$\text{connectivity}\,(i, j) = (D - d(x_i, x_j))/D$$

where i, j denote the indices of brain regions, the feature vector x = (cortical thickness, cortical curvature, surface area, folding index, brain volume), d indicates the Mahalanobis distance and D is the next integer to the maximum of the Mahalanobis distance. The distribution of the Mahalanobis distance could be found in figure 1.1. In this study, D equals 10. In addition to the Mahalanobis distance in the above formula, other metrics of feature distances (i.e., Euclidean, Seuclidean, Cityblock, Minkowski, Chebychev, Pearson correlation) were also analyzed for comparison. The Desikan–Killiany atlas in Freesurfer was applied to segment the individual brain into subregions. The names and abbreviations of the Desikan–Killiany atlas are listed in table 1.2. The illustration of the Desikan–Killiany atlas

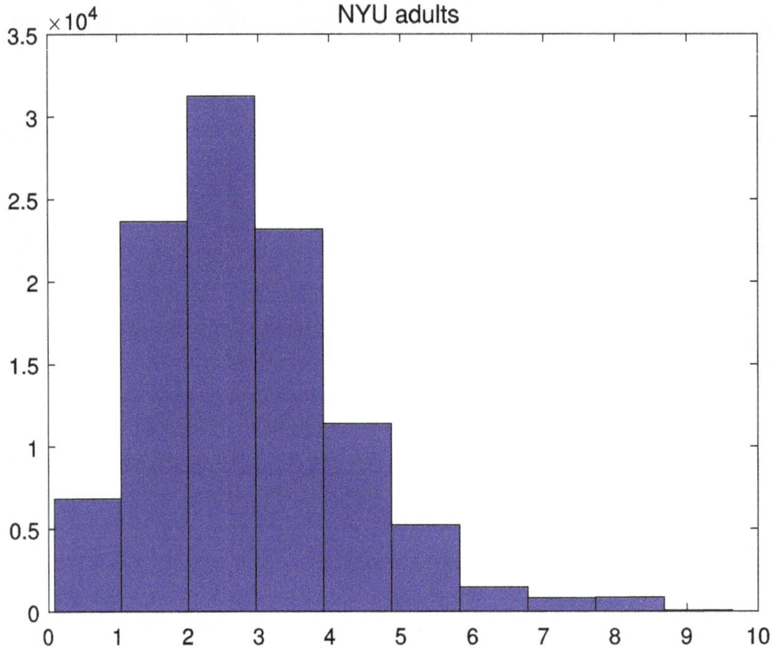

Figure 1.1. Distribution of the Mahalanobis distance.

could be found in figure 1.2. The pipeline of the inter-regional morphological connectivity could be found in figure 1.3.

1.2.4.2 Inter-regional functional connectivity

For each subject, the inter-regional functional connectivity was derived from the pairwise regional functional signals. First, for each subject, the normalized functional volumes were obtained. Then, the Desikan–Killiany atlas in MNI brain space was obtained from The IIT Human Brain Atlas (v.4.1) (https://www.nitrc.org/projects/iit/). Third, the Desikan–Killiany atlas was taken as the mask for each functional volume to obtain the regional signals. Fourth, a 187 × 68 matrix was obtained for each subject as the functional signals. Finally, a 68 × 68 connectivity matrix was obtained for each other based on Pearson correlation

$$r(m_1, m_2) = \frac{\mathrm{cov}(m_1, m_2)}{\delta_{m_1}\delta_{m_2}}$$

Here, m denotes the 187 feature vector within a brain region, cov denotes covariance, and δ denotes the standard deviation of the regional feature vector. The pipeline for functional images preproccesing could be found in figure 1.4.

Table 1.2. Names of brain regions in the Desikan–Killiany atlas.

Brain index	Brain regions	Abbreviation
1, 35	Superior frontal cortex	SFG
2, 36	Caudal middle frontal cortex	CMFG
3, 37	Rostral middle frontal cortex	RMFG
4, 38	Pars orbitalis	PORB
5, 39	Pars opercularis	POPE
6, 40	Pars triangularis	PTRI
7, 41	Lateral orbitofrontal cortex	LOF
8, 42	Medial orbitofrontal cortex	MOF
9, 43	Frontal pole	FP
10, 44	Precentral	PREC
11, 45	Paracentral	PARC
12, 46	Insula	INS
13, 47	Entorhinal cortex	ENT
14, 48	Para hippocampal	PHG
15, 49	Temporal pole cortex	TP
16, 50	Fusiform	FUSI
17, 51	Superior temporal cortex	STG
18, 52	Middle temporal cortex	MTG
19, 53	Inferior temporal cortex	ITG
20, 54	Transverse temporal cortex	TTC
21, 55	Bankssts	BSTS
22, 56	Postcentral cortex	PSTC
23, 57	Supramarginal	SMAR
24, 58	Superior parietal cortex	SPC
25, 59	Inferior parietal cortex	IPC
26, 60	Precuneus	PCUN
27, 61	Lingual	LING
28, 62	Pericalcarine	PERI
29, 63	Cuneus	CUN
30, 64	Lateral occipital cortex	LOCC
31, 65	Caudal anterior cingulate	CACC
32, 66	Rostral anterior cingulate	RACC
33, 67	Posterior cingulate	PCC
34, 68	Isthmus cingulate	ISTC

1.2.5 Diagnostic model for ADHD

Figure 1.2 shows the proposed machine learning approach consisted of feature selection and classification. First, leave-one-out cross-validation (LOOCV) was applied before feature selection and classification. In this study, the LOOCV produced 46 pairs of training and testing datasets. Second, *t*-test was applied on

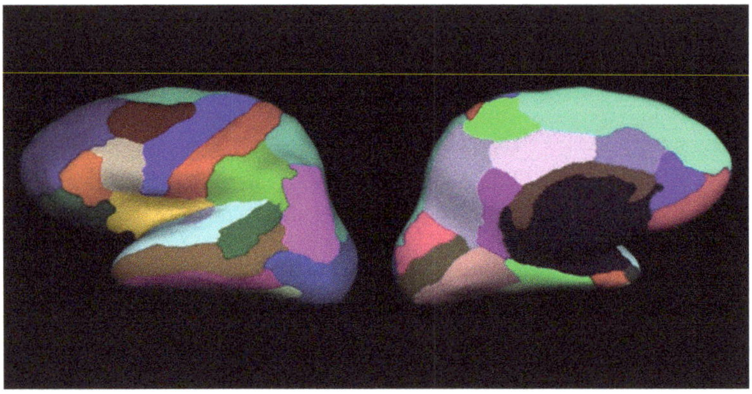

Figure 1.2. The Desikan–Killiany atlas.

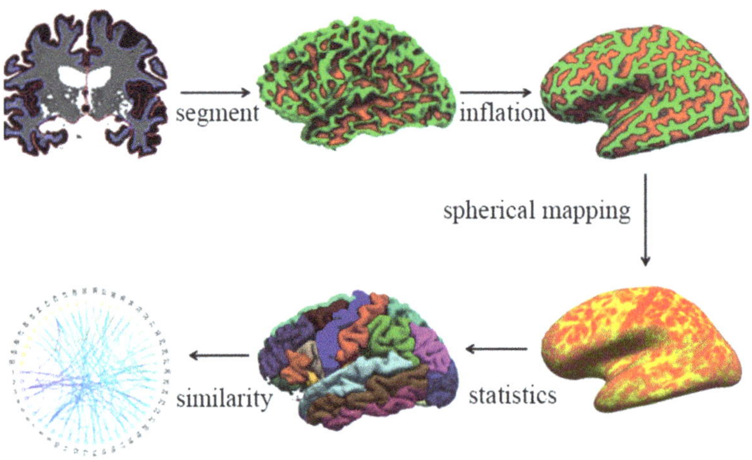

Figure 1.3. The pipeline for inter-regional morphological connectivity.

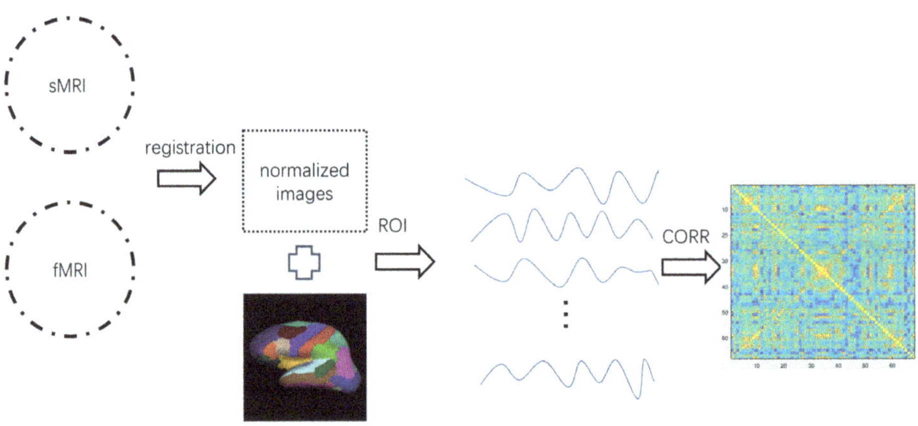

Figure 1.4. The pipeline for inter-regional functional connectivity.

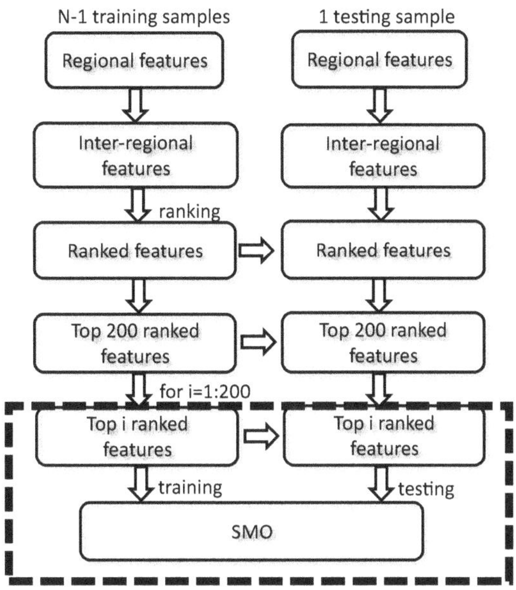

Figure 1.5. The flowchart for machine learning.

the training instances in each fold of the LOOCV. The p-values were rearranged in ascending order for feature selection. Third, support vector machine (SVM) was validated in each fold of the LOOCV after feature selection. Here, the SVMs was based on sequential minimal optimization (SMO) and implanted in WEKA (http://www.cs.waikato.ac.nz/ml/weka/). In addition, the parameter, w, which indicated the weights of the features in SVMs, was derived as the discriminative patterns of brain networks. The detailed procedures of the feature selection and the SMO could be found in [9, 23]. The pipeline for machine learning could be found in figure 1.5.

1.2.5.1 Feature selection

In this study, feature selection was performed based on t-test. For each training dataset, we divided all the datasets into ADHD group and normal control group. Then, two sample t-tests were performed on each feature using the following formula:

$$t = \frac{\bar{X}_1 - \bar{X}_2}{\sqrt{\frac{s_1^2}{n_1} + \frac{s_2^2}{n_2}}}$$

where s_i^2 is the unbiased estimator of the sample variance of each of the two groups and n_i is the number of samples in group i (1 or 2). Finally, the weights of the features were ranked by the p values in ascending order, which means that the most significant features were marked as top-ranked features.

1.2.5.2 Support vector machine

SVMs were applied to establish the predictive model. SVM was proposed by Cortes and Vapnik in 1995 [24]. SVM was one type of neural networks, and has been applied in most of the machine learning domains. SVM was originally designed for identifying two groups. SVM was also designed for machine learning problems based on small instances. The SVM has certain advantages (i.e., high-dimensional pattern recognition, solving small instance problem and nonlinear problem). Using the kernel trick, SVM mapped the original features with lower dimensions into much higher dimensions. The key idea of SVM was finding an optimized hyperplane that can classify two kinds of instances. In this study, the optimized hyperplane was searched by sequential minimal optimization (SMO), which was applied on training and testing datasets. SMO was an iterative and fast-speed algorithm, which could effectively solve the optimizing problems for SVMs [25]. Instead of the original SVMs, the trick of SMO was analytically solving a set of smallest possible sub-problems. SMO significantly improved the performance of SVMs and reduced their computation times. Furthermore, SMO exhibits significantly improved performance with linear SVMs. Here, the diagnostic model was solved by SMO with linear kernels.

1.2.5.3 Cross-validation

The discriminative models were tested using leave-one-out cross-validation (LOOCV). First, all samples were divided ino training group and testing group. Here, 46 pairs of training and testing samples were obtained based on LOOCV. Then, the discriminative models were trained on the training samples, resulting in 46 classifiers. Third, the discriminative models were tested using the testing samples, resulting in 46 testing labels. Finally, the final result was obtained by combining the testing labels as a vector. The performance of machine learning was evaluated by comparing labels and the testing outputs of the LOOCV. In particular, total accuracy, sensitivity and specificity were evaluated as the performance metrics. Here, total accuracy is the proportion of correctly predicted instances. Sensitivity is the proportion of correctly classified positive instances (i.e., patients with ADHD). Specificity is the proportion of correctly classified negative instances (i.e., normal controls). In this study, the total accuracy, sensitivity and specificity were used as evaluation metrics for model comparisons.

1.3 Results

1.3.1 Diagnostic model based on morphological connectivity

1.3.1.1 Performance of diagnostic model

The performance of diagnostic models based on morphological connectivity outperforms that based on regional measures. Figures 1.6 and 1.7 show the curves of accuracy, sensitivity and specificity of the regional feature and morphological connectivity-based classification. The horizontal axis represents the number of selected features during the leave-one-out cross-validation. The total accuracy is higher than 85% from the top 37 to 46 features. The top 45 features are selected to generate optimized discriminative patterns. The optimized accuracy, sensitivity and

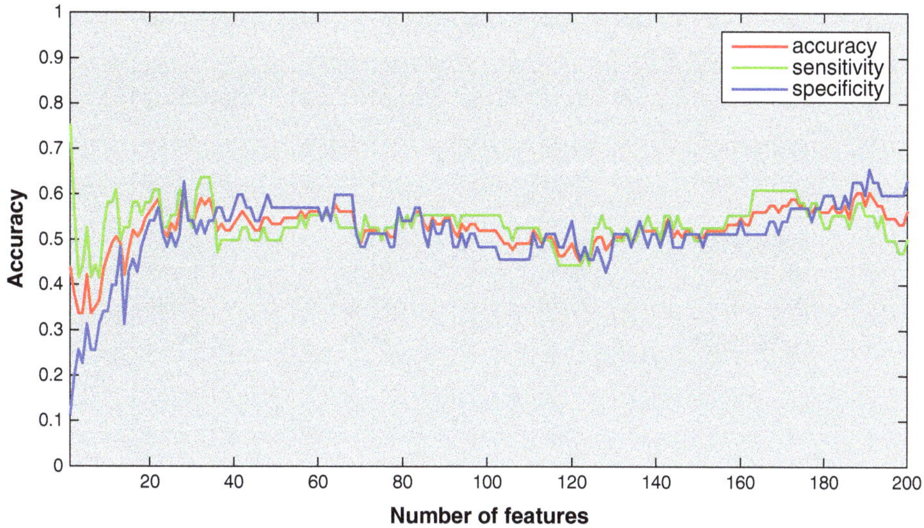

Figure 1.6. Performance of discriminative model based on regional measures.

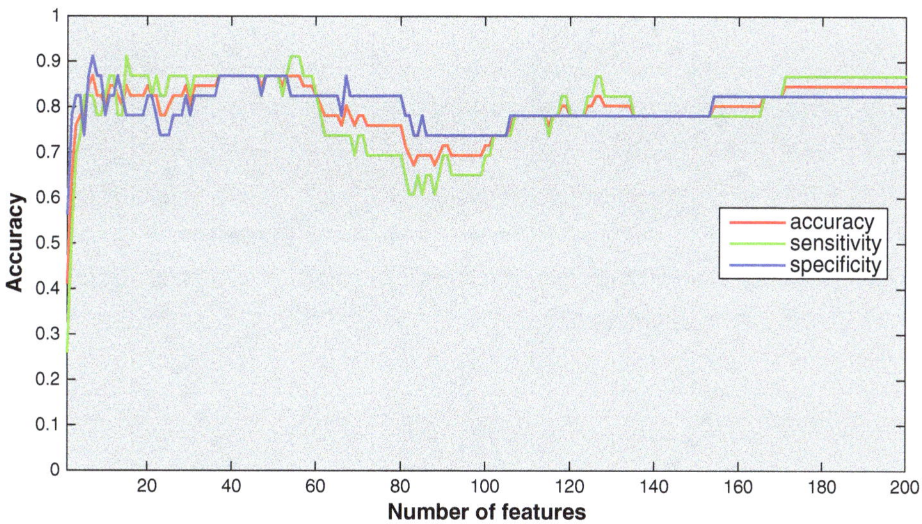

Figure 1.7. Performance of discriminative model based on mahalanobis distance.

specificity with the top 45 features are 86.96%, 86.96%, and 86.96%, respectively. In addition, the performance of classification based on different feature distances is presented in table 1.3.

1.3.1.2 Discriminative patterns of predictive model based on morphological connectivity

In total, 45 discriminative inter-regional morphological connectivities are found in figure 1.8. Adult patients with ADHD exhibit 22 enhanced and 23 decreased

Table 1.3. Performances of the discriminative models based on different metrics of feature distances.

Metric	Accuracy (%)	Sensitivity (%)	Specificity (%)
euclidean	56.52	73.91	39.13
seuclidean	86.96	100	73.91
cityblock	63.04	78.26	47.83
minkowski	56.52	73.91	39.13
chebychev	56.52	56.52	56.52
Pearson	78.26	82.61	73.91
mahalanobis	**86.96**	**86.96**	**86.96**

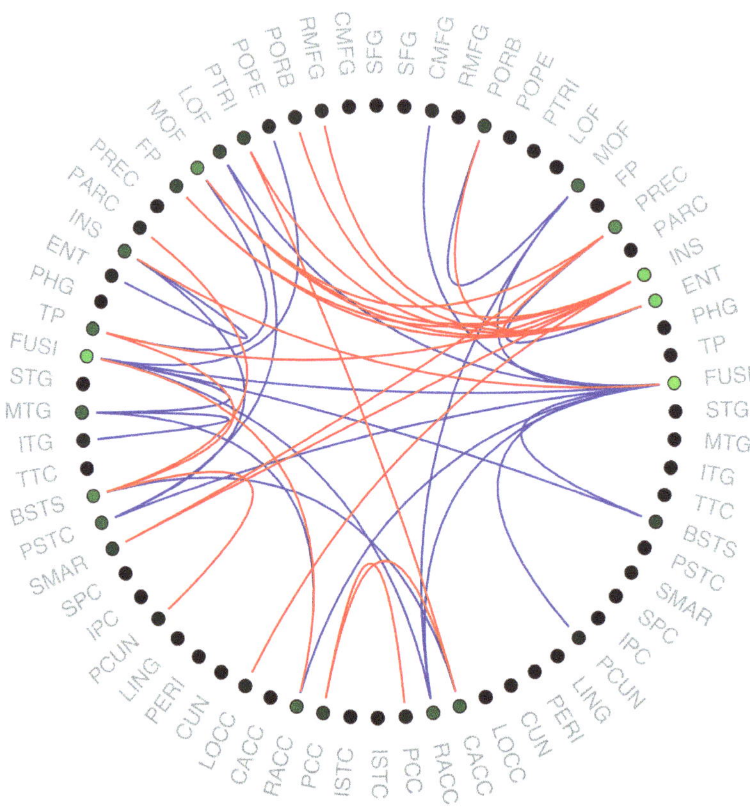

Figure 1.8. Discriminative patterns based on mahalanobis distance.

morphological connections. The altered morphological connectivity exhibits rightward lateralization in ADHD. In particular, the right fusiform gyrus-related connections are decreased to nine brain regions and increased to one brain region. The right insula-related connections are increased to seven brain regions. The right entorhinal cortex-related connections are increased to five brain regions and decreased to one brain region. The left fusiform gyrus-related connections are increased to five brain regions and decreased to one brain region. The right precuneus cortex-related connections are increased to three brain regions and decreased to one brain region.

1.3.1.3 Morphological connectivity and clinical symptoms

Figures 1.9–1.13 show the correlations between the discriminative morphological connectivity and impulsivity. The connection of the right entorhinal cortex and the left medial orbitofrontal cortex was positively related to impulsivity ($r = 0.44, p < 0.05$). The connection of right entorhinal cortex and the left par orbitalis gyrus was positively related to impulsivity ($r = 0.47$, $p < 0.05$). The connection of right entorhinal cortex and the right par orbitalis gyrus was positively related to impulsivity ($r = 0.48, p < 0.05$). The connection of right entorhinal cortex and the left frontal pole was positively related to impulsivity ($r = 0.6, p < 0.05$). The connection of right precuneus cortex and the right fusiform gyrus was positively related to impulsivity ($r = 0.43$, $p < 0.05$).

1.3.2 Predictive model based on functional connectivity

1.3.2.1 Performance of predictive model

Figure 1.14 shows the curves of accuracy, sensitivity and specificity of the functional connectivity-based classification. The diagnostic model based on functional connectivity exhibits the best performance with accuracy of 82.61%, sensitivity of 82.61% and specificity of 82.61%, respectively. The performance of diagnostic model based on functional connectivity was lower than that based on morphological connectivity. According to the number of features in the performance curves, the top eight features are selected to produce the optimized diagnostic model for ADHD.

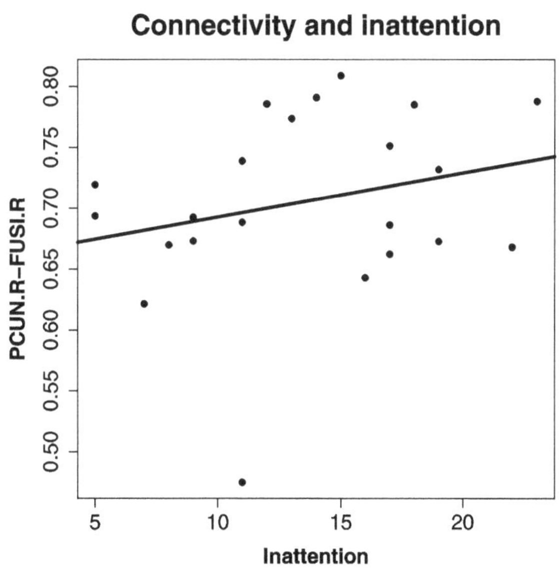

Figure 1.9. Morphological connectivity of PCUN.R−FUSI.R and inattention.

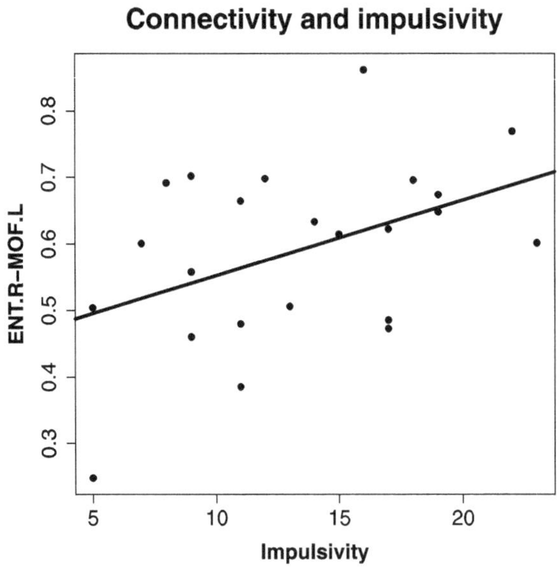

Figure 1.10. Morphological connectivity of ENT.R–MOF.L and impulsivity.

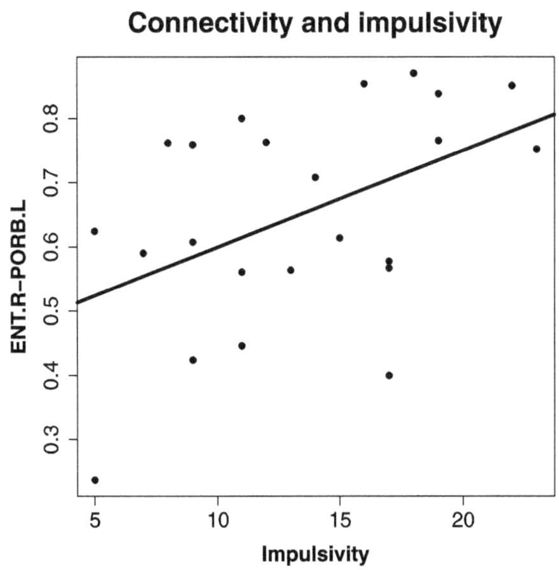

Figure 1.11. Morphological connectivity of ENT.R–PORB.L and impulsivity.

1.3.2.2 Discriminative patterns of predictive model based on functional connectivity

In total, eight discriminative inter-regional morphological connectivities are found in figure 1.15. Adult patients with ADHD exhibit eight enhanced functional connections. The altered morphological connectivity exhibits leftward lateralization

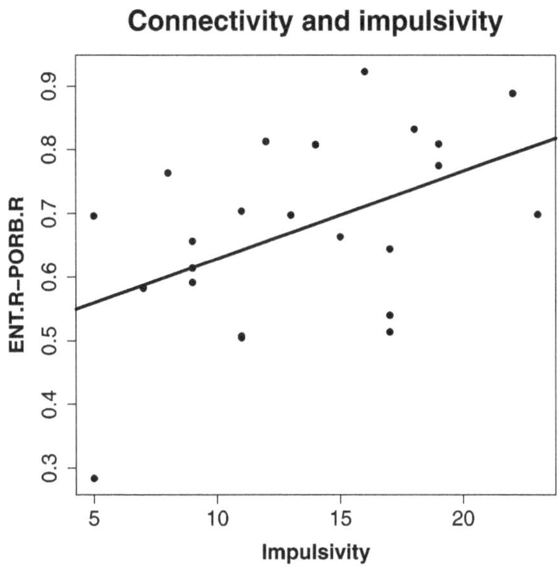

Figure 1.12. Morphological connectivity of ENT.R–PORB.R and impulsivity.

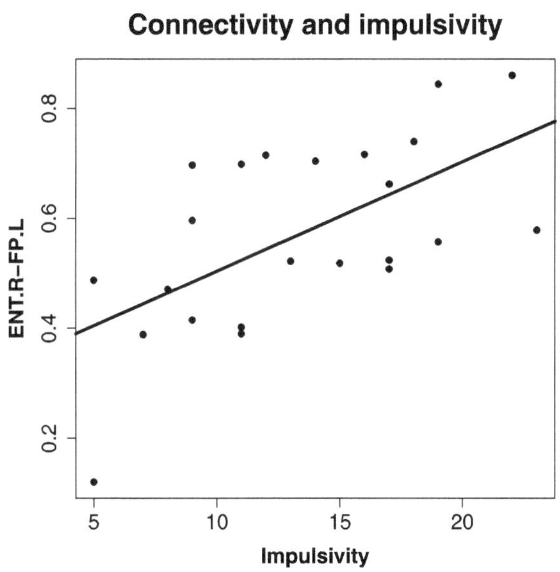

Figure 1.13. Morphological connectivity of ENT.R–FP.L and impulsivity.

in ADHD. Specially, the left entorhinal cortex-related connections are increased to six brain regions (i.e., CMFG.L, SFG.L, CMFG.R, SFG.R, MTG.R, IPC.R, IPC.L). The left hippocampus-related connections are increased to two brain regions (i.e., PREC.R, PARC.R).

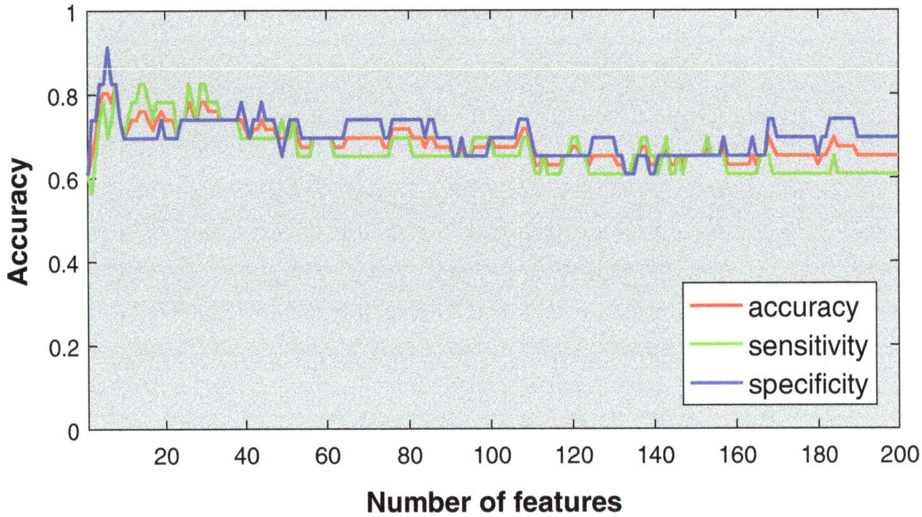

Figure 1.14. Performance of discriminative model based on functional connectivity.

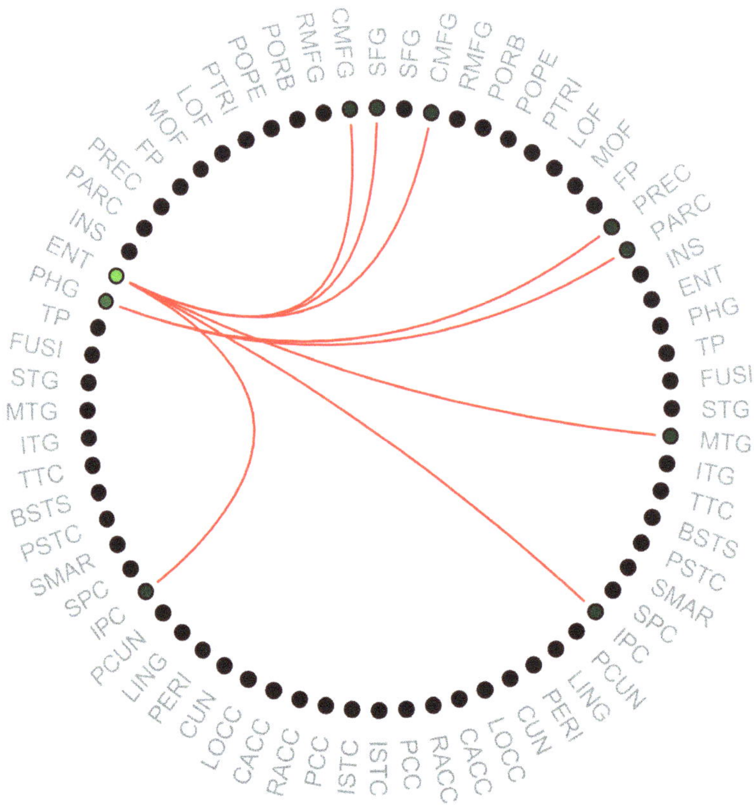

Figure 1.15. Discriminative patterns based on functional connectivity.

1.3.3 Functional connectivity and morphological connectivity

Figures 1.16 and 1.17 show the significant correlations between functional connectivity and morphological connectivity. There are 90 significant relationships ($p < 0.05$). 45 of the significant relationships are negative correlations and the left 45 relationships are positive correlations.

1.4 Discussion

This study proposed novel inter-regional morphological connectivity for a diagnostic model of ADHD and applied machine learning methods to reveal the neural network mechanisms for patients. To the best of our knowledge, this is the first attempt to find altered inter-regional morphological connectivity for adults with ADHD. Compared with the diagnostic model based on functional connectivity, the diagnostic model based on morphological connectivity exhibited high accuracy, sensitivity and specificity of classification. The altered brain network mechanisms in ADHD corresponded to previous findings. In particular, the right entorhinal cortex-related inter-regional morphological connectivity was correlated to the clinical symptoms of ADHD. In addition, the functional connectivity also exhibited

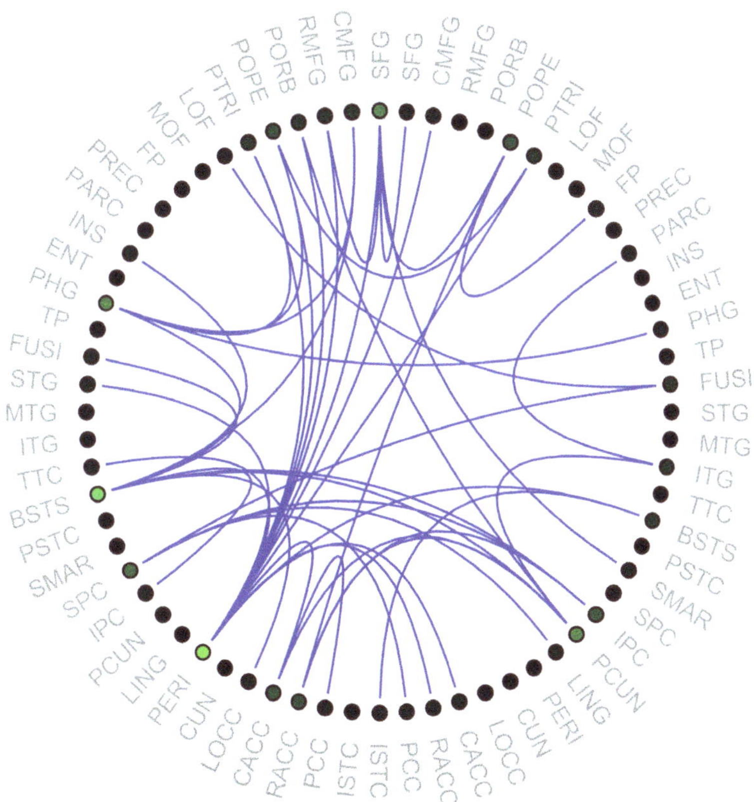

Figure 1.16. Negative correlations between morphological connectivity and functional connectivity.

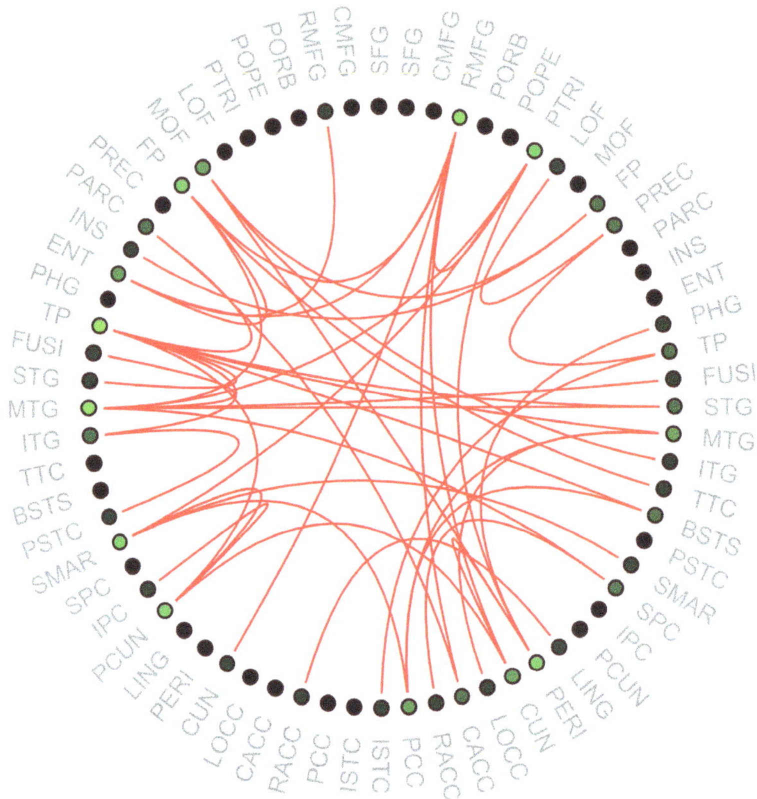

Figure 1.17. Positive correlations between morphological connectivity and functional connectivity.

discrimative power. The predictive patterns of functional connectivity were discovered using machine learning. In summary, the brain morphological network mechanisms and functional network mechanisms were altered in adults with ADHD, and the patients with ADHD could be identified by the morphological connectivity and functional connectivity.

Altered brain structures were found in patients with ADHD. Brain structure-related evidence found that patients with ADHD exhibited decreased whole brain volume, especially in the cerebellar [26]. Different from children, the volumes of hippocampus and amygdala were not decreased in adults with ADHD [27]. Cortical thickness-based evidence found decreased cortical thickness in attention and execution-related brain areas in patients with ADHD. The decreased cortical thickness-based brain areas included inferior parietal lobe, lateral dorsal prefrontal lobe and anterior cingulate cortex [6]. VBM-based evidence found decreased brain volume of bilateral cingulate cortex in adults with ADHD [28]. These results were confirmed with evidence from a large number of samples. However, with family-wise error rate correction, only the putamen nucleus exhibited decreased brain volume [29]. In addition to decreased putamen, the left parts of the bilateral basal ganglia exhibited decreased brain volumes. In particular, compared to normal developed children, boys with ADHD exhibited decreased basal ganglia. However, the brain volume of basal ganglia was not altered in girls with ADHD [7]. Moreover, the basal nucleus in ADHD was related to chronological age. In order to discover the changing patterns of cerebellar volume in patients with ADHD, a two year follow-up study found that the cerebellar volume was not decreased with brain development. However, patients with poor clinical performances exhibited decreased cerebellar volume with brain development [30]. Recently, a big data-based follow-up study (234 ADHDs versus 231 normal controls) found delayed developments of cortical thickness in patients with ADHD. About 50% of the right frontal cortex in patients with ADHD was mature at 14.6 years old. The right frontal cortex in normal controls was mature at 12.7 years old [31]. In addition to anatomical MRI-based results, the diffusion tensor imaging-based evidence found decreased fractional anisotropy (FA) in the right anterior motor region, right striatum, left cerebellum and left occipital region. The results supported the hypothesis that patients with ADHD exhibited altered white matter in frontal cortex and cerebellar [32]. Another study found that decreased FA in frontal-striatum brain areas, and no significant change in developments of myelination [33]. A 33 years follow-up study found that the FA of patients with ADHD was decreased in high functioning brain areas and sensory-motor brain areas [34]. Previous evidence found that the mean diffusivity (MD) of left inferior fasciculus longitudinalis was negatively correlated to clinical symptoms of attention, suggesting that the white matter fibers were related to attention in patients with ADHD [35]. In summary, the brain structures were altered in patients with ADHD, suggesting there were potential changes of brain functions in patients with ADHD.

Altered brain functions were found in patients with ADHD. Using the single-photon emission computed tomography (SPECT), children with ADHD exhibited decreased regional cerebral perfusion in the right middle temporal and lateral prefrontal cortex, both orbital prefrontal cortex as well as both cerebellar cortices [36]. In addition, increased regional cerebral perfusion was found in some parietal and occipital lobes (i.e., posterior brain regions). The magnetoencephalography (MEG)-based evidence found that adults with ADHD exhibited broadband deficits in medial prefrontal cortices (MPFC) [37]. Electroencephalogram (EEG)-based evidence found that the power of EEG signals in patients with ADHD was decreased in the low frequency band (i.e., 0.02–0.2 Hz) [38]. Brain lateralization-related evidence found that the left frontal cortex and middle of the brain exhibited enhanced activity [39]. Resting state fMRI has been applied to investigate the brain mechanisms of ADHD. Patients with ADHD exhibited significant resting state functional connectivities in bilateral dorsal anterior cingulate cortex, bilateral cerebellum, bilateral thalamus, bilateral insula and bilateral brainstem [4]. Functional MRI-based evidences found that the frontal-striatal structures (i.e., lateral prefrontal cortex, dorsal anterior cingulate cortex, caudate, and putamen) was altered in patients with ADHD [40]. Patients with ADHD had decreased amplitude of low-frequency fluctuation (ALFF) in the right inferior frontal cortex, left sensorimotor cortex, and bilateral cerebellum and the vermis as well as increased ALFF in the right anterior cingulated cortex, left sensorimotor cortex, and bilateral brainstem [5]. Patients with ADHD exhibited higher ALFF in the left superior frontal gyrus and sensorimotor cortex (SMC), and lower ALFF in the bilateral anterior, middle cingulate and the right middle frontal gyrus (MFG) [41]. In addition, patients with ADHD exhibited more significant resting-state activities in basic sensory and sensory-related cortices. This finding might reflect the ADHD symptoms of inattention [42]. The results suggested that ADHD might be a brain disorder of excessive approach tendencies. Children with ADHD always exhibited dysfunctions in executive function. Previous evidence found that higher resting baroreflex sensitivity could predict poorer executive function performance in children with ADHD [43]. In summary, the brain functions were altered in ADHD, suggesting there were potential changes of brain topology in patients with ADHD.

Altered brain topologies were found in patients with ADHD. The putamen ROI-based analysis found that the connections between putamen and other brain regions in boys with ADHD was decreased. The negative connection between putamen and default mode network was decreased, while the positive connection between putamen and right frontal cortex was increased [44]. The correlation and coherence-based evidence found decreased connections between the dorsal anterior cingulate cortex and default mode network in patients with ADHD [45, 46]. Another ROI-based evidence found that the connections of cortical-striatum-thalamus was related to working memory in patients with ADHD [47]. The small-worldness evidence found that patients with ADHD exhibited enhanced nodal efficiency and decreased global efficiency [48]. Of note, graph spectral entropy (GSE) was applied to investigate the complex network organizations in patients with ADHD, and found that the hub structures (i.e., bilateral pre and post central cortex, superior temporal gyrus, and inferior frontal gyri) were altered in ADHD [49]. Task-based fMRI found that the brain activities of ADHD patients were missing during attention tasks and working memory tasks, and exhibited poorer and slower performance during tasks [50]. Another study found that the brain activities of ADHD patients were reduced during tasks [51]. Moreover, previous studies found that the brain functional connectivity was related to clinical symptoms [52]. In particular, the dysfunction of default mode network in ADHD has been reported by many studies. The abnormal cingulate-precuneus interactions has been found in patients with ADHD [53]. The abnormal connections between precuneus and other default-mode network components (i.e., ventromedial prefrontal cortex) have been reported. Another study noted that the network homogeneity of precuneus was decreased in patients with ADHD [54]. The coherency of default mode network connectivity was reduced in patients with ADHD [55]. The independent component analysis (ICA) found enhanced coherence of left dorsolateral prefrontal cortex and default mode network [56]. In summary, the functional connectivity of default mode network was altered in patients with ADHD, which might imply the dysfunction of frontal lobe-striatum-cerebellum circuits in ADHD. In addition to default mode network, abnormal frontal-parietal network, attention networks, visual networks and sensory-motor network were found in ADHD. Overall, the brain topologies based on functional connectivity were altered in ADHD. However, the brain topology based on morphological connectivity remains unexplored.

Investigating the individual inter-regional morphological connectivity is an interesting research topic in the field of anatomical MRI. There were few investigations focused on exploring the individual morphological connectivity using anatomical MRI, since each subject had only one volume of T1-weighted MRI images. Thus, it is difficult to derive individual morphological connectivity from anatomical MRI for a single subject. Recently, several groups started to explore individual morphological connectivity using metrics that is based on feature distances. Previous studies suggested that high-order cortical information could be derived from the inter-regional morphological connectivity. The hippocampus-related morphological connectivity exhibited discriminative power for MCI classification [17]. The auditory and language area-related morphological connectivity exhibited significant rightward lateralization in the autistic brain [22]. Moreover, the high-order cortical features, which contains more information than regional features, could be beneficial to a discriminative model of brain disorder. The biological explanations for the inter-regional morphological connectivity remain unexplored. One assumption is that morphologically similar brain regions might be structurally connected to each other according to axon tension theory [18]. Another possible assumption is that the functionally connected brain regions should exhibited similar structures in order to transmit information. In summary, inter-regional morphological connectivity contained high-level cortical information and could be beneficial to probe brain disorder.

The performance of classification is important for a diagnostic model. Our method of classification exhibited excellent accuracy (86.96%), sensitivity (86.96%) and specificity (86.96%). There were a great number of methods to build a diagnostic model for ADHD. Fisher discriminative analysis was applied to identify patients with ADHD based on regional homogeneity of resting state fMRI. The classification accuracy was 85%, and sensitivity was 78% [8]. Feature selection and SVM could discriminate patients with ADHD from normal controls, and achieved prediction accuracy of 80% and sensitivity of 87% [9]. Around 2012, several machine learning methods were applied to classify ADHD. Based on the brain-wise association study, SVM could identify ADHD with classification accuracy of 76.15%, sensitivity of 63.27%, and specificity of 85.11% [13]. Multi kernel learning could classify ADHD with classification accuracy of 67.79%, sensitivity of 38.29%, and specificity 84.08% [11]. Using the multiple support vector machine recursive feature elimination (SVM-RFE) algorithm, SVM could predict ADHD with total accuracy of 55%, sensitivity of 33%, and specificity of 80% [12]. However, most of these studies could not reach satisfactory scores of accuracy, sensitivity and specificity at the same time, which means that those methods were not suitable for clinical applications. In 2013, extreme learning machines (ELMs) were applied to diagnosis of ADHD with total accuracy of 90.18% based on regional features of anatomical MRI [14]. However, the feature selection procedure was out of cross-validation, which means that the performance of the classifiers was overestimated. Recently, an ELM could identify subtypes of ADHD and achieve total accuracy of

60.78% based on regional features [15]. Using multimodal features, an ELM could predict subtypes of ADHD with total accuracy of 76.19% [16]. However, the algorithms of the ELM were complex, thus the implementation of the algorithms was difficult to program. In addition, the algorithms of the ELM were based on random mapping, which means that the results of the ELM were unstable for diagnostic models. Moreover, the procedure of the ELM was a blackbox, thus it could not find the discriminative patterns during machine learning. Of note, our feature selection method based SVM could obtain good performance of total accuracy, sensitivity and specificity at the same time, suggesting potential values in clinical applications. Moreover, the discriminative patterns discovered by the SVMs were more explainable than previous methods.

Several discriminative patterns of the morphological connectivity were related to ADHD, according to the data mining method. In this study, the bilateral fusiform gyrus exhibited decreased morphological connectivity. The right entorhinal cortex and the right insula demonstrated increased morphological connectivity. Moreover, several discriminative patterns of the functional connectivity were related to ADHD, according to the discriminative weights of SVMs. In particular, the left entorhinal-related functional connections were altered in patients with ADHD. The left hippocampus-related functional connections were also altered in the patient group. In previous study, the fusiform-related resting state networks could predict the intelligence quotient (IQ) for ADHD [57]. The altered fusiform-related morphological connectivity might reflect the deficits of facial recognition in patients with ADHD [58]. The altered insula-based morphological connectivity might be related to the dysfunction of emotion regulation in ADHD. The bilateral insula exhibited enhanced resting state functional connectivity in patients with ADHD [4]. The insula also exhibited altered regional homogeneity in adults with ADHD [9]. The altered entorhinal-related connection might reflect the deficits of spatial learning in ADHD [59]. In addition, the right entorhinal cortex-related morphological connections were related to clinical symptoms (i.e., impulsivity). A recent study found that the morphological connectivity could predict individual impulsivity for healthy adults [60], suggesting the potential predictive power of morphological connectivity for behavioral phenotype. In summary, adults with ADHD exhibited distinctive morphological network, which might reflect the clinical behaviors of patients.

Significant relationships between the morphological connectivity and functional connectivity were found in this study. The functional connectivity denoted the functional similarities between the two brain regions. The morphological connectivity might represent the structural similarities between the two brain regions. The morphological connectivity might reflect the functional connectivity in some brain nodes. Both positive and negative relationships were found between morphological connectivity and functional connectivity. The results suggested that a pair of morphologically correlated brain regions might be functionally correlated to each other. Thus, the morphological connectivity might have functional meanings. In summary, the morphological connectivity and functional connectivity were significantly related to each other in some brain regions.

The pairwise functionally connected brain regions might exhibit certain morphological similarities.

One advantage of this study was investigating the individual inter-regional morphological connectivity based on structural MRI, which could not be affected by physiological artifacts. Of note, the anatomical MRI could derive regional features with high test-retest reliability. Thus, the inter-regional morphological connectivity was reliable for a diagnostic model. Another advantage of this study was investigating the neural basis of ADHD based on high-level cortical information, which could capture the brain topology based on anatomical MRI. Thus, the inter-regional morphological connectivity could provide more topology information than regional features. Moreover, the performance of diagnostic model based on morphological connectivity outperformed that based on functional connectivity. The third advantage was applying feature selection before classification in each fold of cross-validation, resulting in unbiased classification. Feature selection could shrink the original raw features into a small subset with lower dimensions. Thus, the selected features were more interpretable than the raw features in original space. The fourth advantage was applying linear kernel with SMO to perform SVMs. The predictive weights discovered by linear kernel in SVM could provide valuable biomarkers for patients with ADHD. The discriminative weights were more interpretable than other machine learning methods (i.e., ELM). In addition, the discriminate patterns of the brain network mechanisms were related to the clinical scores of ADHD. In summary, we proposed novel inter-regional morphological connectivity patterns based on anatomical MRI for ADHD. The proposed inter-regional morphological relationships were beneficial for a diagnostic model of ADHD, and could underlie the brain network mechanisms for patients.

One limitation of this study was the biological meanings of the proposed inter-regional morphological connectivity. Biological interpretability was important for the proposed novel bio-metrics. In this study, functional fMRI was applied in the diagnostic model, suggesting there was a potential functional basis for the morphological connectivity. However, the relationships bewteen morphological connectivity and functional connectivity remains unexplored. Multimodal MRI should be applied to explore the proposed inter-regional morphological connectivity in future study. Another limitation was not considering the subtypes of ADHD, which exhibited different patterns of clinical symptoms. The subtypes of ADHD should be taken into consideration in future study. The third limitation was not considering different kinds of classifiers, although SVM is a well-validated classifier. Neural network-based classifiers should be considered in future study. In addition, the performance of different feature selection methods should be compared in additional studies. The fourth limitation of this study was the population of patients and normal controls. The effects of different ages, different genders, different MRI protocols, and different scanners should be considered in future study. In summary, this perspective study could be expanded in different ways by additional studies.

1.5 Conclusion

In this chapter, we reviewed neuroimaging-related studies for ADHD. In particular, we proposed a novel inter-regional morphological connectivity to classify patients with ADHD. In addition, we also built the predictive model for ADHD based on conventional functional connectivity. The diagnostic model based on inter-regional morphological connectivity outperformed that based on conventional functional connectivity. Predictive patterns were found using the discriminative weights of linear SMO. In summary, patients with ADHD exhibited altered inter-regional morphological connectivity as well as functional connectivity, which could be a potential biomarker for a diagnostic model of ADHD. The predictive features could be beneficial to investigating the neural basis for ADHD.

References

[1] Biederman J 2005 Attention-deficit/hyperactivity disorder: a selective overview *Biol. Psychiatry* **57** 1215–20

[2] Budding D and Chidekel D 2012 ADHD and giftedness: a neurocognitive consideration of twice exceptionality *Appl. Neuropsychol. Child* **1** 145–51

[3] Antshel K M 2008 Attention-deficit hyperactivity disorder in the context of a high intellectual quotient/giftedness *Dev. Disabil. Res. Rev.* **14** 293–9

[4] Tian L *et al* 2006 Altered resting-state functional connectivity patterns of anterior cingulate cortex in adolescents with attention deficit hyperactivity disorder *Neurosci. Lett.* **400** 39–43

[5] Zang Y-F, He Y, Zhu C-Z, Cao Q-J, Sui M-Q, Liang M, Tian L-X, Jiang T-Z and Wang Y-F 2007 Altered baseline brain activity in children with ADHD revealed by resting-state functional MRI *Brain Dev.* **29** 83–91

[6] Makris N, Biederman J, Valera E M, Bush G, Kaiser J, Kennedy D N, Caviness V S, Faraone S V and Seidman L J 2007 Cortical thinning of the attention and executive function networks in adults with attention-deficit/hyperactivity disorder *Cereb Cortex* **17** 1364–75

[7] Qiu A, Crocetti D, Adler M, Mahone E M, Denckla M B, Miller M I and Mostofsky M D 2009 Basal ganglia volume and shape in children with attention deficit hyperactivity disorder *Am. J. Psychiatry* **166** 74–82

[8] Zhu C-Z, Zang Y-F, Cao Q-J, Yan C-G, He Y, Jiang T-Z, Sui M-Q and Wang Y-F 2008 Fisher discriminative analysis of resting-state brain function for attention-deficit/hyperactivity disorder *NeuroImage* **40** 110–20

[9] Wang X, Jiao Y, Tang T, Wang H and Lu Z 2013 Altered regional homogeneity patterns in adults with attention-deficit hyperactivity disorder *Eur. J. Radiol.* **82** 1552–7

[10] Milham M P, Fair D, Mennes M and Mostofsky S H 2012 The ADHD-200 consortium: a model to advance the translational potential of neuroimaging in clinical neuroscience *Front Syst. Neurosci.* **6** 1–5

[11] Dai D, Wang J, Hua J and He H 2012 Classification of ADHD children through multimodal magnetic resonance imaging *Front Syst. Neurosci.* **6** 1–8

[12] Colby J B, Rudie J D, Brown J A, Douglas P K, Cohen M S and Shehzad Z 2012 Insights into multimodal imaging classification of ADHD *Front Syst. Neurosci.* **6** 59

[13] Cheng W, Ji X, Zhang J and Feng J 2012 Individual classification of ADHD patients by integrating multiscale neuroimaging markers and advanced pattern recognition techniques *Front Syst. Neurosci.* **6** 58

[14] Peng X, Lin P, Zhang T and Wang J 2013 Extreme learning machine-based classification of ADHD using brain structural MRI data *PLoS One* **8** e79476
[15] Qureshi M N, Min B, Jo H J and Lee B 2016 Multiclass classification for the differential diagnosis on the ADHD subtypes using recursive feature elimination and hierarchical extreme learning machine: structural MRI study *PLoS One* **11** e0160697
[16] Qureshi M N I, Oh J, Min B, Jo H J and Lee B 2017 Multi-modal, multi-measure, and multi-class discrimination of ADHD with hierarchical feature extraction and extreme learning machine using structural and functional brain MRI *Front Hum. Neurosci.* **11** 157
[17] Zhou L, Wang Y, Li Y, Yap P T, Shen D and Alzheimer's Disease Neuroimaging I Hierarchical anatomical brain networks for MCI prediction: revisiting volumetric measures *PLoS One* **6** e21935
[18] Kong X-Z, Wang X, Huang L, Pu Y, Yang Z, Dang X, Zhen Z and Liu J 2014 Measuring individual morphological relationship of cortical regions *J. Neurosci. Methods* **237** 103–7
[19] Kong X Z, Liu Z, Huang L, Wang X, Yang Z, Zhou G, Zhen Z and Liu J 2015 Mapping individual brain networks using statistical similarity in regional morphology from MRI *PLoS One* **10** e0141840
[20] Wang H, Jin X, Zhang Y and Wang J 2016 Single-subject morphological brain networks: connectivity mapping, topological characterization and test-retest reliability *Brain Behav.* **6** e00448
[21] Wee C Y, Yap P T, Shen D and Alzheimer's Disease Neuroimaging I 2013 Prediction of Alzheimer's disease and mild cognitive impairment using cortical morphological patterns *Hum. Brain Mapp.* **34** 3411–25
[22] Wee C Y, Wang L, Shi F, Yap P T and Shen D 2014 Diagnosis of autism spectrum disorders using regional and interregional morphological features *Hum. Brain Mapp.* **35** 3414–30
[23] Wang X H, Jiao Y and Li L 2018 Diagnostic model for attention-deficit hyperactivity disorder based on interregional morphological connectivity *Neurosci. Lett.* **685** 30–4
[24] Cortes C and Vapnik V N 1995 Support-vector networks *Mach. Learn.* **297** 273–97
[25] Platt J C 1999 Fast training of support vector machines using sequential minimal optimization *Advances in Kernel Methods* (Cambridge, MA: MIT Press) pp 185–208
[26] Kelly a M C, Margulies D S and Castellanos F X 2007 Recent advances in structural and functional brain imaging studies of attention-deficit/hyperactivity disorder *Curr. Psychiatry Rep.* **9** 401–7
[27] Perlov E, Philipsen A, Tebartz van Elst L, Ebert D, Henning J and Maier S *et al* 2008 Hippocampus and amygdala morphology in adults with attention-deficit hyperactivity disorder *J. Psychiatry Neurosci.* **33** 509–15
[28] Amico F, Stauber J, Koutsouleris N and Frodl T 2011 Anterior cingulate cortex gray matter abnormalities in adults with attention deficit hyperactivity disorder: a voxel-based morphometry study *Psychiatry Res.* **191** 31–5
[29] Seidman L J, Biederman J, Liang L, Valera E M, Monuteaux M C, Brown A, Kaiser J, Spencer T, Faraone S V and Makris N 2011 Gray matter alterations in adults with attention-deficit/hyperactivity disorder identified by voxel based morphometry *Biol. Psychiatry* **69** 857–66
[30] Mackie S, Shaw P, Lenroot R, Pierson R, Greenstein D K, Nugent T F, Sharp W S, Jay N, Giedd M D and Rapoport J L 2007 Cerebellar development and clinical outcome in attention deficit hyperactivity disorder *Am. J. Psychiatry* **164** 647–55

[31] Shaw P, Malek M, Watson B, Sharp W, Evans A and Greenstein D 2012 Development of cortical surface area and gyrification in attention-deficit/hyperactivity disorder *Biol. Psychiatry* **72** 191–7

[32] Ashtari M *et al* 2005 Attention-deficit/hyperactivity disorder: a preliminary diffusion tensor imaging study *Biol. Psychiatry* **57** 448–55

[33] de Zeeuw P, Mandl R C W, Hulshoff Pol H E, van Engeland H and Durston S 2012 Decreased frontostriatal microstructural organization in attention deficit/hyperactivity disorder *Hum. Brain Mapp.* **33** 1941–51

[34] Cortese S, Imperati D, Zhou J, Proal E, Klein R G, Mannuzza S, Ramos-Olazagasti M A, Milham M P, Kelly C and Castellanos F X 2013 White matter alterations at 33-year follow-up in adults with childhood attention-deficit/hyperactivity disorder *Biol. Psychiatry* **74** 591–8

[35] Konrad A, Dielentheis T F, Masri D E, Dellani P R, Stoeter P, Vucurevic G and Winterer G 2012 White matter abnormalities and their impact on attentional performance in adult attention-deficit/hyperactivity disorder *Eur. Arch. Psychiatry Clin. Neurosci.* **262** 351–60

[36] Kim B-N, Lee J-S, Shin M-S, Cho S-C and Lee D-S 2002 Regional cerebral perfusion abnormalities in attention deficit/hyperactivity disorder. Statistical parametric mapping analysis. *Eur. Arch. Psychiatry Clin. Neurosci.* **252** 219–25

[37] Wilson T W, Franzen J D, Heinrichs-Graham E, White M L, Knott N L and Wetzel M W 2011 Broadband neurophysiological abnormalities in the medial prefrontal region of the default-mode network in adults with ADHD *Hum. Brain Mapp.* **34** 566–74

[38] Helps S K, Broyd S J, James C J, Karl A, Chen W and Sonuga-Barke E J S 2010 Altered spontaneous low frequency brain activity in attention deficit/hyperactivity disorder *Brain Res.* **1322** 134–43

[39] Keune P M, Schönenberg M, Wyckoff S, Mayer K, Riemann S, Hautzinger M and Strehl U 2011 Frontal alpha-asymmetry in adults with attention deficit hyperactivity disorder: replication and specification *Biol. Psychology* **87** 306–10

[40] Bush G, Valera E M and Seidman L J 2005 Functional neuroimaging of attention-deficit/hyperactivity disorder: a review and suggested future directions *Biol. Psychiatry* **57** 1273–84

[41] Yang H, Wu Q-Z, Guo L-T, Li Q-Q, Long X-Y, Huang X-Q, Chan R C K and Gong Q-Y 2011 Abnormal spontaneous brain activity in medication-naïve ADHD children: a resting state fMRI study *Neurosci. Lett.* **502** 89–93

[42] Tian L, Jiang T, Liang M, Zang Y, He Y, Sui M and Wang Y 2008 Enhanced resting-state brain activities in ADHD patients: a fMRI study *Brain Dev.* **30** 342–8

[43] Dietrich A, Althaus M, Hartman C a, Buitelaar J K, Mindera R B, van den Hoofdakker B J and Hoekstra P J 2012 Baroreflex sensitivity during rest and executive functioning in attention-deficit/hyperactivity disorder. The TRAILS study *Biol. Psychology* **90** 249–57

[44] Cao X, Cao Q, Long X, Sun L, Sui M, Zhu C, Zuo X, Zang Y and Wang Y 2009 Abnormal resting-state functional connectivity patterns of the putamen in medication-naïve children with attention deficit hyperactivity disorder *Brain Res.* **1303** 195–206

[45] Sato J R, Hoexter M Q, Castellanos X F and Rohde L A 2012 Abnormal brain connectivity patterns in adults with ADHD: a coherence study *PLoS One* **7** e45671

[46] Sun L *et al* 2012 Abnormal functional connectivity between the anterior cingulate and the default mode network in drug-naïve boys with attention deficit hyperactivity disorder *Psychiatry Res.* **201** 120–7

[47] Mills K L *et al* 2012 Altered cortico-striatal-thalamic connectivity in relation to spatial working memory capacity in children with ADHD *Front Psychiatry* **3** 2

[48] Wang L, Zhu C, He Y, Zang Y, Cao Q, Zhang H, Zhong Q and Wang Y 2009 Altered small-world brain functional networks in children with attention-deficit/hyperactivity disorder *Hum. Brain Mapp.* **30** 638–49
[49] Sato J R, Takahashi D Y, Hoexter M Q, Massirer K B and Fujita A 2013 Measuring network's entropy in ADHD: a new approach to investigate neuropsychiatric disorders *NeuroImage* **77** 44–51
[50] Stevens M C, Ph D, Pearlson G D and Kiehl K A 2007 An fMRI auditory oddball study of combined-subtype attention deficit hyperactivity disorder *Am. J. Psychiatry* 1737–49
[51] Fassbender C, Schweitzer J B, Cortes C R, Tagamets M a, Windsor T A, Reeves G M and Gullapalli R 2011 Working memory in attention deficit/hyperactivity disorder is characterized by a lack of specialization of brain function *PLoS One* **6** e27240
[52] Mennes M, Vega Potler N, Kelly C, Di Martino A, Castellanos F X and Milham M P 2011 Resting state functional connectivity correlates of inhibitory control in children with attention-deficit/hyperactivity disorder *Front Psychiatry* **2** 83
[53] Castellanos F X *et al* 2008 Cingulate–precuneus interactions: a new locus of dysfunction in adult attention-deficit/hyperactivity disorder *Biol. Psychiatry* **63** 332–7
[54] Uddin L Q *et al* 2008 Network homogeneity reveals decreased integrity of default-mode network in ADHD. *J. Neurosci. Methods* **169** 249–54
[55] Fair D a, Posner J, Nagel B J, Bathula D, Dias T G C, Mills K L, Blythe M S, Giwa A, Schmitt C F and Nigg J T 2010 Atypical default network connectivity in youth with attention-deficit/hyperactivity disorder *Biol. Psychiatry* **68** 1084–91
[56] Hoekzema E *et al* 2014 An independent components and functional connectivity analysis of resting state fMRI data points to neural network dysregulation in adult ADHD *Hum. Brain Mapp.* **35** 1261–72
[57] Wang X H and Li L 2015 Altered temporal features of intrinsic connectivity networks in boys with combined type of attention deficit hyperactivity disorder *Eur. J. Radiol.* **84** 947–54
[58] Ibanez A *et al* 2011 Cortical deficits of emotional face processing in adults with ADHD: its relation to social cognition and executive function *Soc. Neurosci.* **6** 464–81
[59] Terry A V Jr, Hernandez C M, Buccafusco J J and Gattu M 2000 Deficits in spatial learning and nicotinic-acetylcholine receptors in older, spontaneously hypertensive rats *Neuroscience* **101** 357–68
[60] Li J and Kong X Z 2017 Morphological connectivity correlates with trait impulsivity in healthy adults *PeerJ* **5** e3533

IOP Publishing

Neurological Disorders and Imaging Physics, Volume 4
Application to attention deficit hyperactivity disorder
Ayman El-Baz and Jasjit S Suri

Chapter 2

Application of machine learning algorithms to diagnosis attention deficit hyperactivity disorder

Saedeh Tahery and Saeed Farzi

2.1 Introduction

This chapter is going to paraphrase applications of machine learning techniques in diagnosing attention deficit hyperactivity disorder, hereafter, called ADHD. Initially, the overall architecture of the machine learning systems, which consists of three main components, namely, data collection, feature engineering, and learning algorithm, is described. Next, the evaluation criteria of machine learning systems are explained, and eventually, some related research works are presented in more detail.

The data collection is the first component of machine learning which highly affects the system's effectiveness. Effective machine learning is difficult due to the high dependence on the type and amount of data. In recent practices, EEG signal, fMRI, and test-based data have been the most used data types employed by researchers. As to the amount of data, ADHD-200 and Truven are standard and well-known ADHD datasets that work as training and testing data in machine learning systems.

Feature engineering used to identify sophisticated features in the diagnosis of ADHD is the second major component of machine learning systems. This component promotes the quality of machine learning output through the worthless features' removal. Although there are several techniques for feature engineering, in this chapter, PCA and LDA are described as two main methods of linear transformation.

The last and vital component of machine learning systems is the learning algorithm that learns the rules and patterns needed to diagnose ADHD during the training phase. The learning algorithm identifies the rules and patterns of ADHD diagnosis by examining the features and their weights. Exploring the previous

doi:10.1088/978-0-7503-1822-8ch2

related works implies that the most used algorithms are SVM, decision tree, logistic regression, and artificial neural networks, which are explained in more detail.

Once you have prepared your data, identified the sophisticated features, and run the learning algorithm, you need to test and evaluate the system. Sensitivity, specificity, accuracy, and Kappa score are four widely used evaluation measures to assess the performance of a machine learning system output.

This chapter introduces a novel taxonomy of previous works. The related works are studied from two perspectives, i.e., algorithm and data type. The algorithm and data type perspectives divide the related works into 16 and 4 groups, respectively. In the last and important section, the latest and best works of every group are described.

The remaining parts of the chapter are constituted as follows. Sections 2.2 and 2.3 present the system architecture and evaluation criteria, respectively. Recent works are studied in section 2.4.

2.2 System architecture

As shown in figure 2.1, there are three main components: data collection, feature engineering, and learning algorithm in an automatic ADHD diagnosis system using machine learning approaches. The most important question to be answered about collecting data is which type of data should be considered. The most common types of data are images, signals, question forms, and so on. Some research works take into account one type of data, and others use a combination of them.

To provide appropriate features for learning algorithms such as classifiers, feature engineering is embedded as the second component of the system. There are a large number of features in the collected datasets, and it is impossible to consider all of them in classification algorithms due to the curse of dimensionality problem [1]. Therefore, relevant and informative features are gained by feature extraction and feature selection methods.

The learning algorithm is the third component of the system aimed at building a model to distinguish the ADHD-patients from healthy people. There is a wide range of classifier algorithms, including decision trees, neural networks, support vector machines, and so on.

In the following, data types and features are described in more detail.

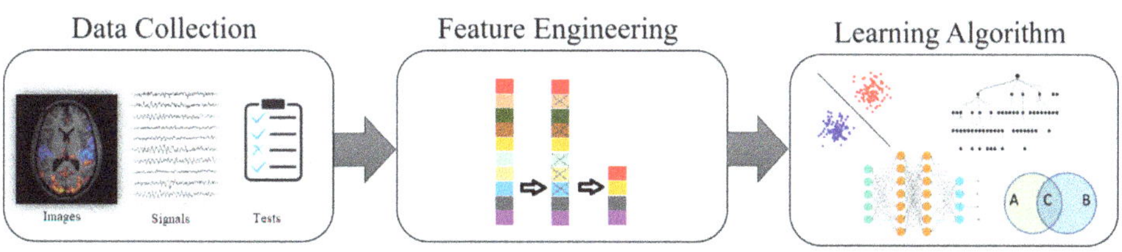

Figure 2.1. The overall architecture of the system.

2.2.1 Data types and features

Table 2.1 reports the reviewed research works in terms of data types. Each data type is briefly described in the rest.

- **EEG signal**
  The brain neuronal activities lead to generating electroencephalography (EEG) signals [2]. They are measured using a scalp electrode and can be divided into a few bands, i.e., gamma, beta, alpha, theta, and delta lying in different frequency ranges [3]. Every frequency band reveals a particular behavior of humans [4]. So, each frequency band's power is considered as a feature. Many researchers also employ the combination of power bands, e.g., alpha/beta ratio [5, 6].

Table 2.1. Data types.

Research work	Year	EEG signal	fMRI/SMRI	Test-based	Others
Marcano *et al* [12]	2016	×			
Bledsoe *et al* [13]	2016			×	
Mohammadi *et al* [14]	2016	×			
Chaim-Avancini *et al* [15]	2017		×		
Garcia *et al* [16]	2017		×		
Duda *et al* [17]	2017			×	
Qureshi *et al* [18]	2017		×		
Alchalabi *et al* [19]	2017	×			
Rahadian *et al* [20]	2017			×	
Duda *et al* [21]	2017			×	
Farzi *et al* [22]	2017		×		
Ustun *et al* [23]	2017			×	
Qureshi *et al* [24]	2017		×		
Yasumura *et al* [25]	2017				×
Khoshnoud *et al* [6]	2018	×			
Alchalabi *et al* [5]	2018	×			
Itani *et al* [26]	2018		×	×	
Fouladvand *et al* [27]	2018				×
Sen *et al* [28]	2018		×		
Karimu *et al* [29]	2018	×			
Riaz *et al* [30]	2018		×		×
Marcano *et al* [31]	2018	×		×	
Emser *et al* [32]	2018			×	×
Shao *et al* [33]	2018		×		
Karimu *et al* [34]	2018	×			
Pereda *et al* [35]	2018	×			
Wang *et al* [36]	2018		×		
Choi *et al* [37]	2018			×	×

The characteristic of an electrode or cortical source of the EEG time series as a spatial feature can be taken into account [7]. There are also some other nonlinear features, including the largest Lyapunov exponent [8], the approximate entropy [9], and dimensions of the multifractal singularity spectrum [10].

- **fMRI**
  Functional magnetic resonance imaging is a technique for quantifying tissue perfusion, neuronal connection of functional brain zones, alteration in brain functionality, and oxygen level condensation [3, 11].
- **Test-based**
  These sorts of data refer to information that can be provided by parents, teachers, and doctors through questionnaires or another tool.
- **Others**
  Research works that follow a particular approach to collect data are considered in this category. This sort of data is collected by either designing and performing a game or using some other type of images or signals information.

2.2.2 Dataset

In this section, some of the popular and well-known datasets that have recently been used in research works are described.

- **ADHD-200**
  ADHD-200 is an international competition in which some fMRI datasets are provided. Table 2.2 reports some information about datasets and universities that collaborate in order to gather them. ADHD-C and ADHD-I show the combined and inattentive type of ADHD, respectively. All of these datasets are apportioned to disjointed training and testing sets. They also contain neuroimaging and non-neuroimaging data, e.g., age, gender, and so on. Each instance is tagged as ADHD or control (non-ADHD) [28].

Table 2.2. ADHD-200[a].

Symbol	Name of university (Country)	#Healthy People	#AHDH-C	#ADHD-I
PU	Peking Univ. (China)	146	46	44
NI	Neuro IMAGE Samples (Netherland)	23	18	1
BU	Brown Univ. (USA)	27	20	3
KKI	Kennedy Krieger Inst. (USA)	61	16	5
NYU	New York Univ. Child Study Center (USA)	99	77	44
OHSU	Oregon Health & Science Univ. (USA)	42	30	5
UP	Univ. of Pittsburgh (USA)	95	0	6
WU	Washington Univ. in St. (USA)	61	0	0

[a] http://fcon_1000.projects.nitrc.org/indi/adhd200/

- **Truven data**
  The Truven dataset is a large-scale dataset that is collected in the Truven MarkScan Commercial Claim dataset between 2009 and 2015 [27]. Fouladvand *et al* [27] elected 254 996 subjects with an International Classification of Disease detection of ADHD (ICD-9 code 314.X) where the count of children (6–12 years) is 136 933, and the count of adolescence (13–20 years) is 18 063. Generally, they elicited 11 778 912 records from Truven.

2.2.3 Feature engineering

Reducing the size of a dataset is important due to removing irrelevant and redundant features. The reduction is carried out through the procedure of feature engineering. The features are mapped into another feature space with lower dimensionality by using feature extraction methods. Principal component analysis (PCA) and linear discriminant analysis (LDA) can be referred to as samples of feature extraction techniques [38].

Decreasing the dimensionality of a dataset is the basic notion of PCA in which the dataset has a huge size of interdependent variables while, as far as is feasible, maintaining the variation existing in the dataset. The reduction is reached through converting to a new group of variables, the principal components that are linearly uncorrelated and regulated, such that the original few, maintain the majority of the variation existing in the entire principal variables [39]. For more about PCA refer to [40].

LDA is also an approach in machine learning to discover a linear combination of features, that determines or disconnects some groups (i.e., classes) of events or objects. It can act either as a linear classifier or before other classification as a dimensionality reduction method[1].

The objective of feature selection is to pick an optimal subset of features that lessen redundancy and increase relevance. Feature selection strategies are incorporated into filter (without using a learning algorithm), wrapper (using learning algorithm), embedding (selecting features during training), and hybrid (a combination of filter and wrapper methods).

Mutual information is one of the popular criteria for filter-based feature selection, which is explained in brief. Information gain is utilized to measure the dependence between features and labels. The information gain between the jth feature, f_j, and the class labels l is computed by equation (2.1), where $H(f_j)$ is the entropy of f_j and $H(f_j|l)$ is the entropy of f_j, given observation l, as shown in equations (2.2) and (2.3), respectively. Thus, if a feature has a high information gain, it will be considered as relevant. Refer to [38], for more information.

$$IG(f_j, l) = H(f_j) - H(f_j \mid l) \tag{2.1}$$

[1] https://en.wikipedia.org/wiki/Linear_discriminant_analysis

$$H(f_j) = -\sum_i p(x_i)\log_2(p(x_i)) \tag{2.2}$$

$$H(f_j \mid l) = -\sum_k p(l_k)\sum_i p(x_i \mid l_k)\log_2(p(x_i \mid l_k)) \tag{2.3}$$

2.2.4 Imbalanced data

Most classifier learning algorithms assume an approximately balanced data. A dataset is imbalanced if the classes are not relatively uniformly represented. In some applications, the correct classification of instances in the small classes is often more remarkable than the contrary one [41]. For example, in the ADHD detection issue where usually the ADHD subjects are infrequent in contrast with non-ADHD subjects, the identification aim is to distinguish cases having ADHD. Therefore, the higher the recognition rate on the ADHD class, the more appropriate a classifier is.

Imbalanced data causes difficulties for learning and detracts from the classifier performance. There are some approaches for addressing imbalanced data such as resampling, using K-fold cross validation, or an ensemble different resampled dataset, and these are described in the next subsections[2].

2.2.4.1 Resampling

Resampling the training dataset is one of the methods to handle imbalanced data. Two main approaches are under-sampling and over-sampling. Under-sampling balances the dataset by decreasing the size of the plentiful class. This method is used when data is of sufficient quantity. A balanced new dataset could be retrieved by retaining total instances in the rare class and arbitrarily choosing the same size of instances in the plentiful class.

In contrast, over-sampling is utilized when the quantity of data is deficient. It balances the dataset by increasing the number of the rare examples. There is not sheer supremacy of one resampling approach over another, but a combination of over- and under-sampling usually has successful results. Note, there is no need to resample the data if the model is suited for imbalanced data.

2.2.4.2 K-fold cross-validation

Cross-validation (CV) should be used in the right manner while using an over-sampling method to handle imbalance problems. Note, CV should always be performed before over-sampling the data, just as how feature selection must be applied. Because, if the CV is done after over-sampling, essentially what is being done is overfitting the model to a particular artificial bootstrapping result. Randomness can be brought into the dataset to make sure that there will not be an overfitting problem by resampling data over and over again.

---

[2] https://www.kdnuggets.com/2017/06/7-techniques-handle-imbalanced-data.html (sections 2.2.4.1–2.2.4.3).

2.2.4.3 Ensemble different resampled dataset

Using more data is a way for generalizing a model. One easy best practice is constructing *N* models that use all the instances of the rare class and *N*-differing instances of the plentiful class. This method is light and perfectly horizontally scalable if there are lots of data since one can train and run the models on various cluster nodes.

In section 2.4, the problem of imbalanced data is raised. The classifiers usually cannot work with imbalanced data, and their performance is decayed. Although there is not a specific list of methods to handle imbalanced data, some conventional techniques are mentioned. Under- or over-sampling using K-fold CV, ensemble different resampled dataset, use of the right evaluation metrics, etc, are some solutions to address this problem. A few common learning algorithms are explained in the rest.

2.2.5 Learning algorithms

Choosing the appropriate machine learning is an important step. So, this section explains a number of machine learning algorithms [42]. The supervised algorithms in this section include decision trees, artificial neural networks (ANNs), support vector machines (SVMs), and statistical and fuzzy approaches.

2.2.5.1 Decision trees

Decision tree is a logic-based technique. In this technique, instances are classified beginning at the root node by sorting trees with respect to feature values. Every node exhibits a feature in an instance to be classified, and every branch exhibits a value the node can suppose [42]. C4.5 is one of the most popular algorithms in literature for constructing decision trees. Refer to [43] for details.

2.2.5.2 Artificial neural networks

Learning will not attain a point wherever the entire instances are classified truly if the instances are not partitionable by a line. ANNs try to address this problem. A multi-layer NN contains a large number of neurons linked in a pattern of linkages. Typically, there are three types of nodes: input nodes, that get information to be processed; output nodes, by which the results of the processing are gained; and hidden nodes between input and output layers. Feed-forward NNs enable signals to move from input to output. Feed-forward NNs are mostly learned by the principal back-propagation algorithm or by some difference. The major obstacle is they are way slow. Thus, for speeding them up, some solutions such as genetic and Bayesian-based methods have so far been proposed [42].

Also, many studies have used the radial basis function (RBF) networks [44]. An RBF network has an architecture with three layers of feedback, in which every hidden node enforces a radial activation function. Moreover, every output node imposes a weighted sum of hidden nodes outputs.

2.2.5.3 Support vector machines

A 'margin' either side of a hyperplane, which segregates two data classes is the most important concept in SVMs. Maximizing the margin and as a result, making the longest probable distance between the disjunctive hyperplane and the instances on another hand can subtract the upper limit for the expected generalization error. When data can be linearly parted, points lying on its margin are assumed as support vectors once the optimal disjunctive hyperplane is determined. Thus, the output is depicted as a linear composition of just these points, whereas others are disregarded.

However, many issues in the real world contain non-separable data for which no hyperplane properly splits the negative from positive instances in the training set. Projecting the data onto a higher-dimensional room (i.e., space) and designating a disjunctive hyperplane there, is a way to address the inseparability issue. *Feature space* is the name of this new room, as resisted to the input space engaged by the training instances.

Each consistent training set can be detached by suitably selecting the feature set of adequate dimensionalities. A linear separation in feature space relates to a non-linear separation in the principal input space. Projecting the data to other Hilbert space H as Φ: $R^d \rightarrow H$. Next, the learning algorithm just pertains to the data via dot products in H. If a 'Kernel Function' K exists where $K(x_i, x_j) = \Phi(x_i). \Phi(x_j)$, it is only necessary to use K in the learning algorithm and there would never be a demand to specify Φ explicitly. Once a hyperplane has been built, the kernel function is employed for projecting new points to the feature space due to classification [42].

2.2.5.4 Statistical approaches

Unlike neural networks, statistical methods are grouped by an express underlying probability model that prepares a probability where an instance is owned in every class. With this standpoint, Bayesian network is one of the approaches that is briefly expressed here.

A Bayesian network (BN) graphically represents the probability relations across a group of features. The BN, B, has a directed acyclic graph (DAG) structure in which the features are in one-to-one correlation with the nodes. Causal influences are displayed by edges between the features, whereas conditional independencies are encoded by the *lack* of feasible edges in B. Furthermore, a feature is conditionally independent of its non-descendants by knowing its parents.

Learning a Bayesian network has two steps: first, the learning of the DAG structural, and second the determination of its parameters. In summary, for training BN these few steps should be followed: (1) let the class features operate as parents; (2) let the whole features be independent; (3) find the dependence for every pair of features; (4) add the edges of dependence relation in the DAG; (5) determine the direction of the edges; (6) obtain the total conditional probability in the DAG.

Naive Bayesian (NB) networks are light Bayesian networks. They are made from DAGs that merely have an unobserved node as a single parent, and some observed children as well. Moreover, independence amid children in the context of their parent is assumed [42].

2.2.5.5 Fuzzy approaches

Fuzzy inference systems (FISs) are rule-based systems having the proper capability to map inputs to outputs. They represent a great part of fuzzy logics. A mixture of expert fuzzy models (MEFM) exerts a supervised ensemble learning to tune its interior parameters. The 'divide and conquer principle' is employed in this system, which is often used to divide an intricate problem into easier ones, whose solutions are integrated to get an ultimate solution [29].

In section 2.5, a few supervised learning algorithms were discussed. The main subject in confronting machine learning classification is this: under which circumstances can a specific algorithm significantly surpass another one on a given application matter? Accordingly, whether a learning algorithm performs better than others or not, should not be considered alone. The criteria and the reviewed recent works are described in the next sections, respectively.

2.3 Criteria

To evaluate a classifier performance and to compare how a classifier works better than the others, some criteria are needed. In this section, most used criteria are mentioned.

Sensitivity or recall, which is shown in equation (2.4), determines the portion of true positives that are correctly classified. The percentage of ADHD subjects who are classified correctly is an example of sensitivity. Indeed, it measures the rate of the count of true positives to the whole number of ADHD subjects in a population.

$$\text{Sensitivity} = \frac{\#\text{True Positive}}{\#\text{True Positive} + \#\text{False Negative}} \tag{2.4}$$

Specificity, which is shown in equation (2.5), calculates the percentages of true negatives that are correctly classified[3]. In an ADHD detection task, specificity is the portion of healthy subjects who are classified as non-ADHD. It measures the rate of the number of true negatives to the whole number of non-ADHD subjects in a population. Equation (2.6), computes accuracy, which is a common criterion. It measures the portion of the number of all true positives and true negatives between the whole number of subjects [45].

$$\text{Specificity} = \frac{\#\text{True Negative}}{\#\text{True Negative} + \#\text{False Positive}} \tag{2.5}$$

$$\text{Accuracy} = \frac{\#\text{True Positive} + \#\text{True Negative}}{\#\text{True Positive} + \#\text{True Negative} + \#\text{False Positive} + \#\text{False Negative}} \tag{2.6}$$

Kappa score shown in equation (2.7), is a robust criterion for evaluation of multi-class classifiers [46], where $P(\text{ra})$ is the relative observer agreement across raters and $P(\text{ca})$ is the hypothetical probability of chance agreement. Refer to [46], for details.

[3] https://en.wikipedia.org/wiki/Sensitivity_and_specificity

$$\text{Kappa} - \text{score} = \frac{P(\text{ra}) - P(\text{ca})}{1 - P(\text{ca})} \tag{2.7}$$

2.4 Recent works

Table 2.3 reports the reviewed research works regarding machine learning algorithms. Algorithms which had the best results are shown by the sign × in each cell. Research works are described briefly in the rest.

2.4.1 EEG-based

Screening and apropos diagnosis of ADHD in childhood help children and parents for growing society mental health [29]. Karimu and Azadi [29] introduced an analysis framework named mixture of expert fuzzy models (MEFM), mixing a group of fuzzy interface systems (FIS). This framework had a great capacity for detecting children having ADHD. By applying features elicited from the continuous wavelet transform scalograms of EEG signals taken from several distinct channels, the MEFM was presented. Then the *genetic algorithm* was used to tune the inner parameters of the MEFM. Moreover, the MEFM classifier exerting the 10-fold CV was evaluated and was compared with SVM and stand-alone FIS. Note, the feature extraction is done employing scalograms of CWT and the features opted by the sequential forward selection (SFS) approach. The data used is as follows:

- examining 40 children in which half of them were healthy;
- every category contained 10 girls and 10 boys between 7 and 10 years old;
- for every child, the EEG signals were recorded in the states of eyes-open resting;
- also, the electroencephalogram data was recorded in a psychiatric clinic supported by the Islamic Azad University, employing a g.USBamp[4] system.

The experimental results showed that RBF-SVM created by the C_z channel had the highest accuracy (98.07%) among classifiers created by an EEG channel, but yet the MEFM classifier accuracy (99.01%) was greater.

Alchalabi *et al* [19] proposed a serious game entitled 'FOCUS' with the aim of increasing the attention of low attention individuals and ADHD subjects. Wireless EEG reading devices employed by brain–computer interface (BCI) works helped read EEG. The BCI-controlled game has to be gamed using the EMOTIV EPOC+ kit.

An avatar must be moved by players using mental commands and focus abilities to stack up the cubical pickups as soon as possible. Two distinct models were utilized based on their attention states for the EEG signals classification. The two labels were *EMOTIV controlled* and *Keyboard controlled.* Note, EMOTIV controlled needs more attention than Keyboard. According to these types of the game, data was labeled. For data pre-processing, data labeling and data wrangling were carried out. Data wrangling included the steps, called frequency bands data filtering, data

[4] http://www.gtec.at/

Table 2.3. Learning algorithms in research works.

Research work	Year	SVM	Decision tree	Logistic regression	LDA	Naive Bayes	KNN	NN	MEFM	GA	GMM	AR model	BN	ELM	AP Clustering	Risk-calibrated supersparse linear integer	Deep belief network
Karimu *et al* [29]	2018								×	×							
Alchalabi *et al* [19]	2017						×										
Marcano *et al* [31]	2018										×	×					
Alchalabi *et al* [5]	2018	×															
Karimu *et al* [34]	2018	×															
Pereda *et al* [35]	2018												×				
Khoshnoud *et al* [5]	2018	×						×									
Marcano *et al* [12]	2016						×					×					
Mohamdi *et al* [14]	2016							×									
Garcia *et al* [16]	2017	×	×			×	×	×									
Shao *et al* [33]	2018	×															
Itani *et al* [26]	2018		×														
Qureshi *et al* [18]	2017													×			
Qureshi *et al* [24]	2017													×			
Riaz *et al* [30]	2018	×													×		
Wang *et al* [36]	2018	×															
Farzi *et al* [22]	2017																×
Duda *et al* [17]	2017	×		×	×												
Duda *et al* [21]	2017	×		×	×												
Rahadian *et al* [20]	2017							×		×							
Ustun *et al* [23]	2017															×	
Bledsoe *et al* [13]	2016	×	×														
Emser *et al* [32]	2018	×															
Choi *et al* [37]	2018			×													
Yasumura *et al* [25]	2017	×															

windowing, feature extraction (extra attributes) and data flattening. The experimental results with healthy subjects illustrated a high accuracy of a maximum of 96% in the EEG data classification at the right attention mood in the course of gameplay.

Marcano *et al* [31] used a universal background model based on a Gaussian mixture model to classify ADHD and non-ADHD individuals in their research, including six-year-old boys. A data collection process was done in which information about ADHD detection was captured through a maternal report. They recorded EEG employing a stretch cap within the developed 10/20 system design. Besides, from more than 20 electrodes placed at equal distances across the scalp, recordings were constructed.

When the EEG electrodes were exerted, subjects took part in eyes closed, eyes open, and quiet VIDEO baseline cases for gathering resting EEG data. Then, the software for analyzing EEG data released by James Long Company helped with data analysis. The EEG data used in this research was for seven subjects, four diagnosed as ADHD and on medication, and three diagnosed as healthy.

Autoregressive (AR) modeling was employed for feature extraction. Gaussian distributions could approximate any optional pdf. That is the primary purpose of utilizing GMMs in classification issues [47]. The expectation maximization (EM) algorithm was utilized for training GMM. Universal background models were found by diverse compositions of features extracted from subjects without ADHD. Also, models were found to coordinate the class of subjects with ADHD. Figure 2.2 shows how the classification was accomplished in [31] using the log-likelihood ratio (LLR). A subject is classified as ADHD if the LLR is bigger than or equal to zero; otherwise as non-ADHD.

The efficacy of the proposed method was considered in the traditional detector performance measures such as the equal error rate and the area under the curve. Based on results, a low probability of equal error and a high probability of diagnosis were attained at the same time with this strategy while utilizing EEG prepared throughout an attention network task (ANT). Furthermore, the use of contaminated data efficacy is perused. Inferior discrimination performance results at training and testing were performed with rest-derived data, with eyes closed, indicating the hypothesis from which the performance of ADHD diagnosis is related to the task.

Serious games (games with nonentertainment aims), could help to measure the patient's brain activity while playing a game by using an EEG recording device. The volume of information in EEG signals is enormous, and detecting abnormalities is too hard for humans. Therefore, machine learning is used here [5].

Alchalabi *et al* [5] used machine learning for detecting ADHD using EEG signals. Playing a serious game will appreciably diminish the 'white coat effect' that prevents detections in established pen-and-paper screening trials, particularly for children interpreting a doctor's act as a penalty. The environment of the game helps the flow of detection. Moreover, removing the 'training effect' by making a training step before concrete measurements becomes possible. They put these two things alongside and studied incorporating a serious game controlled by the EEG while using machine learning to predict the level of patient attention. The game can be played using the

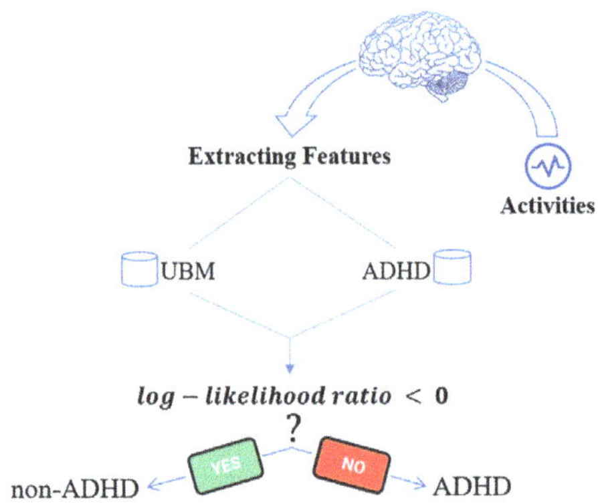

Figure 2.2. ADHD subjects classification.

EMOTIV EPOC+ kit. In this work, participants were requested to use two game control modes: (i) directing the character with keyboard arrows, and (ii) directing the character utilizing the EEG apparatus. They employed SVMs models for classification so that a vector of features represents a data sample. The experimental results indicated that ADHD classification had an accuracy of up to 98%.

Research works which studied the effects of ADHD on brain signals are divided into three categories: (i) those that analyzed the efficacy of ADHD symptoms on the potentials related to the event, employing persistent performance tests, and revealed a distinct activity level on the frontal and parietal lobes; (ii) those that studied ADHD influences on the slow cortex potentials; and (iii) those that utilized EEG signals in data mining and neurofeedback. Many research works on the children with ADHD that used the EEG signals to examine the effects of ADHD on brain activity noticed the EEG signals as a chaotic or random procedure regardless of the impression of the opposites in brain activity [34].

Karimu *et al* [34] showed that the EEG signals, biotic processes, do not have a random nature. Through determining the dual transitions sets among states in quantized EEG complement plots, they analyzed the ADHD influence on brain activity. They compared the accuracy of SVMs with the RBF kernel and for every feature of the entire dataset. The t-test analysis could just test the division of features in one dimension, so they applied an SFS algorithm. They found the optimal features and then used the RBF-SVM classifier with a 10-fold CV. They also compared the EEG-based studies and showed that their proposed approach had the most accuracy (98.25%) among the previous studies.

Pereda *et al* [35] utilized the Bayesian network classifier to categorize 33 children into two classes of ADHD and control using EEG signals. For dimensionality reduction, they selected the fast correlation based filter, and the population-based Scatter Search algorithm to capture non-linear relations among features and use a reference set consisting of high-quality and scattered solutions, which elaborates by bringing them together. Two classes of children with ages of 6–10 years were examined, including 19 boys with ADHD and 14 non-ADHD boys. The dataset was a subset of a larger one, which is stated in [48].

Instead of using a wrapper approach, the correlation feature selection measure which is the novation feature was utilized with *K*-fold and leave-one-out CV. They investigated the specificity and sensitivity attained by different search methods for Bayes network structure learning. Indeed, they proposed a solution for confronting the curse of dimensionality and turned it into a blessing. So, the combination of an exact selection of the data sections, a good technique for feature selection and an algorithm like Bayesian network classifier was offered.

Khoshnoud *et al* [6] used a dataset collected at the Atieh Comprehensive Centre [49]. The dataset contains 24 EEG records of right-handed children between 7 and 12 years. The aim of this work was to classify the patients and healthy people. They used PCA to reduce the feature space. Then they employed SVM and RBFNN (radial basis function neural network) to classify data. SVM provided 83.33% accuracy using fourfold CV testing.

Marcano *et al* [12] employed autoregressive (AR) models for ADHD classification. The participants in the study were the children between the ages of 8 and 10 years. EEG signals were seized utilizing a stretch cap. For inspection of EEG signals, they considered the usage of AR parameterization for classifying control and ADHD children. Since two classes were separable in AR parameters, they reached a high accuracy and confidence. Indeed, they showed a KNN classifier could be used to achieve high performance.

Mohammadi *et al* [14] performed feature extraction to get non-linear features from EEG signals, then employed two approaches for feature selection, namely, double input symmetrical relevance (DISR) and minimum redundancy maximum relevance (MRMR). The participants in the study were 30 ADHD subjects (8 girls and 22 boys) and 30 controls (5 girls and 25 boys) with the age of 9.62 ± 1.75 and 9.85 ± 1.77 years, respectively. Experimental results showed that *MLP with DISR* and *MLP with mRMR* had an accuracy of 93.65% and 92.28%, respectively.

2.4.2 MRI-based (fMRI/SMRI)

Garcia *et al* [16] collected four different rs-fMRI datasets from various places to provide independent datasets for experiments. These four datasets are called KKI (58 No, 20 Yes), NeuroImage (22 No, 17 Yes), NYU (91 No, 96 Yes) and Peking (93 No, 57 Yes). There are 17 955 features in all datasets. All datasets exist in ADHD-200.

They aimed at comparing multiple feature selection algorithms to overcome the curse of dimension issue and comparing several well-known machine learning algorithms. First, every dataset was partitioned with leave-one-out CV. Then, five feature selection algorithms (PCC, Wilcoxon, LASSO, RFE, and MRMD) were applied to each training fold. Next, the ranking of the feature component was used for evaluation. In the end, various classifiers (Naïve Bayes, Perceptron, C4.5, SVM, and KNN) was run into the reduced training data.

They used criteria defined as (sensitivity + specificity)/2. They did the experiments with all features and with reduced features of each selection algorithm. The feature selection for the Peking dataset did not work. The results showed the Wilcoxon in the KKI dataset, MRMD in NeuroImage dataset, and LASSO in NYU dataset improved the result of classifiers. However, none of these methods could not increase the quality of classifiers in the Peking dataset.

A bi-objective ADHD classification system was introduced by Shao *et al* [33] with the help of *L1 Norm* SVM. The objectives, i.e., the empirical error and the margin of separation, were assumed simultaneously. In order to work out the bi-objective optimization issue, the Normal Boundary Intersection technique of Das and Dennis was applied.

They used the resting-state fMRI data from the Neuron Bureau ADHD-200 competition. KKI and PU-1, PU-2, and PU-3 (from PU) datasets were used. Additionally, they generated the PU-joint dataset made from PU-1, PU-2, and PU-3 and a large one named KKI-PU-joint made from PU-joint and KKI. Their approach's experimental validations were accomplished on PU-1, PU-joint, KKI, and KKI-PU-joint datasets.

DPARSF toolbox[5] was employed for data preprocessing, and statistical analysis was used for showing the disparity of the brain between control and ADHD subjects. Reducing dimensionality was necessary as the initial brain features had a higher dimension than the number of instances. They compared PCA, Isomap [50], and LLE [51] methods and chose PCA for reducing the dimensionality of initial features. Comparative results showed that the proposed approach (bi-objective optimization scheme) gave more accuracy than traditional classifiers like SVM and NN.

Itani *et al* [26] used the ADHD-200 collection dataset to conduct experiments. There are 947 people in this dataset. Decision tree, as a well-known machine learning algorithm, was applied to the dataset. Figure 2.3 shows that they extracted four types of features to execute the algorithm on them. Brain features were obtained from fMRI images, and there were some phenotypic features such as age, gender, IQ, and so on [26].

They obtained different results with various features. Figure 2.4 shows one of them trained on the New-York set [26]. Note, the type of ADHD-HI (hyperactive-impulsive) was not estimated, as the related population in the training data was pretty slight.

To classify the multi-class data, Qureshi *et al* [18] applied the global connectivity features based on maps having more differentiated power from resting-state fMRI images. They adopted selective fMRI images of the ADHD-200 dataset and preprocessed them via software called analysis of functional neuroimages[6] [52].

They employed a hierarchical extreme learning machine (H-ELM) classifier, which is introduced by Tang *et al* [53]. Some count of hyperparameters of the mentioned classification framework was set to get the best classification accuracy, and a greedy search method was employed for tuning them. They attained a nested CV accuracy of 71.11% and a multi-class kappa score of 0.57.

Qureshi *et al* [24] used two classifications: ELM and SVM having RBF and linear kernels. They used the ADHD-200 dataset, which has three categories of ADHD-I, ADHD-C, and typically developing. The relation between functional and structural

[5] http://www.restfmri.net/forum/DPARSF/

[6] http://afni.nimh.nih.gov/afni/

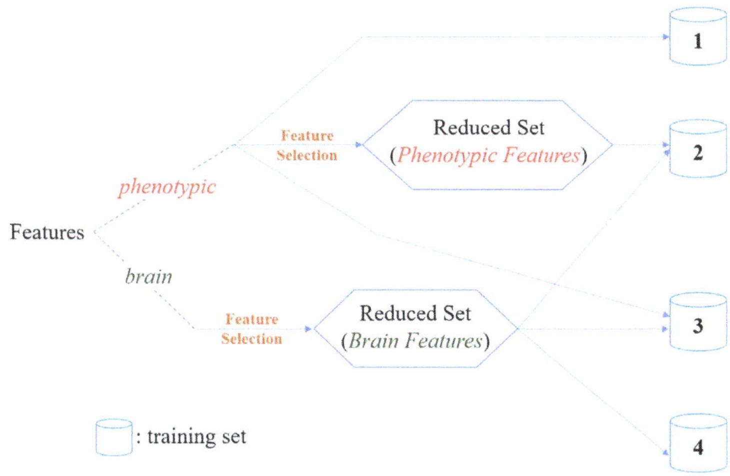

Figure 2.3. Four training sets for ADHD classification.

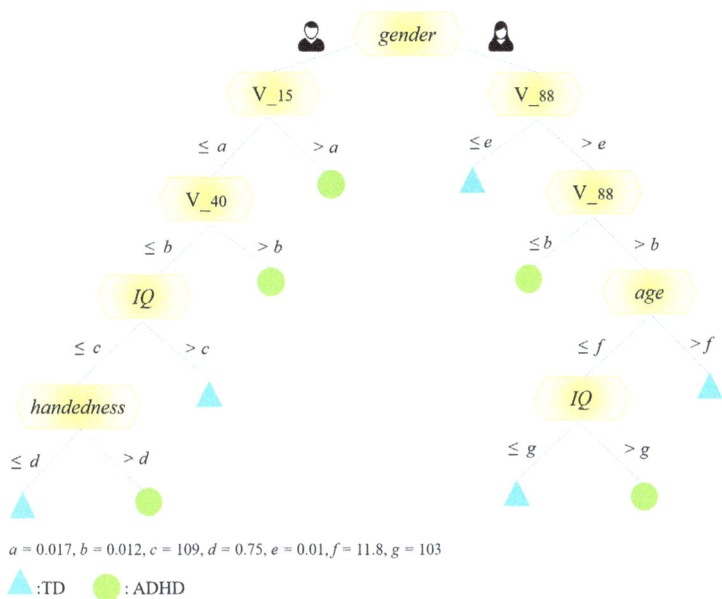

Figure 2.4. A model trained on the New-York set (TD: typically developing).

measures and also symptom severity score, IQ, and age were studied. An ELM carried out binary and multi-class classifications, where 76.190% and 92.857% accuracy were obtained in multi- and binary-class, respectively.

Riaz *et al* [30] proposed a machine learning framework to study functional connectivity alteration amongst ADHD and non-ADHD individuals. Imaging and non-imaging features were brought together to create a univalent feature vector utilized for classifying the subjects as ADHD or non-ADHD.

The framework had several phases. Firstly, the functional connectivity of brain zones was specified by employing the affinity propagation (AP) clustering algorithm. They designed a method for initializing the AP by using the density peaks approach. In the second phase, they chose diacritical features via elastic net incorporated variable shrinkage with an assorted range of variables. Lastly, for classifying ADHD and non-ADHD subjects, an SVM classifier was used. They used ADHD-200 dataset. The data included both the resting-state fMRI and various non-imaging data for every individual. Datasets were from four sites of KKI, NI, NYU, and PU.

Wang *et al* [36] used the ADHD-200 dataset, which contains 35 patients and 25 healthy people. All MRI images were preprocessed by FreeSurfer[7] tool that passed some stages such as motion rectification, intensity standardization, segmentation of white matter, etc.

They applied a hybrid machine learning algorithm constituted of classification and feature selection algorithms as well. First, leave-one-out CV and then, SVM recursive feature elimination were used in the training set. Next, they employed 200 features to build a model. They used two types of features, including regional feature and morphological connectivity-based, and built two distinct models for each of them. The results for the top 45 features from morphological connectivity-based were 74.65%, 75%, and 74.29% regarding the accuracy, sensitivity, and specificity, respectively. In conclusion, using morphological connectivity-based features instead of regional features improved the diagnosis result.

Farzi *et al* [22] suggested a deep belief network as a model of deep learning to diagnosis ADHD. Figure 2.5 shows a structure of the deep belief network constructed by Stacked Restricted Boltzmann Machines. Refer to [54] for details.

Two common datasets of ADHD-200 including, NeuroImage, and NYU were used, and different features such as IQ measure, gender, and fMRI features were considered. They employed a greedy learning algorithm to train the model. The result of comparing their method with common ones such as SVM and decision tree showed the supremacy of the proposed model.

2.4.3 Test-based

Autism spectrum disorder (ASD) and ADHD have similar behavioral symptoms. Since there is no test for screening to discern these disorders, methods with fast and accurate distinguishing of ADHD from ASD are needed [17].

To tackle this issue, Duda *et al* [17] studied improved machine learning algorithms employing just a mini subset of objects from the Social Responsiveness Scale. They also extended their work with the help of a crowdsourced dataset of responses to the prelimited top-15 Social Responsiveness Scale questions taken from parents of subjects suffering from ADHD or ASD. They procured Stanford

[7] http://surfer.nmr.mgh.harvard.edu

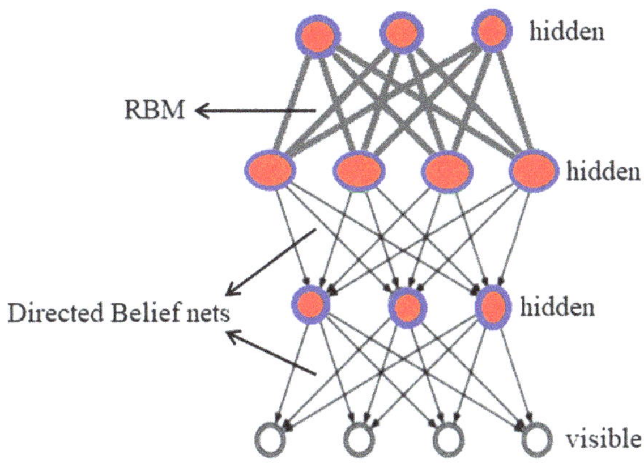

Figure 2.5. Deep belief network structure.

institutional review board confirmation to roll up questionnaire data from parents of children aged between 2 and 17.

Crowdsource service manner and mainstream social media networking platforms were used. The parents electronically were inquired about the child's general demographic features, how the child learned about a study, and whether or not he/she had a history of any clinical identification of neuropsychiatric or developmental disease. Moreover, the parents answered 15 questions concerning the daily behavior of their child noticed from the Social Responsiveness Scale analysis of machine learning. SVM, LDA, Logistic Regression with l_1 regularization[8], Logistic Regression with l_2 regularization[9], and Elastic Net[10] were used in this work.

Every algorithm was trained on a hundred random archival data sub-samples and tested in a trial on the same review sample. In another trial, each method was trained one time on the whole review sample and tested on a hundred random sub-samples archival data sub-samples. Lastly, all algorithms were learned and tested over 50 turns of the two-fold CV with sub-sampling. As stated, they developed a classification algorithm that fulfills the area under the curve (AUC) equal to 0.89 ± 0.01.

As there are overlaps between symptoms of autism and ADHD, which make it complicated to differentiate for doctors, Duda *et al* [21] utilized some experiments to classify two groups of ASD and ADHD. They used the Social Responsiveness Scale data based on 65 questions from parents. The dataset also contains 2925 instances. First, they used the 10-fold CV. Then, they ranked 65 features based on mutual information, calculated with the mRMR algorithm [55]. Next, they used 10 random under-samplings to come up with the imbalanced datasets. After that, they implemented forward feature selection with ranked features for training and testing algorithms.

[8] Lasso.

[9] Ridge.

[10] A logistic regression considering both l_1 and l_2 regularization.

They applied various algorithms of machine learning on a dataset. They made a comparison between different classifiers and trained dataset with Linear Discriminant Analysis, Categorical Lasso, Logistic Regression, SVC, Random Forest, and Decision Trees. The experimental results showed that Linear Discriminant Analysis, Categorical Lasso, Logistic Regression, and SVC had high AUC.

Rahadian *et al* [20] implemented a Genetic Algorithm Learning Vector Quantization two Neural Network (GA-LVQ2NN). LVQ is an approach in NN algorithms which classifies via computing the vector distance weights applying Euclidean Distance, and it is usually adopted for solving non-linear and complex issues. Optimization was the goal of the proposed method by combining GA and LVQ2. Indeed, first, GA produced some weight vectors. Then LVQ2 used them for training the network. The best weight vectors having the highest fitness value were chosen.

Released issues of screening scales in an ADHD diagnosis task are calibrated to DSM-5 criteria [23, 56]. Ustun *et al* [23] introduced a sort of the extensively consumed Adult ADHD Self-Report Screening Scale [57, 58] for *DSM-5* criteria updating. They presented 10-fold cross-validated AUC (10-CV-AUC) and mean calibration accuracy (10-CV-CAL) regarding the count of questions in the screening scale. A monotonous growth of 10-CV-AUC was found as the number of questions increased, whereas a nonmonotonic trend was seen in 10-CV-CAL. Thus, the 6-question model was chosen due to the best-in-class result in both.

They indicated that Risk Calibrated Supersparse Linear Integer Model could be used to construct a screening scale for *DSM-5* adult ADHD, utilizing optimum rules for scoring integer. The new scale was examined in a 2011–2012 clinical instance of patients that sought assessment at NYU Langone and 2015–2016 preliminary treatments.

Bledsoe *et al* [13] utilized neuropsychological features. A forward selection approach was followed to find the best features for SVM and Decision tree. They achieved high performance, as 100% accuracy of ADHD and non-ADHD subjects was observed. Moreover, one hundred percent specificity and sensitivity were obtained in Decision Trees considering subjects with and without ADHD-C.

2.4.4 Others

Emser *et al* [32] used objective measures instead of subjective measures to distinguish ADHD patients and controls because subjective measures have a lot of error bias. Objective criteria were two well-known tests called battery of attention and the quantified behavior test. Their sample contains 136 people that they divided into 76 adults and 60 children.

First, every person was given two mentioned tests and features were extracted from the results. Then SVM was applied to these features. They did two various experiments with just objective measures and with mixed up subjective and objective methods. The experimental results showed that when the subjective and objective measures were used, diagnosing was more accurate.

Choi *et al* [37] extracted features from RBG and 3D sensors in the robot. Also, they preprocessed and analyzed data with the Point Cloud Library (PCL) [59]. They filtered noise and resampling PCL to five-hundred pixels via the method of uniform sampling. They used KNN to define objects. There are three possible labels for each instance; ADHD, ADHD at risk, and healthy. They extracted 19 features after the test for clustering, 13 features from robot measurements, three features from success information at the level and three features from a question-based test.

A dataset used in [37] was collected from all primary school students grade 3rd and 4th in Seoul from April to May 2016 and February to May 2017. There were 3226 participants in this collecting data. The data gathered from a robot test game tracked the children active during the test. Each test took about 10–12 min

They employed four well-known machine learning algorithms, including Logistic Regression, SVM, Random Forest, and Gradient Tree Boosting. They performed three different experiments, including balanced data with all features, imbalanced data with all features, and imbalanced data with a robust-measure feature only. They also compared between classifier results. LRC had the best result in the third phase of the experiment.

Near-infrared spectroscopy (NIRS), is an alternative imaging approach which is employed for measuring brain blood flow, even when the patients move their heads [25]. Yasumura *et al* [25] utilized NIRS to measure variation in oxygenated hemoglobin levels. Data were collected from six facilities in Japan in which there were 62 ADHD children and 37 typically developing children. SVM with RBF kernel was used as a machine learning algorithm with high sensitivity and specificity.

References

[1] Bellman R E 2003 *Dynamic Programming* (Princeton, NJ: Princeton University Press)

[2] Sanei S and Chambers J A 2007 *EEG Signal Processing* (Chichester: Wiley)

[3] Sridhar C, Bhat S, Acharya U R, Adeli H and Bairy G M 2017 Diagnosis of attention deficit hyperactivity disorder using imaging and signal processing techniques *Comput. Biol. Med.* **88** 93–9

[4] Tenev A, Markovska-Simoska S, Kocarev L, Pop-Jordanov J, Müller A and Candrian G 2014 Machine learning approach for classification of ADHD adults *Int. J. Psychophysiol.* **93** 162–6

[5] Alchalabi A E, Shirmohammadi S, Eddin A N and Elsharnouby M 2018 FOCUS: detecting ADHD patients by an EEG-based serious game *IEEE Trans. Instrum. Meas.* **67** 1512–20

[6] Khoshnoud S, Nazari M A and Shamsi M 2018 Functional brain dynamic analysis of ADHD and control children using nonlinear dynamical features of EEG signals *J. Integr. Neurosci.* **17** 17–30

[7] Lenartowicz A and Loo S K 2014 Use of EEG to diagnose ADHD *Curr. Psychiatry Rep.* **16** 498

[8] Stam C J 2005 Nonlinear dynamical analysis of EEG and MEG: review of an emerging field *Clin. Neurophysiol.* **116** 2266–301

[9] Pincus S M 1991 Approximate entropy as a measure of system complexity *Proc. Natl Acad. Sci.* **88** 2297–301

[10] Kantelhardt J W, Zschiegner S A, Koscielny-Bunde E, Havlin S, Bunde A and Stanley H E 2002 Multifractal detrended fluctuation analysis of nonstationary time series *Physica* A **316** 87–114

[11] Konrad K and Eickhoff S B 2010 Is the ADHD brain wired differently? A review on structural and functional connectivity in attention deficit hyperactivity disorder *Hum. Brain Mapping* **31** 904–9916

[12] Marcano J L L, Bell M A and Beex A L 2016 Classification of ADHD and non-ADHD using AR models *Engineering in Medicine and Biology Society (EMBC) 2016 (Orlando, FL)* 363–6

[13] Bledsoe J C, Xiao D, Chaovalitwongse A, Mehta S, Grabowski T J, Semrud-Clikeman M, Pliszka S and Breiger D 2016 Diagnostic classification of ADHD versus control: support vector machine classification using brief neuropsychological assessment *J. Attention Disorders* https://doi.org/10.1177/1087054716649666

[14] Mohammadi M R, Khaleghi A, Nasrabadi A M, Rafieivand S, Begol M and Zarafshan H 2016 EEG classification of ADHD and normal children using non-linear features and neural network *Biomed. Eng. Lett.* **6** 66–73

[15] Chaim-Avancini T, Doshi J, Zanetti M, Erus G, Silva M, Duran F, Cavallet M, Serpa M, Caetano S and Louza M 2017 Neurobiological support to the diagnosis of ADHD in stimulant naïve adults: pattern recognition analyses of MRI data *Acta Psychiat. Scand.* **136** 623–36

[16] Garcia R, Paraiso E C and Nievola J C 2017 Comparative study of dimensionality reduction methods using reliable features for multiple datasets obtained by rs-fMRI in ADHD prediction *Canadian Conf. on Artificial Intelligence (Edmonton, AB, Canada)* pp 97–102

[17] Duda M, Haber N, Daniels J and Wall D 2017 Crowdsourced validation of a machine-learning classification system for autism and ADHD *Transl. Psychiat.* **7** e1133

[18] Qureshi M N I, Jo H J and Lee B 2017 ADHD subgroup discrimination with global connectivity features using hierarchical extreme learning machine: resting-state FMRI study *2017 IEEE 14th Int. Symp. on Biomedical Imaging (ISBI 2017) (Rochester, MN)* pp 529–32

[19] Alchalabi A E, Elsharnouby M, Shirmohammadi S and Eddin A N 2017 Feasibility of detecting ADHD patients' attention levels by classifying their EEG signals *Proc., 12th Annu. IEEE Int. Symp. Med. Meas. Appl.* pp 314–9

[20] Rahadian B A, Dewi C and Rahayudi B 2017 The performance of genetic algorithm learning vector quantization. 2. Neural network on identification of the types of attention deficit hyperactivity disorder *2017 Int. Conf. on Sustainable Information Engineering and Technology (SIET) (Malang, Indonesia)* pp 337–41

[21] Duda M, Ma R, Haber N and Wall D 2017 Use of machine learning for behavioral distinction of autism and ADHD *Transl. Psychiat.* **6** e732

[22] Farzi S, Kianian S and Rastkhadive I 2017 Diagnosis of attention deficit hyperactivity disorder using deep belief network based on greedy approach *2017 5th Int. Symp. on Computational and Business Intelligence (ISCBI) (Dubai, United Arab Emirates)* pp 96–9

[23] Ustun B, Adler L A, Rudin C, Faraone S V, Spencer T J, Berglund P, Gruber M J and Kessler R C 2017 The World Health Organization adult attention-deficit/hyperactivity disorder self-report screening scale for DSM-5 *JAMA psychiatry* **74** 520–6

[24] Qureshi M N I, Oh J, Min B, Jo H J and Lee B 2017 Multi-modal, multi-measure, and multi-class discrimination of ADHD with hierarchical feature extraction and extreme learning machine using structural and functional brain MRI *Front. Human Neuroscience* **11** 157

[25] Yasumura A, Omori M, Fukuda A, Takahashi J, Yasumura Y, Nakagawa E, Koike T, Yamashita Y, Miyajima T and Koeda T 2017 Applied machine learning method to predict

children with ADHD using prefrontal cortex activity: a multicenter study in Japan *J. Attention Disorders* **24** 2010–20

[26] Itani S, Lecron F and Fortemps P 2018 A multi-level classification framework for multi-site medical data: application to the ADHD-200 collection *Exp. Syst. Appl.* **91** 36–45

[27] Fouladvand S, Hankosky E R, Henderson D W, Bush H, Chen J, Dwoskin L P, Freeman P R, Kantak K, Talbert J and Tao S 2018 Predicting substance use disorder in ADHD patients using long-short term memory model *2018 IEEE Int. Conf. on Healthcare Informatics Workshop (ICHI-W)* pp 49–50

[28] Sen B, Borle N C, Greiner R and Brown M R 2018 A general prediction model for the detection of ADHD and autism using structural and functional MRI *PLoS One* **13** e0194856

[29] Karimu R Y and Azadi S 2018 Diagnosing the ADHD using a mixture of expert fuzzy models *Int. J. Fuzzy Syst.* **20** 1282–96

[30] Riaz A, Asad M, Alonso E and Slabaugh G 2018 Fusion of fMRI and non-imaging data for ADHD classification *Comput. Med. Imaging Graphics* **65** 115–28

[31] Marcano J L, Bell M A and Beex A L 2018 Classification of ADHD and non-ADHD subjects using a universal background model *Biomed. Signal Process. Control* **39** 204–12

[32] Emser T S, Johnston B A, Steele J D, Kooij S, Thorell L and Christiansen H 2018 Assessing ADHD symptoms in children and adults: evaluating the role of objective measures *Behav. Brain Funct.* **14** 11

[33] Shao L, Xu Y and Fu D 2018 Classification of ADHD with bi-objective optimization *J. Biomed. Inform.* **84** 164–70

[34] Karimui R Y, Azadi S and Keshavarzi P 2018 The ADHD effect on the actions obtained from the EEG signals *Biocybern. Biomed. Eng.* **38** 425–37

[35] Pereda E, García-Torres M, Melián-Batista B, Mañas S, Méndez L and González J J 2018 The blessing of dimensionality: feature selection outperforms functional connectivity-based feature transformation to classify ADHD subjects from EEG patterns of phase synchronisation *PLoS One* **13** e0201660

[36] Wang X-H, Jiao Y and Li L 2018 Diagnostic model for attention-deficit hyperactivity disorder based on interregional morphological connectivity *Neurosci. Lett.* **685** 30–4

[37] Choi M-T, Yeom J, Shin Y and Park I 2019 Robot-assisted ADHD screening in diagnostic process *J. Intell. Robot. Syst.* **95** 351–63

[38] Tang J, Alelyani S and Liu H 2014 Feature selection for classification: A review *Data classification: Algorithms and applications* ed C C Aggarwal (Boca Raton, FL: CRC Press) p 37

[39] Jolliffe I T 1989 *Principal Component Analysis.* (New york: Springer)

[40] Smith L I 2002 A tutorial on principal components analysis *Available:* http://csnet.otago.ac.nz/cosc453/student_tutorials/principal_components.pdf

[41] Sun Y, Wong A K and Kamel M S 2009 Classification of imbalanced data: A review *Int. J. Pattern Recog. Artif. Intell.* **23** 687–719

[42] Kotsiantis S B, Zaharakis I D and Pintelas P E 2006 Machine learning: a review of classification and combining techniques *Artif. Intell. Rev.* **26** 159–90

[43] Quinlan J 1993 *C4. 5: Programs for Machine Learning* (San Francisco, CA: Morgan Kaufmann)

[44] Howlett R J and Jain L C 2013 *Radial Basis Function Networks 2: New Advances in Design* (Berlin: Springer)

[45] Metz C E 1978 Basic principles of ROC analysis *Semin. in Nucl. Med.* **8** 283–98

[46] Cohen J 1960 A coefficient of agreement for nominal scales *Educ. and Psychol. Meas.* **20** 37–46

[47] Reynolds D 2009 *Gaussian Mixture Models, Encyclopedia of Biometrics* (Berlin: Springer) pp 659–63

[48] González J J, Méndez L D, Mañas S, Duque M R, Pereda E and De Vera L 2013 Performance analysis of univariate and multivariate EEG measurements in the diagnosis of ADHD *Clin. Neurophysiol.* **124** 1139–50

[49] Ahmadlou M and Adeli H 2010 Wavelet-synchronization methodology: a new approach for EEG-based diagnosis of ADHD *Clin. EEG Neurosci.* **41** 1–10

[50] Tenenbaum J B, De Silva V and Langford J C 2000 A global geometric framework for nonlinear dimensionality reduction *Science* **290** 2319–23

[51] Roweis S T and Saul L K 2000 Nonlinear dimensionality reduction by locally linear embedding *Science* **290** 2323–6

[52] Cox R W 1996 AFNI: software for analysis and visualization of functional magnetic resonance neuroimages *Comput. Biomed. Res.* **29** 162–73

[53] Tang J, Deng C and Huang G-B 2016 Extreme learning machine for multilayer perceptron *IEEE Trans Neural Netw. Learn. Syst.* **27** 809–21

[54] Hinton G E, Osindero S and Teh Y-W 2006 A fast learning algorithm for deep belief nets *Neural Comput.* **18** 1527–54

[55] Peng H, Long F and Ding C 2005 Feature selection based on mutual information criteria of max-dependency, max-relevance, and min-redundancy *IEEE Trans. Pattern Anal. Mach. Intell.* **27** 1226–38

[56] Adler L A, Spencer T J and Wilens T E 2015 *Attention-Deficit Hyperactivity Disorder in Adults and Children* (Cambridge: Cambridge University Press)

[57] Kessler R C, Adler L, Ames M, Demler O, Faraone S, Hiripi E, Howes M J, Jin R, Secnik K and Spencer T 2005 The World Health Organization Adult ADHD Self-Report Scale (ASRS): a short screening scale for use in the general population *Psychol. Med.e* **35** 245–56

[58] Kessler R C, Adler L A, Gruber M J, Sarawate C A, Spencer T and Van Brunt D L 2007 Validity of the World Health Organization Adult ADHD Self-Report Scale (ASRS) Screener in a representative sample of health plan members *Int. J. Methods Psychiat. Res.* **16** 52–65

[59] Rusu R B and Cousins S 2011 3d is here: Point cloud library (pcl) *2011 IEEE Int. Conf. Robotics and automation (ICRA) (Shanghai, China)* pp 1–4

IOP Publishing

Neurological Disorders and Imaging Physics, Volume 4
Application to attention deficit hyperactivity disorder
Ayman El-Baz and Jasjit S Suri

Chapter 3

Classification of attention deficit hyperactivity disorder (ADHD) by using statistical features of MR images

Gulay Cicek and Aydin Akan

3.1 Introduction

Attention deficit hyperactivity disorder (ADHD), one of the most common chronic disorders of our times, is a neuropsychiatric disorder in which individuals experience degradation in personal, academic, and social functioning due to excessive hyperactivity, inattention and concentration disorder and impulsivity symptoms [1]. Attention deficit or inattention, hyperactivity, and impulsivity are the main symptoms of ADHD [2]. Inattention expresses that a person has difficulty focusing on details and organizing. People with attention deficit are easily distracted, and lose their belongings. They have difficulty performing tasks that require mental effort. Hyperactivity refers to the state of the individual being in constant motion. People with hyperactivity usually cannot stay steady for a long time, and talk intensively. Impulsivity is the problem of self-control. People with impulsivity act hastily, decide without thinking, and have problems waiting in a queue.

Studies have shown that 80% of people with ADHD have another psychiatric disorder [3]. Among these, depression, anxiety and obsessive compulsive disorder are at the forefront. Disorders accompanying ADHD make the diagnosis difficult.

Studies reveal that 7.9% of the adolescent population are diagnosed with ADHD, with an increased rate of 10.2% between 2015 and 2016 [4]. The prevalence of ADHD varies with age and gender. Especially in children between 6 and 16 years, ADHD is more common, and 2–3 times higher in males than females.

Diagnosis of ADHD is not as easy as with other physical diseases. Symptoms of ADHD differ from person to person. Sometimes, the symptoms of attention deficit, impulsivity and hyperactivity are observed together, but sometimes two of them are more dominant [5]. This makes the diagnosis of ADHD difficult. For ADHD diagnosis, the patient begins a routine visit to a physician where the patient's

doi:10.1088/978-0-7503-1822-8ch3

complaints are listed, necessary clinical examinations are performed, and some required tests are done. Many different tests are performed to determine the symptoms that do not occur in clinical interviews. By using ADHD rating scales, tests are conducted to understand the behaviour of individuals in different situations and times. Besides the standard intelligence test, a broad spectrum scales screen is applied to determine problems of social, emotional and psychiatric condition of individuals. Information about language development, vocabulary set, memory capacity, and motor skills of individuals are also determined by using special tests. However, these tests are not objective, and give different results at different times and situations. Hence, the diagnosis of ADHD becomes difficult due to the above stated reasons.

In recent decades, magnetic resonance imaging (MRI) of the brain has been used to examine anatomical differences. Differences such as total cerebral volume, prefrontal regions, basal ganglia, cerebellum, and the ratio of grey and white matter between individuals diagnosed with ADHD and healthy controls were investigated. In many studies, it is observed that children with ADHD had smaller brain volume in all regions and less grey matter than healthy controls [6, 7]. In addition, white matter abnormalities were also observed in individuals with ADHD [8].

The presence of many psychiatric disorders associated with ADHD, the subjectivity of the tests used in the diagnosis, the variation of symptoms among subjects make the diagnosis of ADHD difficult. As such, there exist cases of misdiagnosis and non-diagnosis. Our aim is to develop an objective, and reliable computer aided diagnosis method for ADHD that minimizes the human effort, and eliminates the above mentioned shortcomings.

3.1.1 Objective

3.1.1.1 General

The aim of this study is to minimize the human effort in the diagnosis of ADHD, and to develop an objective and reliable tool that can help physicians. Towards this direction, a model has been proposed by utilizing MRI data obtained from NPIstanbul Hospital.

3.1.1.2 Specific

Main steps of the proposed method are:

- create a different dataset with statistical features extracted from magnetic resonance images;
- determine the key features and select the most important ones;
- classify the features using K-nearest neighbour, and decision tree classification algorithms for the diagnosing of ADHD;
- MR images consist of several slices. Slices are combined and a new texture is obtained. Utilize this texture for diagnosis as well;
- analyse and select the best model that helps physicians to diagnose.

3.2 Methodology

The brain images of 30 individuals were obtained from NPIstanbul Neuropsychiatric Hospital. Statistical features are extracted to characterize the brain images. First and second order statistical features are used to create the dataset. Principal component analysis (PCA) is used to determine the most important features. Extracted features from patients diagnosed with ADHD and control MR images are classified using the k-nearest neighbour (kNN) and decision tree algorithms. The performance is evaluated by using 10-fold, and hold-out cross validation methods. Accuracy, sensitivity, specificity, true positive rate, false positive rate, recall and f-measure were calculated to evaluate the algorithm. In addition, receiver operating curve (ROC) is obtained. A flowchart of the proposed method is shown in detail in figure 3.1.

3.2.1 The application domain

The main symptoms of ADHD are attention deficit, hyperactivity and impulsivity. Sometimes, one and two of the symptoms may occur at a time, but sometimes two of them are more dominant. At NPIstanbul Hospital, clinical examinations and psychometric tests on patients are done by experts. Diagnosis of ADHD can be very time consuming and requires intensive attention. In addition, psychometric tests are not objective. Hence, misdiagnosis and non-diagnosis case are common.

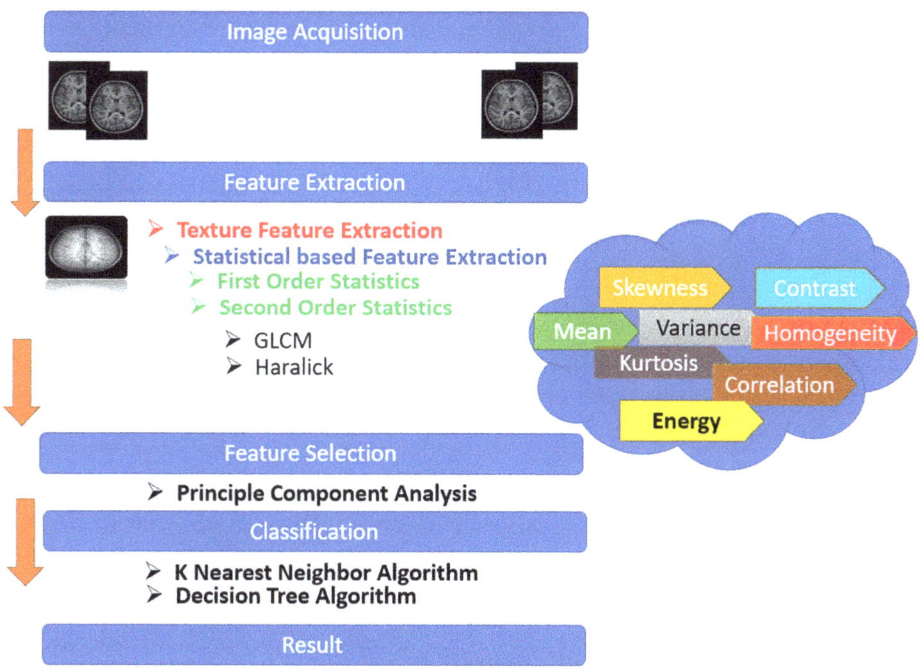

Figure 3.1. Research methodology.

In this study, we developed an accurate, objective, and reliable computer aided tool for the diagnosis of ADHD using MR images.

3.2.2 Selecting and creating the target dataset

MR images from 30 subjects, 15 with ADHD and 15 controls, were obtained from NPIstanbul Neuropsychiatric Hospital, Istanbul, Turkey. Images are collected using a 1.5 Philips Acheiva MRI scanner. T1-weighted high-resolution, fast magnitude of the slope prepared by 3D magnetization was obtained by using gradient eco method. The parameters of the magnetic resonance images are as follows: acquisition matrix: $256 \times 256 \times 140$; TR: 2.8 s; T.E: 4.0 s; flip angle: 8°; field of view: 240 mm; voxel size = $0.937 \times 0.937 \times 1.2$ mm resolution.

3.2.3 Feature extraction

Feature extraction is the process of selecting a set of parameters that best characterizes the whole image. On the other hand, the whole image intensity values may also be used as an attribute. In that case, the computational complexity of the algorithm increases. In this study, however, the minimum number of statistical features that best characterize MR images was determined and used in the classification process.

Texture Features:

Texture, one of the key features used to identify relevant regions of an object, describes repetitive patterns of local variations in image density. Many definitions have been given for texture in the literature. Some of these definitions are as follows:

- Texture is characterized as a spatial distribution at the grey level of the image, it cannot be defined in a single point. Texture used in areas such as computer vision, image processing and pattern recognition plays an important role in the extraction of surface attributes in an image [9].
- Defined as the collection of elements that resemble an image [10].
- Defined as a regular pattern of pixel values in an image. There are patterns with sub-patterns such as color, shape, and size in each image. Each of these patterns forms the texture of the image [10].

Methods of texture analysis are categorized into four groups: *statistical*, structural, model based, and transform based methods. The statistical method was utilized in our study to extract the features for diagnosing ADHD.

3.2.4 Statistical texture features

The statistical method extracts a series of statistical information from the distribution of local characteristics at each point, taking into account the spatial distribution of each element [10]. This method is categorized into *first order, second order*, and higher order statistical method. In this study, first and second order statistical methods were used to extract attributes from MR images.

3.2.4.1 First-order statistical texture analysis

The first-order statistical method utilizes the image histogram, or each pixel using frequency information in the image, making a series of statistical calculations regardless of the relationship of each pixel value to the adjacent pixel value. Mean, variance, skewness, and kurtosis are extracted as attributes of each MR image. Thus, we have created the first feature set, called **first order feature set**, containing the following attributes obtained with this method.

First-order texture attributes are as follows:

Mean: The average is known as the sum of elements in the data set divided by the number of elements.

$$\text{Mean} = \frac{1}{N}\sum\nolimits_{j=1}^{N} x_j \tag{3.1}$$

Variance: It measures each element in data set how spread out.

$$\text{Var}(x_1, ,x_N) = \frac{1}{N-1}\sum\nolimits_{j=1}^{N}(x_j - \mu) \tag{3.2}$$

Skewness: It is a measure of the asymmetry of the data around the sample mean.

$$\text{Skew}(x_1, ,x_N) = \frac{1}{N}\sum\nolimits_{j=1}^{N}\left(\frac{x_j - \mu}{\sigma}\right) \tag{3.3}$$

Kurtosis: Indicates how flat or steep the normal distribution curve is.

$$\text{Kurt}(x_1, ,x_N) = \left\{\frac{1}{N}\sum\nolimits_{j=1}^{N}\left(\frac{x_j - \mu}{\sigma}\right)\right\} - 3 \tag{3.4}$$

First order statistical feature set:

The brain images of 30 individuals, 15 with ADHD and 15 healthy individuals, were obtained from NPIstanbul Neuropsychiatry Hospital. Thus, a balanced dataset was created by selecting the equal number of samples between classes. Each MR image consist of 256 slices. However, 60 slices of interest, between 141 and 200 containing white and grey area, of each MR image were used in this study. These 60 slices are added together to obtain a combined slice. In figures 3.2, 60 slices of an MRI image is given.

In figure 3.3, each slice is added with the previous slice. Attributes were extracted from the texture of the last image which is the sum of all 60 slices. The first feature set was created by extracting the attributes of the 30 MRI images using the first order statistical method.

The mean, variance, skewness, and kurtosis attributes were calculated from the texture obtained by adding all 60 slices of each image. As an example, attributes of six images are given in table 3.1. The first three rows of the table show the features obtained from MR images of individuals diagnosed with ADHD, while the last three rows indicate the features of healthy individuals' MR images.

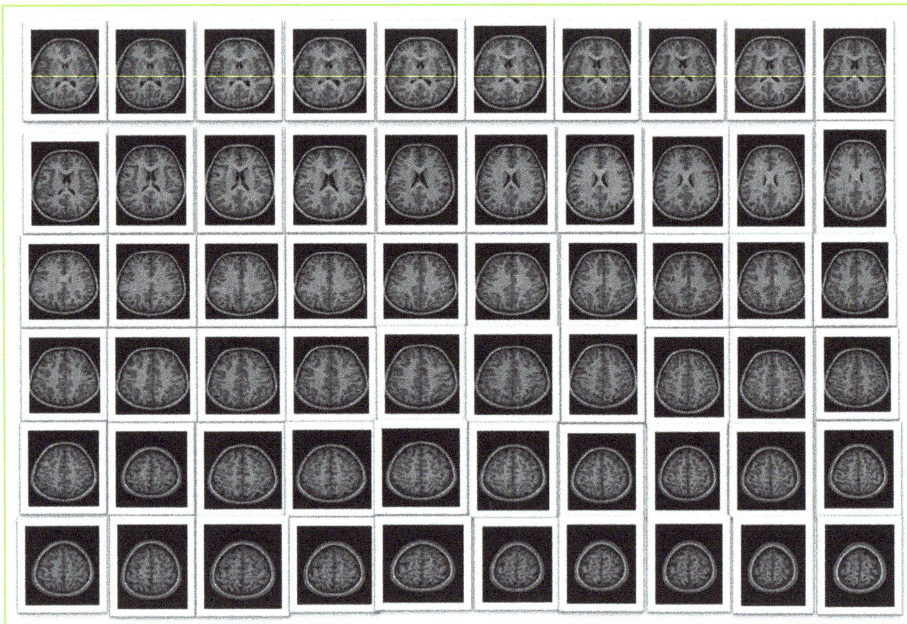

Figure 3.2. Slices of a magnetic resonance imaging.

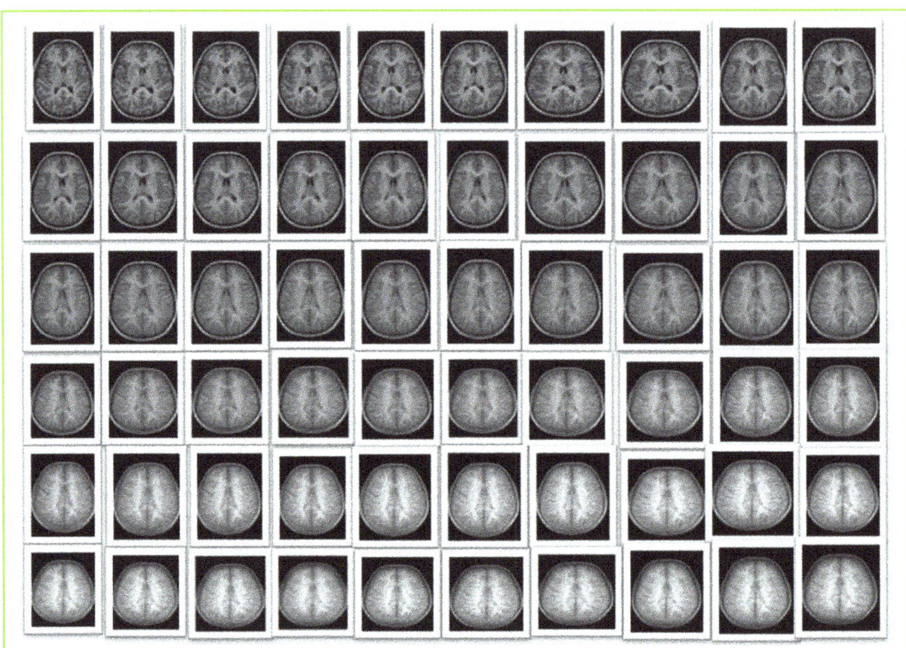

Figure 3.3. An image of the sum of slices of a magnetic resonance image.

Table 3.1. Examples of first order dataset.

Mean	Variance	Skewness	Kurtosis
68.6450	3.1118e+05	0.0064	0.0251
83.3716	3.4305e+05	0.0019	0.0235
58.7414	2.4672e+05	0.0087	0.0278
63.3492	2.6193e+05	0.0056	0.0238
65.9540	2.4467e+05	0.0035	0.0234
63.4313	2.7936e+05	0.0081	0.0271

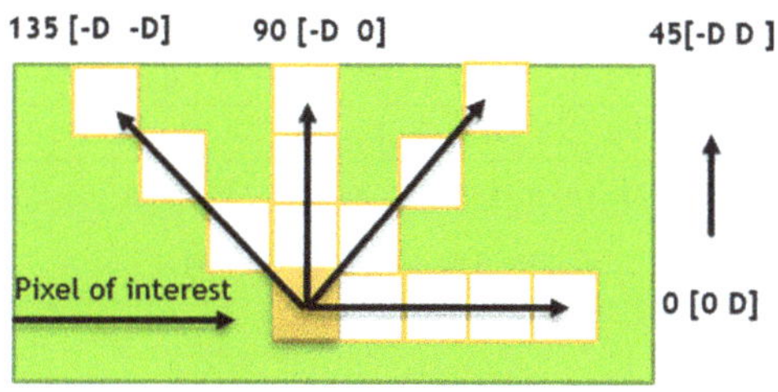

Figure 3.4. Directional analysis.

3.2.4.2 Second-order statistical texture analysis

The second-order statistical method provides information about the relative positions of grey levels. It makes a series of statistical calculations, considering the relationship of one pixel to another [11]. In this study, gray-level co-occurrence, and Haralick methods are used to generate two feature sets.

3.2.4.2.1 Gray-level co-occurrence method

The relationship of pixel positions with each other is an important parameter when extracting attributes to characterize data. The gray-level co-occurrence method (GLCM) makes it possible to access this parameter. GLCM is a matrix that describes the frequency information of specific pixel pairs in given spatial relationships. The attributes, namely energy, contrast, correlation, and homogeneity that will characterize the magnetic resonance image have been extracted with this method. The co-occurrence matrix is created using distance and direction parameters between the pixels (figure 3.4). For each pixel, four GLCM matrices were calculated in 0°, 45°, 90°, and 135° directions. Thus, four different GLCM matrices for the same image are obtained as clearly seen in figure 3.5.

Assume that the intensity values of an input image are as shown in the figure. GLCM matrices are created in four directions for each pixel. The number of pixel pairs are counted and written in GLCM matrices. These show the GLCM for 0°, 45°, 90°, and 135°, respectively. That is, as shown clearly in the figure, the knowledge that two adjacent pixels repeat each other is held in the co-occurrence matrices, which are created with different angles of the images. In this study, energy,

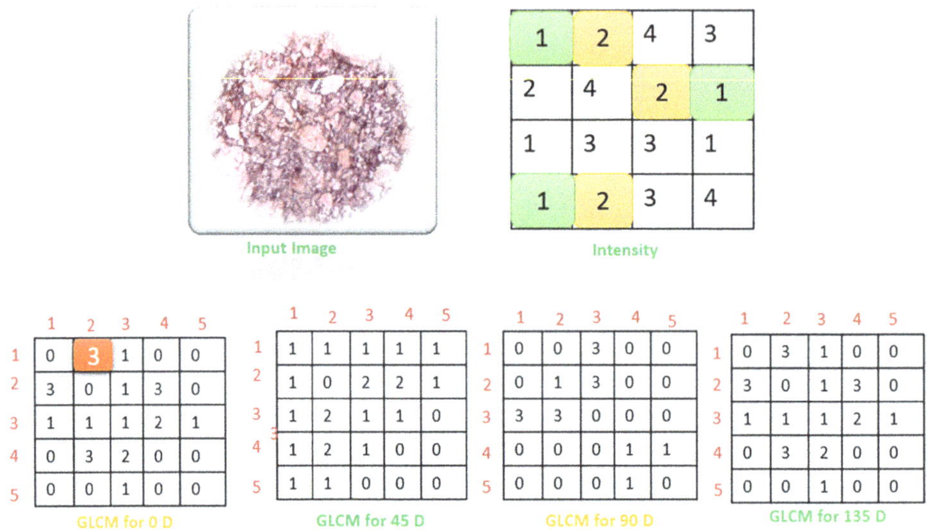

Figure 3.5. Creating GLCM.

contrast, correlation, and homogeneity have been extracted by using GLCM matrices.

Contrast: Measures local variations in the gray-level co-occurrence matrix.

$$\text{Contrast} = \sum_{i,\,j=0}^{N-1} P_{ij}(i-j)^2 \tag{3.5}$$

Correlation: Measures linear dependence between an image's gray level value and the specified color on a whole image.

$$\text{Correlation} = \sum_{i,\,j=0}^{N-1} P_{ij}\frac{(i-\mu)(j-\mu)}{\sigma} \tag{3.6}$$

Energy: This term, known as the angular second momentum, is calculated as the sum of the squares of the elements in the GLCM matrix.

$$\text{Energy} = \sum_{i,\,j=0}^{N-1} (P_{ij})^2 \tag{3.7}$$

Homogeneity: It is a measure of the similarity in different regions of the image.

$$\text{Homogeneity} = \sum_{i,\,j=0}^{N-1} \frac{P_{ij}}{1+(i-j)} \tag{3.8}$$

In the above equations (3.5–3.8), i and j are the indices of row and column, p is element of matrix, μ represents the mean, σ is the standard deviation of the co-occurrence matrix.

In our study, contrast, correlation, homogeneity, and energy attributes were extracted from the texture obtained from the sum of 60 slices of MR images. As an example, attributes calculated from six MR images are given in table 3.2. Thus, we

Table 3.2. Examples of GLCM dataset.

Mean	Variance	Skewness	Kurtosis
68.6450	3.1118e+05	0.0064	0.0251
83.3716	3.4305e+05	0.0019	0.0235
58.7414	2.4672e+05	0.0087	0.0278
63.3492	2.6193e+05	0.0056	0.0238
65.9540	2.4467e+05	0.0035	0.0234
63.4313	2.7936e+05	0.0081	0.0271

have created the GLCM dataset containing these attributes for all subjects. The first three rows of table 3.2 show the features obtained from MR images of individuals with ADHD, and the last three rows give the features of healthy individuals' MR images.

3.2.4.2.2 Haralick texture feature

Haralick texture attributes, which are one of the second-order statistical feature extraction techniques, are one of the well-known mathematical methods. They have been used in the diagnosis of Alzheimer's disease [12]. The aim is to determine the most prominent features in the determination of attention deficit hyperactivity disorder. For this purpose, Haralick texture feature, one of the statistical texture extraction methods, was used. Extracted features are as follows: *angular second moment, contrast, correlation, sum of squares, variance, inverse difference moment, sum average, sum variance, Eentropy, difference variance, difference entropy, information measure of correlation I, information measure of corrrelation II*, and *maximal correlation coefficient*. Definitions of these features are given in table 3.3.

Here, σ is the standard deviation, μ represents the mean, $\mathrm{HXY} = -\Sigma_i\Sigma_j p(i, j)\log(p(i, j))$, HX and HY are the enropies of p_x and p_y, $\mathrm{HXY1} = -\Sigma_i\Sigma_j p(i, j)\log\{p_x(i)p_y(j)\}$, $\mathrm{HXY2} = -\Sigma_i\Sigma_j p_x(i)p_y(j)\log\{p_x(i)p_y(j)\}$, Max Correlation is the square root of the second largest eigenvalue of Q where $Q(i,j) = \frac{p(i,k)p(j,k)}{p_x(i)p_y(k)}$.

In this study, the above Haralick attributes are extracted from the texture of the images, which is the sum of all 60 slices of the MR images. As an example, the attributes extracted from six structural MR images are given in table 3.4 where the first three columns show samples of ADHD, and the last three columns give the samples of healthy individuals' MR images.

3.2.5 Feature selection using principal component analysis

Feature selection is the process of selecting a sub-data set from the existing dataset to reduce the computational complexity. There may be attributes that make the classification difficult. In addition, irrelevant attributes may adversely affect the

Table 3.3. Texture features obtained with Haralick method.

Feature Name	Formula	Feature Name	Formula
Angular Second Moment	$\Sigma_i \Sigma_j p(i,j)^2$	Correlation	$\sum_{i,j=0}^{N-1} P_{ij} \frac{(i-\mu)(j-\mu)}{\sigma}$
Contrast	$\sum_{i,j=0}^{N-1} P_{ij}(i-j)^2$	Sum of Squares	$\Sigma_i \Sigma_j (i-j)^2 p(i,j)$
Inverse Difference Moment	$\Sigma_i \Sigma_j \frac{1}{1+(i-j)^2} p(i,j)$	Sum Average	$\sum_i^{2N} i\, p_{x+y}(i)$
Sum Variance	$\sum_{i=2}^{2N} (i - (- \sum_{i=2}^{2N} p_{x+y}(i) log\{p_{x+y}(i)\}))^2 p_{x+y}(i)$	Sum Entropy	$- \sum_{i=2}^{2N} p_{x+y}(i) log\{p_{x+y}(i)\}$
Entropy	$-\Sigma_i \Sigma_j p(i,j) \log (p(i,j))$	Difference Variance	$\sum_{i=0}^{N-1} i^2 p_{x-y}(i)$
Difference Entropy	$- \sum_{i=2}^{N-1} p_{x-y}(i) log\{p_{x-y}(i)\}$	Info. Measure of Corr. I	$\frac{HXY-HXY1}{\max(HX,HY)}$
Info. Measure of Correlation II.	$(1\text{-}\exp[(2(HXY2 - HXY))^{\frac{1}{2}}])$	Max. Correlation Coeff.	$Q(i,j) = \frac{p(i,k)p(j,k)}{p_x(i)p_y(k)}$

Table 3.4. Examples of Haralick dataset.

	1. ADHD	2.ADHD	3.ADHD	1. CONTROL	2.CONTROL	3.CONTROL
Angular Second Moment	0,6583	0,6624	0,6740	0,7292	0,7081	0,7034
Contrast	1,2256	1,2710	1,2595	1,2744	1,2155	1,2104
Correlation	0,9212	0,9169	0,9146	0,8941	0,9074	0,9094
Variance	51,3507	51,5915	52,1640	54,7549	53,7625	53,5503
Inverse Difference Moment	0,9755	0,9746	0,9748	0,9745	0,9757	0,9758
Sum Avearge	13,2310	13,2888	13,4170	13,9942	13,7709	13,7214
Sum Variance	204.9325	205,9281	208,2459	218,6206	214,6612	213,7752
Sum Entropy	0,5911	0,5875	0,5731	0,5038	0,5293	0,5351
Entropy	0,8777	0,8735	0,8525	0,7528	0,7885	0,7667
Difference Variance	1,1974	1,2412	1,2302	1,2445	1,1877	1,1828
Difference Entropy	0,1169	0,1203	0,1195	0,1206	0,1162	0,1158
Information Measure of Corr.I	-0,7760	-0,7680	-0,7641	-0,7299	-07529	-0,7560
Information Measure of Corr.II	0,8197	0,8146	0,8072	0,7610	0,7838	0,7880
Maximal Corr Coeff.	0,2087	0,2058	0,1979	0,1645	0,1763	0,1789

classification performance. In other words, the process of selecting the attributes is used to facilitate the fitting of the model, to find the attributes that best represent the data, to improve the classification performance, to reduce the computational cost. In this study, principal component analysis, one of the well-known and widely used methods, was utilized to determine the irrelevant features.

Principal component analysis (PCA), which is a useful statistical technique, helps to reduce the dimension of the feature set. It extracts relevant information from a confusing dataset. Some of data can be lost during the dimensionality reduction. The aim is to preserve the relevant information as much as reducing the dimension. The following operations are performed in order to apply the basic component analysis method. The following operation is done in order to find principal component of the dataset. Covariance matrix of the dataset is calculated, eigenvectors and eigenvalues of the matrix are obtained. Then the eigenvalues are sorted to find the maximum eigenvalue which corresponds to the main component of the dataset.

3.2.6 Classification

There are two classes of MR images obtained from NPIstanbul Neuropsychiatry Hospital. These are (i) healthy controls, and (ii) ADHD classes. K-nearest neighbour and decision tree classification algorithm were used to detect ADHD images.

3.2.6.1 K-nearest neighbour algorithm

The K-nearest neighbour (K-NN) algorithm is a simple and successful classification algorithm. When a new sample comes, the object's similarity to all objects in the training set is computed. Generally, Manhattan, Euclidean, Minkowski, and Hamming distances are used to find similarity between the objects. We utilized Euclidean distance to find similarity between the features of MR images.

$$E(x, y) = \sqrt{\sum_{i=0}^{n}(x_i - y_i)^2} \tag{3.9}$$

3.2.6.2 Decision tree algorithm

Decision tree is a powerful classification algorithm that is easy to understand and interpret. The decision tree continually divides the search space by a certain parameter. This parameter is equal to the attribute that best distinguishes the samples from the training set. The best distinguishing attribute in the training set is found by calculating the information gain for each attribute. Thus, the first node of the tree, called root node, is found. The search space shrinks as the process continues. The information gain is calculated over all samples in the data set, and child nodes are determined. This procedure lasts until we find the leaves of the tree, meaning that there are no samples left. The tree consists of root node, child nodes, and leaves. Leaves represent the classes of the data. In the second phase of the algorithm, the samples are applied to the model, and classes of all samples are determined. Figure 3.6 is an example of a binary tree.

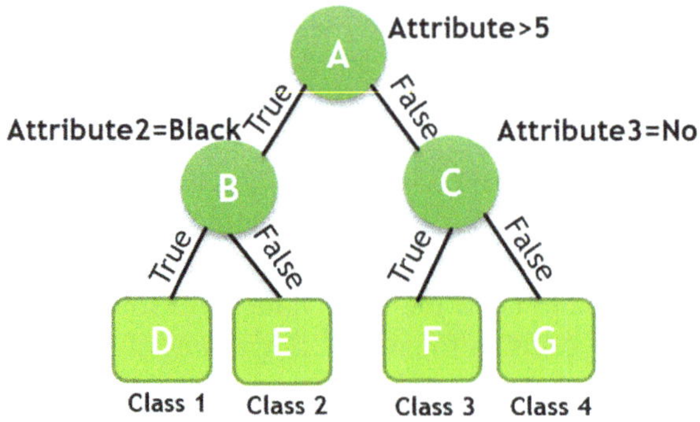

Figure 3.6. Binary tree.

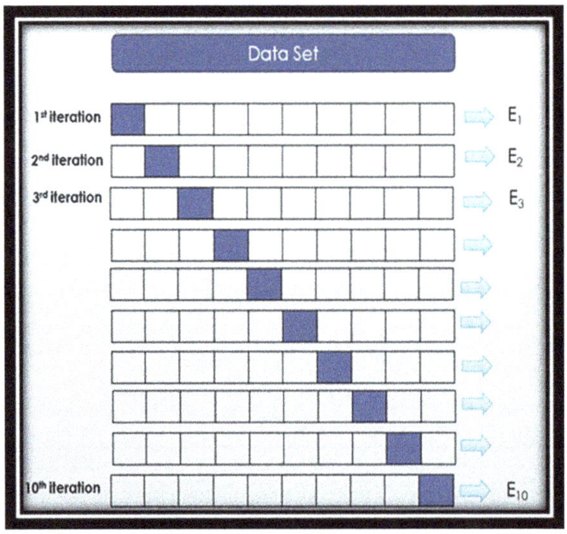

Figure 3.7. 10-Fold cross validation.

3.3 Performance measures

Cross validation is a statistical method used to evaluate and compare the performance of classification algorithms. Data is divided into parts for training and test purposes. The partition format is varied according to the evaluation method chosen. In our study, we used 10-fold cross validation, and hold-out cross validation methods to calculate the performance of our proposed method.

3.3.1 K-fold cross validation

It is one of the statistical methods which is used commonly to evaluate and compare the performance of classifiers with training phase (figure 3.7).

The following steps are performed in order to apply a 10-fold cross validation.

1. Data is divided into 10 equal size partitions.

2. One part is used as test and the other parts used for training. Performance of the classifier is calculated for this case.
3. The second step is repeated for each of the 10 parts. Then, average accuracy is calculated for the model by

$$E = \frac{1}{10}\sum\nolimits_{i=0}^{10} E_i \tag{3.10}$$

3.3.2 Hold-out cross validation

The second performance measure we employed is the hold-out cross validation. In this approach, the data is divided into two parts. One piece is used for training and the other part is used for testing the classifier. The disadvantage of this method is that the performance depends on the section of the data chosen, i.e., a large difference may be observed in the performance ratios of the model. This does not always give accurate information about the robustness of the model (figure 3.8).

In our study, 75% of the data were used for training purposes, and the remaining 25% were used for testing purposes.

3.3.3 Confusion matrix

Confusion matrix is one of the methods used to measure classification performance. *Accuracy, sensitivity, specificity, true positive rate, false positive rate, recall*, and *F-measure* parameters are computed by using this matrix (figure 3.9). Each of them reveals information about the performance of a classification system (table 3.5).

3.4 Experimental results

The features extracted from MR images by using first- and second-order statistical methods were used for the detection of ADHD images. Three different datasets were generated from the same MR images, namely *first order dataset*, *GLCM dataset*, and *Haralick dataset*. The principle component analysis algorithm was applied in order to determine the dominant attributes. These three datasets were used as input to K-NN, and decision tree classification algorithms. Two different scenarios were designed for each classifier using:

i. all extracted attributes;
ii. only selected attributes.

10-fold cross validation, and hold-out cross validation were adopted for randomly training and testing the algorithms in order to evaluate the performance metrics. In addition, *accuracy, specificity, sensitivity, true positive rate, false positive*

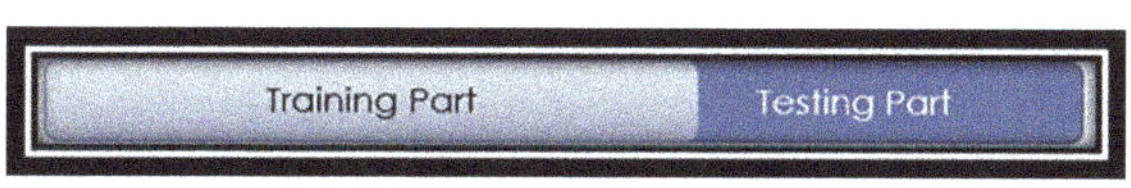

Figure 3.8. Hold-out cross validation.

Actual Class \ Predicted Class	ADHD	HEALTHY
ADHD	True Positive (TP)	False Negative (FN)
HEALTHY	False Positive (FP)	True Negative (TN)

Figure 3.9. Confusion matrix.

Table 3.5. Performance measures.

$$Accuracy = \frac{(TP + TN)}{(TP + FN + FP + TN)}$$

$$Sensitivity(Recall) = \frac{(TP)}{(TP + FN)}$$

$$Specificity = \frac{(TN)}{(TN + FP)}$$

$$True\ Positive\ Rate(Precision) = \frac{(TP)}{(TP + FP)}$$

$$True\ Negative\ Rate = \frac{(TN)}{(TN + FN)}$$

$$False\ Positive\ Rate = \frac{(FP)}{(FP + TN)}$$

$$Recall = \frac{(FP)}{(FP + TN)}$$

$$FMeasure = 2 * \frac{(Precision * Recall)}{(Precision + Recall)}$$

rate, F-measure, and *receiver operating characteristic (ROC) curve* (the true positive rate as a function of the false positive rate) were calculated to evaluate the classification performance.

In our experiments, the following models were generated, and the performance of ADHD classification was evaluated using *first order dataset*, *GLCM dataset*, and *Haralick dataset*:

Model 1: Decision tree algorithm with all attributes.
Model 2: Decision Tree algorithm with selected attributes.
Model 3: K-NN algorithm with all attributes.
Model 4: K-NN algorithm with selected attributes.

First order dataset classification results:
We evaluated the performance of the above four models by using first order dataset, and confusion matrices and ROC curves are shown in table 3.6 for both 10-fold and hold-out cross validation cases.

Performance of all four models was evaluated using both 10-fold, and hold-out cross validation methods and performance metrics are given in table 3.7.

Table 3.6. Confusion matrix and ROC curves for first order dataset.

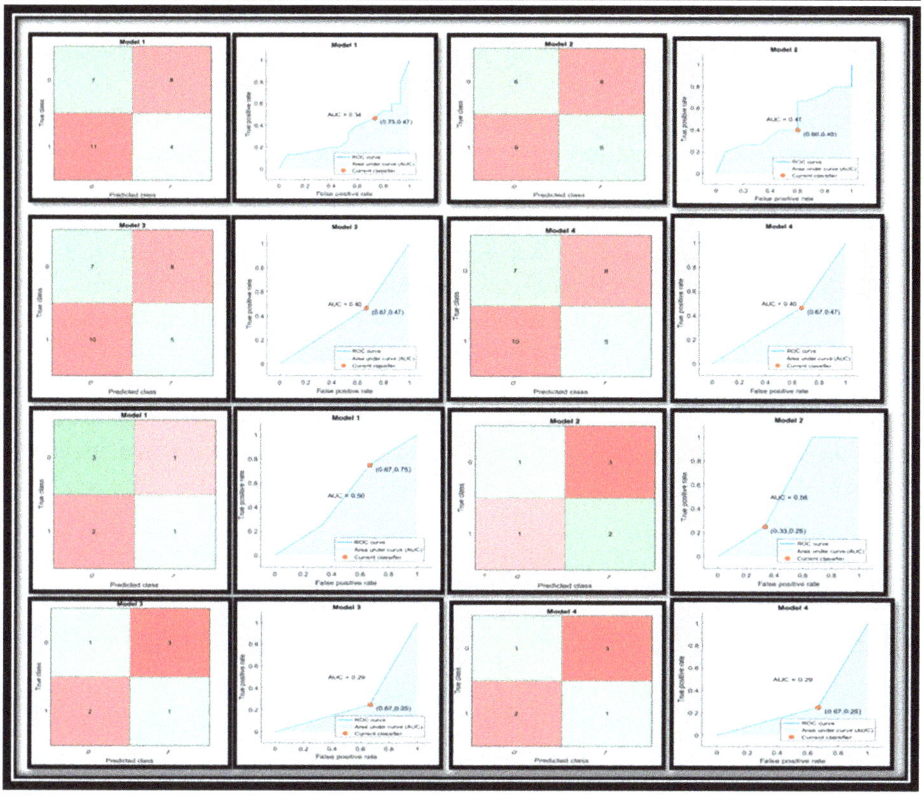

Table 3.7. Detailed performance measures for first order dataset.

	10 Fold Cross Validation			
	Decision Tree		K Nearest Neighbor	
	All attributes	Selected Attributes	All Attributes	Selected Attributes
Accuracy	0.36	0.40	0.40	0.40
Sensitivity	0.38	0.40	0.41	0.41
Specificity	0.33	0.40	0.38	0.38
TP Rate	0.46	0.60	0.46	0.46
FP Rate	0.66	0.40	0.61	0.61
Recall	0.46	0.40	0.46	0.46
F-Measure	0.46	0.40	0.46	0.46
	Hold Out Cross Validation			
	Decision Tree		K Nearest Neighbor	
	All attributes	Selected Attributes	All Attributes	Selected Attributes
Accuracy	0.57	0.42	0.28	0.28
Sensitivity	0.60	0.50	0.33	0.33
Specificity	0.50	0.40	0.25	0.25
TP Rate	0.75	0.25	0.25	0.25
FP Rate	0.50	0.60	0.75	0.75
Recall	0.75	0.25	0.25	0.25
F-Measure	0.75	0.25	0.25	0.25

GLCM dataset classification results:
Classification performance of the four models were evaluated by using the second order GLMC dataset, and confusion matrices and ROC curves are shown in table 3.8.

Detailed performance of all four models was evaluated using both 10-fold, and hold-out cross validation methods and performance metrics are given in table 3.9.

Haralick dataset classification results:
Performance of the four models in the ADHD detection were evaluated using the Haralick dataset, and confusion matrices and ROC curves are given in table 3.10.

Detailed performance measures of all four models are also given in table 3.11, using both 10-fold, and hold-out cross validation methods.

Table 3.12 provides a summary of the performances of all three datasets, two classification algorithms, advantage or disadvantage of feature selection, and two cross validation approaches. The highest classification performance was achieved by using the Haralick dataset, and all extracted features.

Table 3.8. Confusion matrix and ROC curves for GLMC dataset.

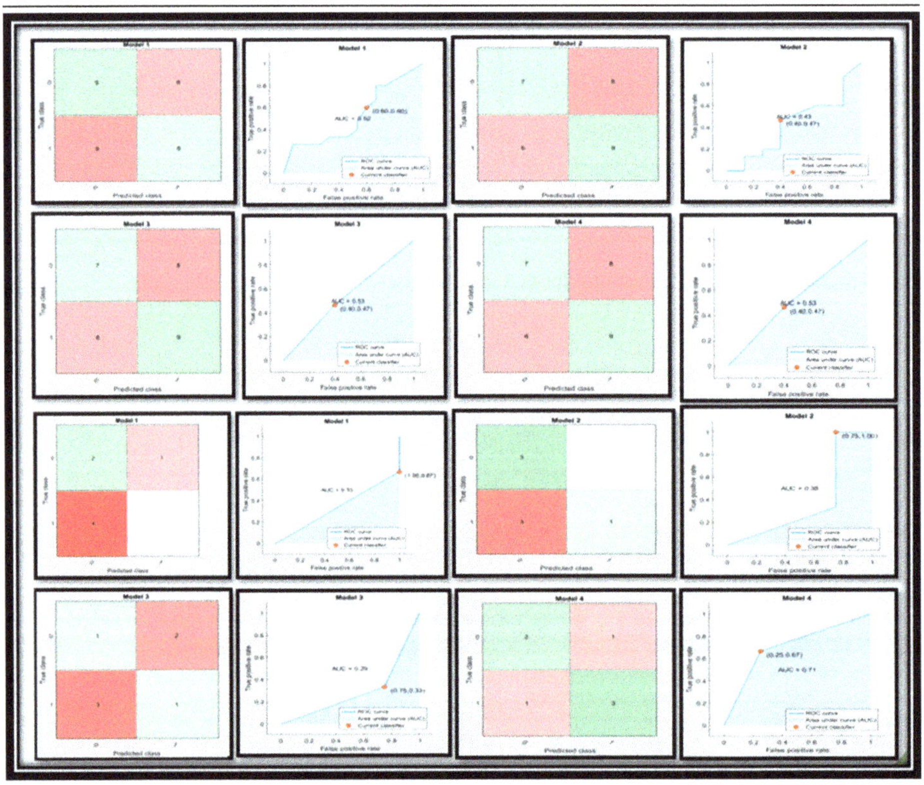

Table 3.9. Detailed performance measures for the GLCM dataset.

	10 Fold Cross Validation			
	Decision Tree		K Nearest Neighbor	
	All attributes	Selected Attributes	All Attributes	Selected Attributes
Accuracy	0.50	0.53	0.53	0.53
Sensitivity	0.50	0.53	0.53	0.53
Specificity	0.50	0.52	0.52	0.52
TP Rate	0.60	0.46	0.46	0.46
FP Rate	0.50	0.47	0.47	0.47
Recall	0.60	0.46	0.46	0.46
F-Measure	0.60	0.46	0.46	0.46
	Hold Out Cross Validation			
	Decision Tree		K Nearest Neighbor	
	All attributes	Selected Attributes	All Attributes	Selected Attributes
Accuracy	0.28	0.57	0.28	0.71
Sensitivity	0.33	0.50	0.25	0.66
Specificity	0.0	1	0.33	0.75
TP Rate	0.66	1	0.33	0.66
FP Rate	1	0	0.66	0.25
Recall	0.66	1	0.33	0.66
F-Measure	0.66	1	0.33	0.66

Table 3.10. Confusion matrix and ROC curves for Haralick dataset.

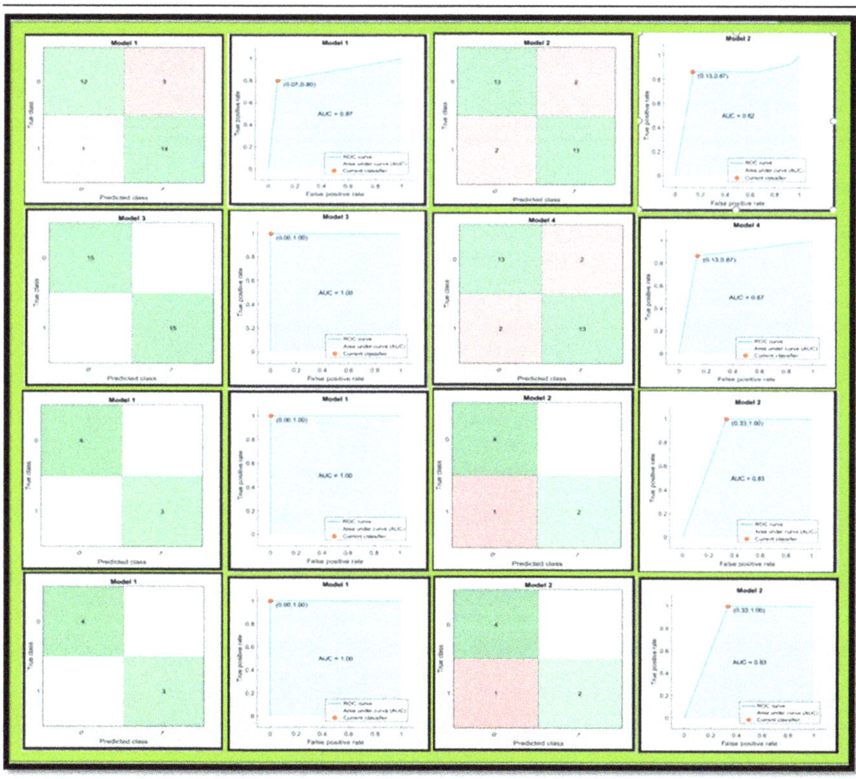

Table 3.11. Detailed performance measures for Haralick dataset.

	10 Fold Cross Validation			
	Decision Tree		K Nearest Neighbor	
	All attributes	Selected Attributes	All Attributes	Selected Attributes
Accuracy	0.86	0.86	1	0.86
Sensitivity	0.92	0.86	1	0.86
Specificity	0.82	0.86	1	0.86
TP Rate	0.80	0.86	1	0.86
FP Rate	0.17	0.13	0	0.13
Recall	0.80	0.86	1	0.86
F-Measure	0.80	0.86	1	0.86
	Hold Out Cross Validation			
	Decision Tree		K Nearest Neighbor	
	All attributes	Selected Attributes	All Attributes	Selected Attributes
Accuracy	1	0.85	1	0.85
Sensitivity	1	0.80	1	0.80
Specificity	1	1	1	1
TP Rate	1	1	1	1
FP Rate	0	0	0	0
Recall	1	1	1	1
F-Measure	1	1	1	1

Table 3.12. Classification performances of all three datasets.

DataSet	Performance Measure	Number of Features	Classification Algorithm	Accuracy
First Order DataSet	10 Fold Cross Validation	All Attributes	Decision Tree	36 %
First Order DataSet	10 Fold Cross Validation	Selected Attributes	Decision Tree	40 %
First Order DataSet	10 Fold Cross Validation	All Attributes	K Nearest Neighbor	40 %
First Order DataSet	10 Fold Cross Validation	Selected Attributes	K Nearest Neighbor	40 %
First Order DataSet	Hold Out Cross Validation	All Attributes	Decision Tree	57 %
First Order DataSet	Hold Out Cross Validation	Selected Attributes	Decision Tree	42 %
First Order DataSet	Hold Out Cross Validation	All Attributes	K Nearest Neighbor	28 %
GLCM	10 Fold Cross Validation	All Attributes	Decision Tree	50 %
GLCM	10 Fold Cross Validation	Selected Attributes	Decision Tree	53 %
GLCM	10 Fold Cross Validation	All Attributes	K Nearest Neighbor	53 %
GLCM	10 Fold Cross Validation	Selected Attributes	K Nearest Neighbor	53 %
GLCM	Hold Out Cross Validation	All Attributes	Decision Tree	28 %
GLCM	Hold Out Cross Validation	Selected Attributes	Decision Trees	57 %
GLCM	Hold Out Cross Validation	All Attributes	K Nearest Neighnor	28 %
GLCM	Hold Out Cross Validation	Selected Attributes	K Nearest Neighbor	71 %
Haralick	10 Fold Cross Validation	All Attributes	Decision Tree	86 %
Haralick	10 Fold Cross Validation	Selected Attributes	Decision Tree	86 %
Haralick	10 Fold Cross Validation	All Attributes	K Nearest Neighbor	100 %
Haralick	10 Fold Cross Validation	Selected Attributes	K Nearest Neighbor	86 %
Haralick	Hold Out Cross Validation	All Attributes	Decision Tree	100 %
Haralick	Hold Out Cross Validation	Selected Attributes	Decision Tree	85 %
Haralick	Hold Out Cross Validation	All Attributes	K Nearest Neighbor	100 %
Haralick	Hold Out Cross Validation	Selected Attributes	K Nearest Neighbor	85 %

3.5 Results

The dataset in our study consists of 30 MR images, 15 of them are of ADHD, and the other 15 of healthy controls; hence a balanced dataset was used. Each MR image consists of 256 slices. Sixty slices of interest of MR images were added to generate a new texture from which statistical features are extracted. The first dataset was created by using first-order statistical features. Attributes of this dataset were mean, variance, skewness, and kurtosis. Second and third datasets were created using second-order statistical features.

The second dataset contains GLCM features which are contrast, correlation, homogeneity, and energy. The third dataset is generated using Haralick features including angular second moment, contrast, correlation, sum of squares, variance, inverse difference moment, sum average, sum variance, entropy, difference variance, difference entropy, info. measure of corr. I, and info. measure of corr. II. PCA was used in order to find irrelevant features. Extracted features are applied to K-NN, and decision tree classification algorithms. 10-fold cross validation accuracy on the Haralick dataset using all attributes using K-NN classification algorithm was 100%. Another very successful model is obtained by the Haralick dataset using all attributes, and decision tree classifier with 100% hold-out cross validation accuracy.

References

[1] Adesman A 2001 The diagnosis and management of attention-deficit/hyperactivity disorder in pediatric patients *Prim. Care Companion J. Clin. Psychiatry* **3** 66–77

[2] Miller D, Derefinko K, Lynan D and Milich R 2001 Impulsivity and attention deficit-hyperac tivity disorder: subtype classification using the UPPS impulsive behavior scale *Prim. Care Companion J. Clin. Psychiatry* **32** 323–32

[3] Waxmonsky J 2003 Assesment and treatment of attention deficit hyperactivity disorder in children with comorbid psychiatric illness *Curr. Opin. Pediatry* **15** 476–82

[4] Martin K, Timoty B, Pratap C, Angelo F and Larry K 2017 Adult ADHD and comorbid disorders: clinical implications of a dimensional approach *BMC Psychiatry*

[5] Gentile J, Atig R and Gilig M 2006 Adult ADHD: diagnosis, differential diagnosis, and medication management *Psychiatry(Edgmont)*

[6] Martin B, Elizabeth B, Alain P and Gaia S 2010 Cortical gray matter in attention-deficit/hyperactivity disorder: a structural magnetic resonance imaging study *J. Am. Acad. Child Adolesc. Psychiatry*

[7] Castellanos F, Lee P, Sharp W and Greenstein D 2002 Developmental trajectories of brain volume abnormalities in children and adolescents with attention-deficit/hyperactivity disorder *J. Am. Med. Assoc.* **288** 1740–8

[8] Kelly A, Margulies D and Castellanos F 2007 Recent advances in structural and functional brain imaging studies of attention-deficit/hyperactivity disorder *Curr. Psychiatry Rep.* **9** 401–7

[9] Ramesh J, Rangachar K and Brian G 1995 *Machine Vision* (New York: McGraw-Hill)

[10] Ershad S 2011 Color texture classification approach based on combination of primitive patterns units and statistical features *Int. J. Multimedia Appl.*
[11] Srinivisan G and Shobba G 2008 Statistical texture analysis *Proc. World Acad, Sci. Eng. Technol.*
[12] Rajeesh J and Palanikumar S 2012 Discrimination of Alzheimer's disease using hippocampus texture features from MRI *Asian Biomed*

IOP Publishing

Neurological Disorders and Imaging Physics, Volume 4
Application to attention deficit hyperactivity disorder
Ayman El-Baz and Jasjit S Suri

Chapter 4

The new methods of application to attention deficit hyperactivity disorder

Yunhee Shin and Won-Seok Kang

4.1 Introduction

Attention deficit hyperactivity disorder (ADHD) is a neurodevelopmental disorder, one of the common childhood behaviour disorders, and it is possible to diagnose for ages between 5 and 12 by doctors and psychologists. Professionals mainly use the guidelines in the American Psychiatric Association's *Diagnostic and Statistical Manual of Mental Disorders* 5th edn (DSM-5) [1], to help diagnose ADHD. This shows a persistent pattern of inattention, and/or hyperactivity-impulsivity.

Recently, the prevalence of ADHD and autism in children has been on the rise, but they often vary widely due to changes in the environment and social development. According to [1], ADHD is estimated to affect 5% of the population in childhood within and between countries. Thomas *et al* reported for ADHD an overall pooled estimate of 7.2% from 175 eligible studies by review and meta-analysis [2]. Whether ADHD is over-diagnosed or under-diagnosed, it has been controversy to diagnosis ADHD. Wolraich *et al* reported that within the current ADHD diagnosis there does not exist biological evidence to confirm ADHD clearly, and the current test or checklist does not make a clear boundary between proper or inappropriate behaviours [3].

There is also often a dependence on environment or stimulation, for example, people with ADHD pay attention to a game they like. Most checklists consist of three ADHD diagnosis traits—inattention, hyperactivity, and impulsivity using DSM criteria [4, 5]. Behavior data is more easily collected and it is possible to handle the statistical process. At the first line of ADHD diagnostic process, their parent's report is a very important source because behaviour should be observed over two scenes of a child's life (e.g. home and school), and over six months. In the educational field, many teachers want to take a doctor's note to arrange their class, and to consult their parent. The parent has a valuable role as mediator between doctors, teachers and their child in

doi:10.1088/978-0-7503-1822-8ch4

the educational or medical field. It is a natural process for diagnosis of ADHD even though it does not take account of the parent's psychological condition [6].

ADHD screening tests are mostly in the form of checklists using Likert-scale by parent's and teacher's reports. Many researchers try to improve reliability through standardization or agreement between parents and teacher. It might be time-consuming or stressful for the parent and teacher because there is often disparity between parents' and teachers' reports of behaviour. Also, as many as 80% of adults with ADHD have at least one comorbid psychiatric disorder including autism spectrum disorders, mood and anxiety disorders, substance use disorders (USDs), and personality disorders [7]. Someone might be re-diagnosed due to the rules of diagnostic criteria or reliability of the checklist result.

Researchers have tried to make new approaches for assessments and diagnosis of ADHD using technology, as many studies published have shown that ADHD is related to frontal lobe brain damage. In order to make a solution, neuro-psychological tests converted to computer-based test like CPT, WCST, are collected and analyzed data using CT, MRI, PET, and fMRI [8, 9]. The brain imaging technology has development rapidly with physics and neuroscience, however, it is rare to be used for ADHD diagnosis due to cost issues. This is a reason the EEG device is used by the therapist and psychologist in the field due to relatively lower cost, although it is difficult to wear an EEG device without actually moving. In this chapter, we will describe the currently used ADHD assessment methods and tools in the clinical situation and introduce two new approaches. One is focused on behaviour observation with text-based data and on the brain signal. Another is focused on behaviour observation by kinetic sensor using a game with a robot.

4.2 Textual based and brain signal based method

Teachers of special education have recorded the monitored behaviour data in order to make use of diagnosis methods to classify or cluster the spectrum disorder. However, teachers only use the recorded data in historical views of the children due to IT-based processing limitation of the large-scale monitored data. There are so many valuable and meaningful features which teachers may miss on the database.

For the ADHD children disorder spectrum analysis in the special education field, '1. Data for special education' in figure 4.1, which is collected and written by teachers and others, should be prepared for ADHD assessments. Then, pre-processing such as de-noising for signal data and sentence segmentation for text data is performed according to the data type. After doing the features-modelling included in the refined data is performed, the features are extracted. Finally, the classification scheme is processed for ADHD disorder spectrum classification.

This section describes two major IT-based techniques for ADHD classification. One is a text-based approach and the other is a brain signal (especially, EEG)-based approach.

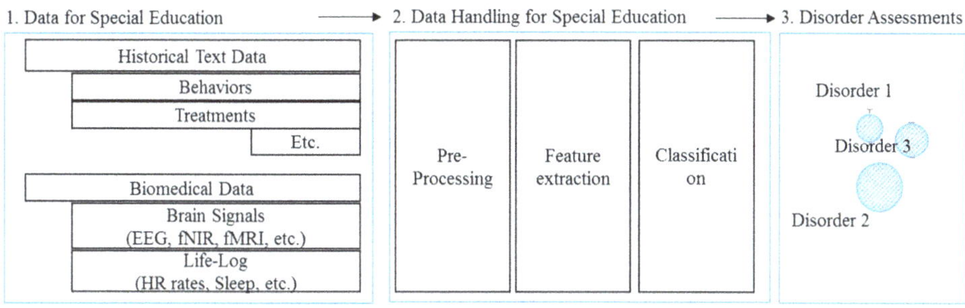

Figure 4.1. General method for analysis.

Table 4.1. An example of the behavior text (written in Korean).

Class	Categorized Korean terminology
Aggression	'때리기(Beating)', '물기(Biting)', '꼬집기(Pinching)', '할퀴기 (Scratching)', '밀기(Pushing)'
Depression–anxiety	'공포(Fear)', '불안(Anxiety)', '갑작스런 감정변화(감정기복)(Emotional changes suddenly)'
Self-mutilation	'벽에 머리 찧기(Beating one's head against the wall)', '머리 때리기 (Beating one's head)', '머리 뜯기(Pick one's hair)'
Abnormal sleep behaviour	'수면곤란(Sleeping difficulty)', '수면과다(Hypersomnia)', '수면부족(Lack of sleep)'
Problems with concentration	'허공 응시(Staring into the air)', '헷갈림(Confusability)', '긴장(Tension)', '불안한 몸짓(Anxious motion)', '안절부절

4.2.1 Textual data-based method

It is impossible for every teacher to inspect all of the specific features on the database in detail [10–16]. Natural language processing and data mining are an adequate approach to find out, cluster and classify the disorder features in the whole recorded data. One method is to use observed behaviour text-data which a special educator or rehabilitation scientist have saved, in order to cluster ADHD and autism disorder.

The special educator has categorized 11 disorder classes for ADHD and autism children [17]. The disorder groups are 'aggression', 'depression-anxiety', 'self-mutilation', 'antisocial behaviour', 'stereotyped behaviour', 'sexually abnormal behaviour', 'physical symptoms', 'abnormal feeding behaviour', 'abnormal sleep behaviour' and 'problems with concentration' as presented in table 4.1. The Korean terminology features which have meanings of disorder level are assigned to each disorder group by special educators. The features described here are words or phrases. In table 4.1, the specific morphological analyser can be used for extracting the textual behaviour features in English, Japanese, Chinese and so on.

Morphology analyzers have been used in natural language processing for several decades to analyse text-based languages. A morphology analyzer is useful to observe the terminologies of the disorders from the text-typed data of specific behavior of ADHD and autism children. In Korean, the morphological analysis can employ an open distributed software program, called HAM, downloaded on the website [18].

In general, a method for ADHD disorder spectrum classification technology is to process the procedure as shown in figure 4.2. Proactively, the behaviour textual data (behavior textual database in figure 4.2) must be collected by a special educator, medical doctor and so on.

The next step is to perform morph-analysis and extract the predefined behaviour word or phrase for each language. A classification processing that can perform classification after features-extraction is performed to derive ADHD disorder spectrum results. There are many ways to do a classification processing, but this section describes frequency-based approaches as an example.

Figure 4.3 shows a sample result after morphology processing. The ‘Column 1: Observed date, Column 2: Recorded date and Column 3: ID of disorder children’ data is a historical behaviour text data written by special educators, automatic writing software tools and so on. The morphology analyser can generate the ‘Column 4: Morphology analysis data’ for each language.

In the next step, ‘features extraction’ extracts the terminologies tagged with N (noun) and V (verb, adjective) in order to cluster the disorder. The terminologies N, V are features sets which can be defined by software developers or special educators in advance. The ‘classification processing’ can use the conventional classification algorithms such as K-nearest neighbor (KNN), support vector machine (SVM), artificial neural network (ANN) and so on. Also, new algorithms such as frequency-based processing can be newly constructed for ADHD disorder classification. This section provides an example of a frequency-based approach.

The frequency-based approach can perform the frequency of the terminologies tagged with N and V like equation (4.1) where $\boldsymbol{T}$ is a set of the terminologies extracted from features extraction. $\text{freq}_{\text{local}}(T)$ is the occurrence frequency with children identification information for a specific term. $\text{freq}_{\text{total}}(T)$is the occurrence frequency without the identification information.

$$\text{freq}(T) = \frac{\text{freq}_{\text{local}}(T)}{\text{freq}_{\text{total}}(T)} \tag{4.1}$$

where

$$\text{freq}_{\text{local}}(T) \neq 0$$

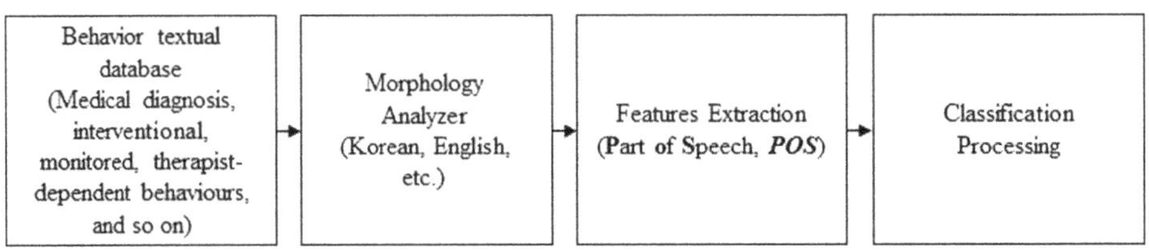

Figure 4.2. Disorder classification procedure based on textual data.

Observed Date	Recored Date	ID of disorder Children	Morphology analysis Data
정상적인 배변을 한다.	09-Dec-02	6	정상적/N + 이/c + ㄴ/e + 배변/N + 을/j + 하/V + ㄴ다/e + ./q +
정상적인 배변을 한다.	11-Dec-02	6	정상적/N + 이/c + ㄴ/e + 배변/N + 을/j + 하/V + ㄴ다/e + ./q +
정상적인 배변을 한다.	23-Jan-02	6	정상적/N + 이/c + ㄴ/e + 배변/N + 을/j + 하/V + ㄴ다/e + ./q +
정상적인 배변을 한다.	24-Jan-02	6	정상적/N + 이/c + ㄴ/e + 배변/N + 을/j + 하/V + ㄴ다/e + ./q +
소변을 볼 때 양이 많다.	08-Apr-06	6	소변/N + 을/j + 보/V + ㄹ/e + 때/V + 어/e + 양/N + 이/j + 많/V + 다/e + ./q +
대변을 볼 때 양이 적다.	21-Oct-06	6	대변/N + 을/j + 보/V + ㄹ/e + 때/V + 어/e + 양/N + 이/j + 적/V + 다/e + ./q +

Figure 4.3. Morphology analysis results in Korean.

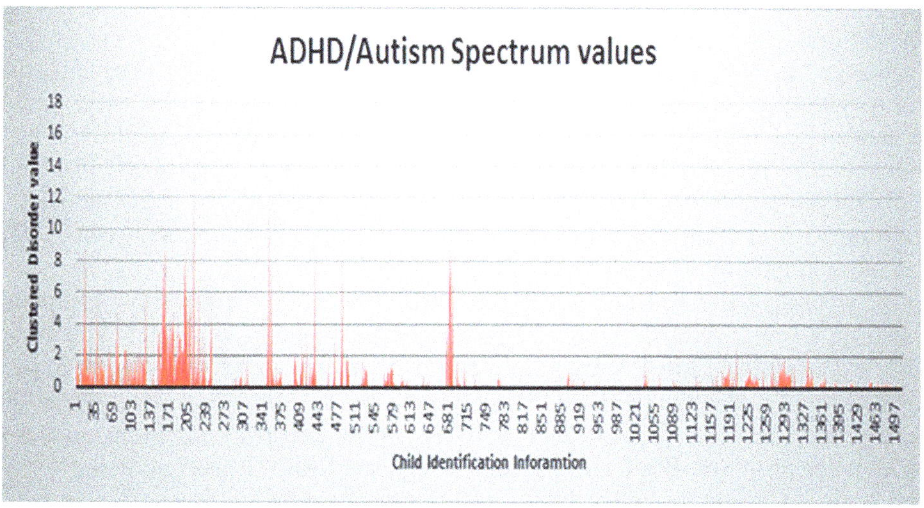

Figure 4.4. ADHD classification visualization.

Using equation (4.2), the accumulated specific behaviour frequency can generate historically

$$f(T, t_s, t_e) = \prod_{t=t_s}^{t_e} \frac{\text{freq}_{\text{local}}(T)}{\text{freq}_{\text{total}}(T)} \times \alpha_t \tag{4.2}$$

where

$$\text{freq}_{\text{local}}(T) \neq 0$$

Finally, a software developer or special educator can make up the final ADHD disorder spectrum data like figure 4.4. using equation (4.3). This method has a problem that high precision cannot be guaranteed by performing software processing on a database without expert verification

$$F(T, t_s, t_e) = \sum_{\text{child}_{\text{id}}=1}^{N} f(\text{child}_{\text{id}}, t_s, t_e) \tag{4.3}$$

4.2.2 Brain signal-based method

Recently, brain–computer interface (BCI) research has been employed as tools for assistive approaches of rehabilitation, medicine and special education fields. The electroencephalogram (EEG) is one of the biomedical signals mostly used in BCI. However, EEG is complicated with various noises which make it difficult to make precise the important information retrievals [19, 20]. Furthermore, EEG depends on the subject's situation such as testing environment, mood of the day, mental activity patterns and so on. Although EEG has many drawbacks, it is the most popular material which is used in BCI research with easy usability, and mobility. In addition, it costs less than other non-invasive devices such as functional near-infrared spectroscopy (fNIRS), magnetic resonance imaging (MRI), positron emission tomography (PET), and magnetoencephalography (MEG) [21].

Researches on ADHD disorder investigate the brain functions using various brain activity recording techniques. In particular, EEG, one of the advantageous methods, is non-invasive, economical and long-time recordable. ADHD is not a psychological problem but a kind of encephalopathy where there occurs imbalance of brain development. Recently, many countries studied the EEG activity of children with and without ADHD to understand the differences between ADHD and normal children with EEG data [22].

In general, a method for ADHD disorder spectrum classification technology based on a brain signal is to use the procedure as shown in figure 4.5. The devices such as EEG, fMRI must be prepared for classifying the disorder spectrum in order to analyse a brain signal with ADHD children. Brain stimulation programs should be provided for specific disorders analysis. Many researchers call it a stimulus protocol or program. Brain signals must be collected with the stimulation protocols and brain-acquisition devices. Once the three phases (device selection, stimulation protocol, and brain signal database) are ready, you can analyse the ADHD disorder spectrum with software processing.

Similar to the text-based processing method, brain signal data can be processed automatically by performing the feature modelling, pre-processing and analysis procedures. The brain signals as shown in figure 4.6 can be obtained by the brain acquisition equipment and the stimulation protocol.

Many software algorithms have been proposed for brain signal processing. Recently, the most popular method is the discrete wavelet transform (DWT)-based approaches for brain signal filtering, classification and clustering processing. Traditionally, the brain signal event-related potential (ERP), frequency and

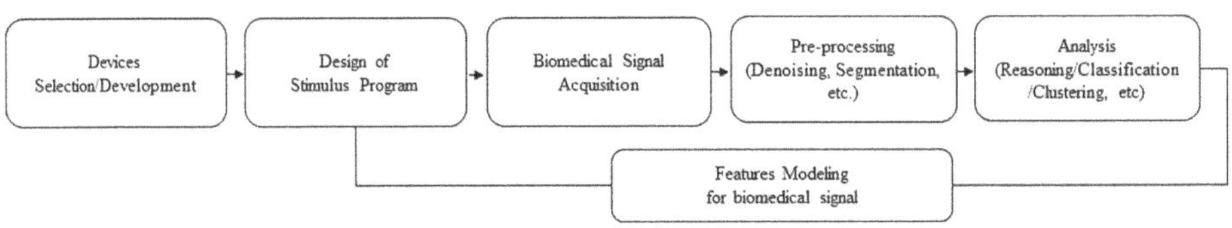

Figure 4.5. Disorder classification procedure based on brain signal.

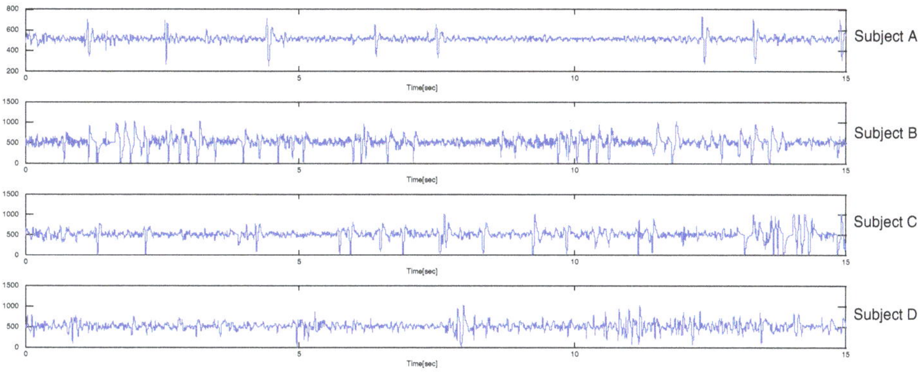

Figure 4.6. Examples of EEG data from four ADHD children belonging to several disorders.

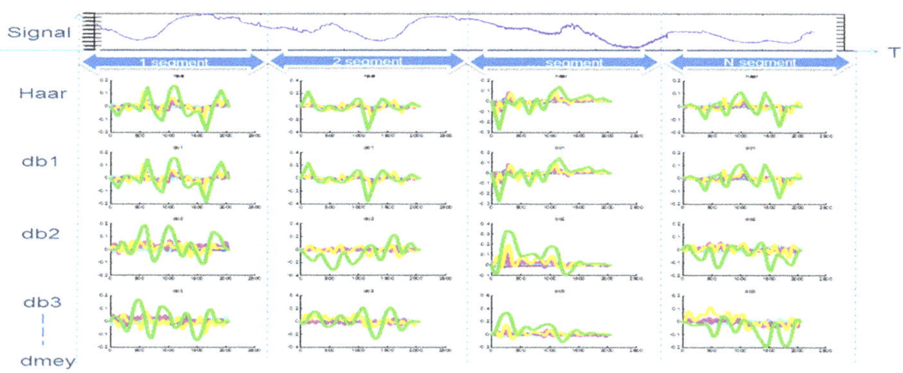

Figure 4.7. Detailed coefficients calculated by decomposition level based on DWT.

frequency's amplitude have been performed. The fast Fourier transform (FFT) which is one of the frequency and amplitude analysis methods, is applied to translate the EEG data to delta band (1–4 Hz), theta band (4–7 Hz), alpha band (8–14 Hz), beta band (14–30 Hz), and gamma bands (30 Hz–) in EEG data.

In the case of feature modelling based on DWT, DWT's coefficient variables are used. figure 4.7 shows the result of DWT's coefficients through the discrete wavelet transform with the acquired brain signal data. Wavelet analysis methods have been used widely in the area of biomedical signal processing [23–25].

In the pre-processing step, the de-noising processing is very important to increase accuracy. There are several techniques to reduce noise in the signal. Many researchers have used wavelet-based techniques as a denoising approach. The previous literature of wavelet-based analysis is focused on semi-auto optimal wavelet selection or manual optimal wavelet selection after evaluating the performance test or comparing the shape of EEG signals with the shape of a mother wavelet function. Software developers and special educators can choose to use the appropriate noise-cancelling methods [26–28].

Similar to the text-based classification methods, The 'analysis' can also use the conventional classification algorithms such as KNN, SVM, ANN, k-means clustering, self-organizing map (SOM) and so on. This section provides an example of an SOM-based approach.

SOM is one of the clustering methods based on ANN. Figure 4.8 shows the conceptual structure. It is a statistical analysis which is split into several groups according to similarity of input data [29]. The purpose is to increase the similarity of objects belonging to the group and the differences of objects between other groups, then clustering becomes clear.

The 'analysis' modules can generate a trial result like figure 4.9. Software developers or special educators can confirm the final ADHD disorder spectrum data.

4.3 Method based on kinetic data by game with a robot

The game with a robot test is designed to help professional diagnosis of ADHD children; this is mainly targeted for children aged 5–12 years. The motive for this game with a robot comes from the European fairy tale, called *Le Petit Chaperon Rouge* written by Charles Perrault and the Grimm brothers. The main story is that a girl called Little Red Riding Hood walks through the woods to deliver food to her sickly grandmother (figure 4.10). This test is edited to fit game activities for which children follow correct paths on the grid floor by remembering the robot's path, also including interceptions with indications of bad wolf or neighbourhood appears to check whether children would show correct responses or not during the walk.

The robot use in this test is a personal care robot called Silbot [26]. This robot has various expressions by graphic avatar, and the body of this robot has a touch sensor for interacting contents with a 360-degree omni-directional mobile platform. The CCD camera for face recognition helps with interaction and location estimation to the user (figure 4.11).

Generally, DSM-criterion is widely used for diagnosis of ADHD, and three core factors are inattention, hyper-activity, impulsivity included the criteria. Nowadays,

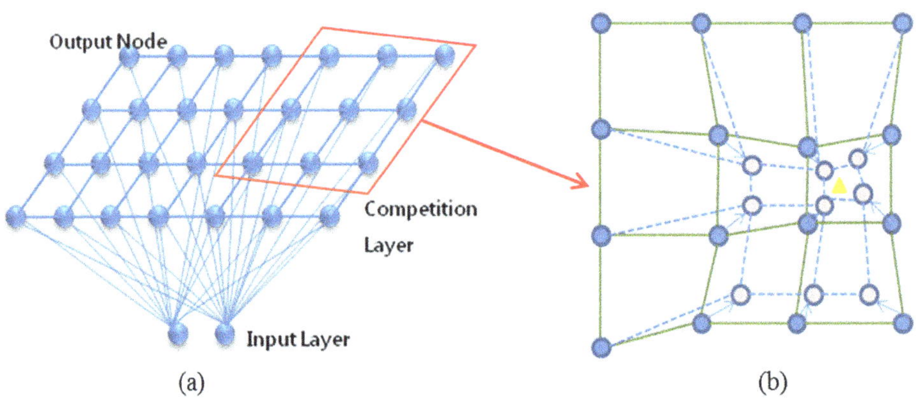

Figure 4.8. Self-organizing maps: (a) structure of SOM; and (b) update of weighting vector.

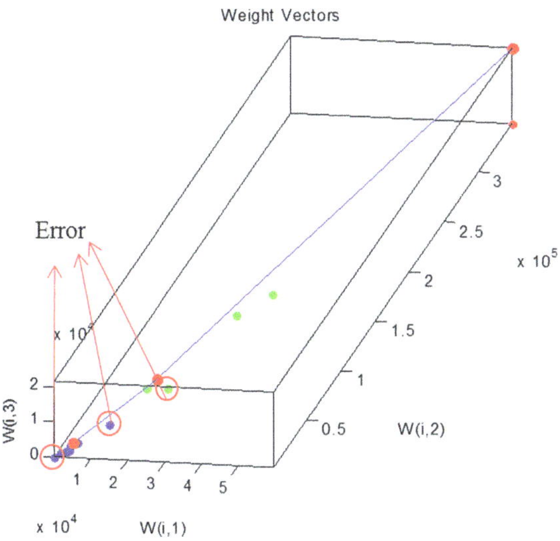

	Clinical diagnosis
Normal	5
Mental retardation	1
ADHD	7

Figure 4.9. ADHD disorder analysis using DWT and SOM. Copyright Robocare.

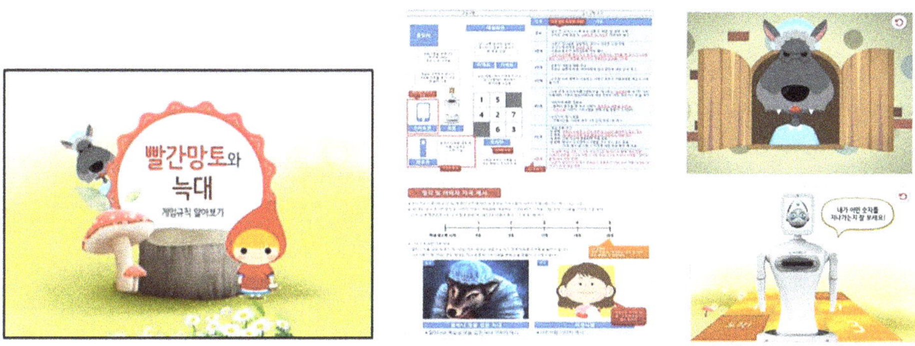

Figure 4.10. Little Red Riding Hood and Wolf Game. Copyright Robocare.

many studies reported that working memory is the important factor of ADHD diagnosis [30, 31], so this test tries to measure three factors of ADHD diagnosis: inattention, hyperactivity-impulsivity and working memory deficits in executive function (table 4.2).

The participants are elementary school students from third to fourth years in accordance with Korean conditions and most prevalent ADHD by age. We also excluded intellectual disabilities under IQ 75. The total number of children is 328, of which 35 children were diagnosed with ADHD by doctors in hospital. 26 children were categorized ADHD at risk by CBCL and K-ADHDDS (Korean ADHD Diagnostic Scale). Their score is between 65–69 T-score (93%–98%tile) by attention and DSM-ADHD scales, and 70–79 T-score by K-ADHDDS. K-ADHDDS is one of the standard tests for ADHD diagnosis in Korea. This test provides dimensional scores of ADHD symptoms using Likert scales of three factors.

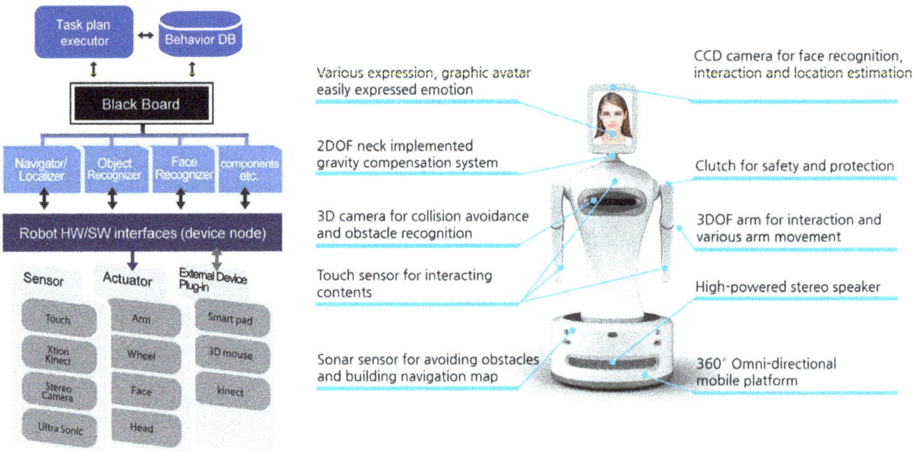

Figure 4.11. Silbot's features. Copyright Robocare.

Table 4.2. Measurement during game with robot test.

Measurement of behaviour	Description	
Route	Success[c]	Step on the route from start point to finish point by following robot's suggestion
	Failure[c]	Time out or step on the incorrect route from start point to finish point by route to robot's suggestion
Response behavior	Correct response score[a]	Number of correct responses to stimulus (wolf/ neighbor)
	Commission error score[b]	Number of commission errors to stimulus (wolf/ neighbor)
	Omission error score[a]	Number of omission errors to stimulus (wolf/ neighbor)
Deviant behavior	Move before start instruction[b]	Record the behavior of attempting to move before the start instruction of the robot
	Attempting commission error before correct response[b]	Frequency of attempting to comission error before correct response
	Attempting a deviated route[c]	Frequency of attempting a deviated route
	Attempting to move before move alarm[b]	Record the behavior of attempting to move before move alarm

[a] Inattention.
[b] Hyperactivity-impulsivity.
[c] Working memory.

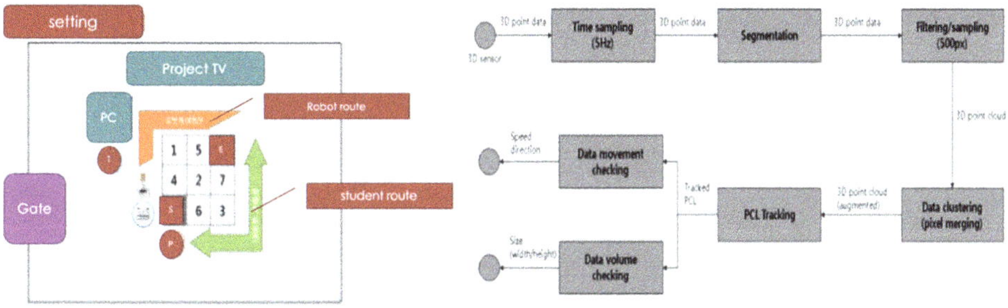

Figure 4.12. Setting of game with robot and data analysis. Copyright Robocare.

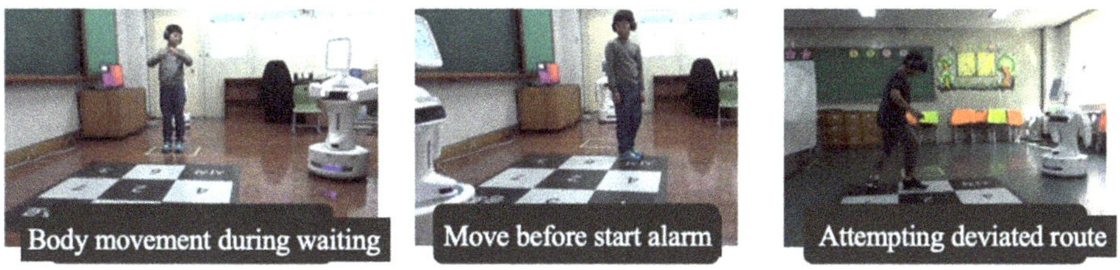
Body movement during waiting
Move before start alarm
Attempting deviated route

Figure 4.13. Silbot's feature. Copyright Robocare.

Under the instructor's guidance, all participants undertook this test. However, instructors were not to respond to the questions of children. They were only to help the participant for safety reasons; the session is fully-automated in the task. For this test, it takes about 10 min or more, depending on the participant's ability (figure 4.12).

In the test, the robot starts to say 'hello, my name is enkey (silbot's name), nice to meet you' and first moves along a path on the numbered mat, showing a certain sequence of numbers from 3 to 5 digits on each level (figure 4.13). While the robot moves, the participant should remember the robot's pathway and therefore the sequence of numbers. After the robot arrives at the finish point, the participant should follow the exact path taken by the robot. When the robot says, 'let's start', the participant stands on the start point to move. the participant should move to the next point after the moving alarm is detected by the system. When stepping on the digit, a stimulus is suddenly given during the move with a voice sound from the TV, calling an auditory stimulus, 'Red Riding Hood!', and then a visual stimulus, a person or a wolf appears on the TV screen. If a person shows, the subject should shake their hand over their head. On the other hand, if a wolf shows, the subject should squat down. After reacting to the stimulus, the participant finishes the remaining path.

If the participant misses what they are supposed to do for a given stimulus, the commission error is counted and recorded in this case. The time allowed is 5 s on each digit in order to account for task completion time. When a participant has one

Table 4.3. Success and fail rates among the group on each stage unit, n(%).

Level		ADHD	ADHD at risk	Normal	Sum	x^2
stage 1	S[a]	25 (71.4)	11 (45.8)	224 (83.6)	260 (79.5)	20.839*** ($df = 2$, $p = .000$)
	F[a]	10 (28.6)	13 (54.2)	44 (16.4)	67 (20.5)	
	Sum	35 (100)	24 (100)	268 (100)	327 (100)	
stage 2	S[a]	10 (40.0)	5 (45.5)	160 (71.4)	175 (67.3)	12.588** ($df = 2$, $p = .002$)
	F[a]	15 (60)	6 (54.5)	64 (28.6)	85 (32.7)	
	Sum	25 (100)	11 (100)	224 (100)	260 (100)	
stage 3	S[a]	6 (60)	2 (40)	109 (68.1)	117 (66.9)	1.956 ($df = 2$, $p = .376$)
	F[a]	4 (40)	3 (60)	51 (31.9)	58 (33.1)	
	Sum	10 (100)	5 (100)	160 (100)	175 (100)	

[a] Working memory.S = Success. F = Fail.

omission error, the task completion adds 5 s (1-digit × 5 s). In the pilot study, children with intellectual disability usually take a time over 5 s in a simulation.

The results of this study were that there was a significant difference of success/fail on route per stage level among the group; ADHD children failed on the first level, an easier level than ADHD at risk and normal children (table 4.3). In the response behavior of the stimulus, data of the participants following the successful route was analyzed.

In this data, there was a significant difference among the participants on the first stage level. Half of ADHD children had an incorrect response, and more ADHD at risk children failed than normal children. There was also a significant difference among participants on two deviant behaviours—attempting an incorrect (commission/omission error) reaction before the correct reaction and attempting to move before the moving alarm because the participants' attention and control skills were different (table 4.4).

ADHD children showed the lowest performance, and also their performance was different from ADHD at risk and normal children(table 4.5). They failed more on the easier stage with difficulties on working memory test. They also had many more errors against sudden stimulus on each stage, particularly having omission errors. In deviant behaviors, they had many instances of attempting an incorrect reaction before the correct reaction, and attempting to move before the move alarm (table 4.6). ADHD children showed impulsive behaviors from the beginning and

Table 4.4. Correct/commission error/ommission error rates Unit: n(%).

Level		ADHD	ADHD at risk	Normal	Sum	x^2
stage 1	C[a]	18 (52.9)	15 (68.2)	236 (91.1)	269 (85.4)	53.249*** ($df = 4$, $p = .000$)
	Co[b]	0 (0)	2 (9.1)	2 (0.8)	4 (1.3)	
	O[a]	16 (47.1)	5 (22.7)	21 (8.1)	42 (13.3)	
	Sum	34 (100)	22 (100)	259 (100)	315 (100)	
stage 2	C[a]	9 (27.3)	11 (73.3)	206 (97.6)	226 (87.3)	132.588*** ($df = 4$, $p = .000$)
	Co[b]	2 (6.1)	1 (6.7)	0 (0)	3 (1.2)	
	O[a]	22 (66.7)	3 (20)	5 (2.4)	30 (11.6)	
	Sum	33 (100)	15 (100)	211 (100)	259 (100)	

[a] Inattention.
[b] Hyperactivity-implusiveness. C = Correct. Co = Commission error, O = Ommission error.

Table 4.5. Descriptive statistics of behavior rate among the groups.

Behaviors		Group	*N*	*M*	*SD*
Deviant behavior	Move before start instruction[b]	ADHD	35	0.286	.169
		ADHD at risk	24	.2500	.531
		Normal	269	.2454	.591
	Total		328		
	Attempting incorrect reaction before correct reaction[b]	ADHD	34	.6765	.911
		ADHD at risk	23	.3043	.470
		Normal	263	.0760	.265
	Total		320		
	Attempting deviated route[c]	ADHD	34	.2941	.629
		ADHD at risk	24	.1250	.448
		Normal	269	.1190	.357
	Total		327		
	Attempting to move before move alarm[b]	ADHD	35	.6571	.998
		ADHD at risk	24	.5417	1.141
		Normal	269	.1524	.535
	Total		328		

[a] Inattention.
[b] Hyperactivity-Impulsiveness.
[c] Working memory.

Table 4.6. ANOVA result on behavior rates among the group.

Behaviors			Sum of squares	df	Mean square	*F*	Post hoc test
Deviant behavior	Move before start instruction[b]	Between groups	1.475	2	.737	2.367	-
		Within groups	101.278	325	.312	(p = .095)	
		Total	102.753	327			
	Attempting incorrect reaction before correct reaction[h]	Between groups	11.398	2	5.699	35.569***	a > b > c
		Within groups	50.790	317	.160	(p = .000)	
		Total	62.188	319			
	Attempting deviated route[c]	Between groups	.930	2	.465	2.905	-
		Within groups	51.877	324	.160	(p = .056)	
		Total	52.807	326			
	Attempting to move before move alarm[b]	Between groups	10.32	2	5.164	11.938***	a,b > c
		Within groups	140.595	325	.433	(p = .000)	
		Total	150.924	327			

[a] Inattention.
[b] Hyperactivity-Impulsiveness.
[c] Working memory. a = ADHD. b = ADHD at risk. c = Normal.

chose wrong decisions on sudden situations, with lower working memory during the active game with the robot, and a different performance from other groups.

4.4 Conclusion

In conclusion, a new approach of methods using technology will provide easier and more accurate diagnosis for ADHD by data processing and big data in the future. Studies have been performed in neurocognitive tests for ADHD diagnosis like CPT, Stroop test, WISC, symbol digit tests.

These tests have developed computerized versions from hand-writing tests and using monitors, with the child sitting in front of them for 10–15 min. The stimulus of the test was usually a simple and single design; these tests did not record the child's behaviors, instead focusong on the response on the screen during the test [32–34]. In the educational field, there are many issues for ADHD diagnosis testing. Despite the efforts to diagnose ADHD, this has been controversial for parents and teachers [35, 36]. Serious problems of ADHD can be found by teachers and parents, however, children at risk might be misdiagnosed or re-diagnosed by disagreement between teacher and parents. This could delay providing intervention to children at risk due to delayed diagnosis. Therefore, a new technological approach to the method for ADHD diagnosis will help agreement between parent and teacher to make more efficient decisions from reliable and objective data directly, rather than relying on the Likert scale test by report on the screening. Also, the school setting is one of the familiar environments for children unlike the clinical setting, and can help alleviate stress for the educational assessment.

References

[1] American Psychiatric Association 2013 *Diagnostic and Statistical Manual of Mental Disorders* 5th ed (Arlington, VA: APS)

[2] Thomas R, Sanders S, Doust J, Beller E and Glasziou P 2015 Prevalence of attention-deficit/hyperactivity disorder: a systematic review and meta – analysis *Pediatrics* **135** 1–8

[3] Wolraich M L, Bard D E, Neas B, Doffing M and Beck L 2013 The psychometric properties of the vanderbilt attention-deficit hyperactivity disorder diagnostic teacher rating scale in a community population *J. Dev. Behav. Pediat.* **34** 83–93

[4] Barkley R A 1997 Behavioral inhibition, sustained attention, and executive functions: constructing a unifying theory of ADHD *Psychol. Bull.* **121** 65–94

[5] Barkley R A 1998 *Attention-Deficit Hyperacitivity Disorder: A Handbook for Diagnosis and Treatment* 2nd ed (New York: Guilford Press)

[6] Shin Y 2012 The study on parents' perception according to diagnostic and educational history of children with attention deficits and hyperactivity problems (in Korean) *J. Spec. Educ. Rehab. Sci.* **51** 21–44

[7] Katzman M A, Bilkey T S, Chokka P R, Fallu A and Klassen L J 2017 Adult ADHD and comorbid disorders: clinical implications of a dimensional approach *BMC Psychiatry* **17** 302

[8] Cortese S, Kelly C, Chabernaud C, Proal E, Martino A D, Milham M and Castellanos X 2012 Toward systems neuroscience of ADHD: a meta-anlaysis of 55 fMRI studies *Am. J. Psychiatry* **169** 1038–55

[9] Frodl T and Skokauskas N 2012 Meta-analysis of structural MRI studies in children and adults with attention deficit hyperactivity disorder indicates treatment effects *Acta Psychiatr. Scand.* **125** 114–26
[10] Achenbach T M and Edelbrock C S 1983 *Manual for the Child Behaviour Checklist and Revised Child Behaviour Profile* (Burlington, VT: University of Vermont)
[11] Barnes G M and Farrell M P 1992 Parental support and control as predictors of adolescent drinking, delinquency, and related problem behaviors *J. Marriage Family* **54** 763–76
[12] Carr E G 1977 The motivation of self-injurious behavior. A review of some hypotheses *Psychol. Bull.* **84** 800–16
[13] Miltenberger R G 2001 *Behavior Modification — Principles and Procedures* (Belmont, CA: Wadsworth/Thomson Learning)
[14] Hutchins W J 1986 *Machine Translation: Past, Present, Future* (Chichester: Ellis Horwood)
[15] Wang P, Hu J, Zeng H-J and Chen Z 2009 Using wikipedia knowledge to improve text classification *Knowl. Inf. Syst.* **19** 265–81
[16] Quay H C, Morse W C and Cutler R L 1966 Personality patterns of pupils in special classes for the emotionally disturbed *Exceptional Children* **32** 297–301
[17] Lee S B, Naa W W, Shin Y, Bae M J and Ku H J 2010 A study on development and application of intervention for challenging behavior and linguistic skills for preschoolers with developmental disabilities *J. Spec. Educ. Rehab. Sci.* **49** 285–307
[18] Kang S-S *et al* HAM: Hangul Anaysis Module http://nlp.kookmin.ac.kr/HAM/kor/index.html
[19] Hinterberger T, Kubler A, Kaiser J, Neumann N and Birbaumer N 2003 A brain computer interface (BCI) for the locked-in: comparison of different EEG classifications for the thought translation device *Clin. Neurophysiol.* **114** 416–25
[20] Subasi A 2007 EEG signal classification using wavelet feature extraction and a mixture of expert model *Expert Syst. Appl.* **32** 1084–93
[21] Abibullaev B, Lee S H, Kang W-S, An J and Seo H D 2010 Funtional brain activity during cognitive tasks *IEEE SENSOR 2010 Conf.* 542–7
[22] Lee B D, Jeong S H, Lee M G, Chang S M, Baek J Y and Rim H D 2002 Altered quantified EEG activity following administration of methylphenidate in children with attention deficit hyperactivity disorder *J. Korean Soc. Biol. Ther. Psychiatry* 118–27
[23] Akay M 1995 Introduction: wavelet transforms in biomedical engineering *Ann. Biomed. Eng.* **23** 529–30
[24] Frisch M and Masser H 1992 The use of the wavelet transforms in the detection of an unknown transient signal *IEEE Trans. Inform. Theory* **38** 892–7
[25] Erdol N 1999 Multiscale detection Wavelets *Subband and Block Transforms in Communications and Media* (Dordrecht: Kluwer)504 183–205
[26] Elena M M, Quero J M and Borrego I 2006 An optimal technique for ECG noise reduction in real time applications *Comput. Cardiol.* **33** 225–8
[27] Rodney Tan H G, Tan A C, Khong P Y and Mok V H 2007 Best wavelet function indentification system for ECG signal denoise applications *ICIAS* 631–4
[28] Phinyomark A 2010 Optimal wavelet functions in wavelet denoising for multifunction myoelectric control, ECTI Trans *Electrical Eng., Electron. Commun.* **8** 43–52
[29] Kohonen T 1995 *Self-Organizing Maps* (Berlin, Heidelberg: Springer)

[30] Tillman C, Eninger L, Forssman L and Bohlin G 2011 The relation between working memory components and ADHD symptoms from a developmental perspective *Dev. Neuropsychol.* **36** 181–98
[31] Kokkalia G K and Drigas A S 2015 Working memory and ADHD in Preschool education. The role of ICT's as a diagnostic and intervention tool: an overview *Int. J. Emerg. Technol. Learn.* **10** 4–9
[32] Greenberg L M and Waldmant I D 1993 Developmental normative data on the test of variables of attention (TOVA) *J. Child Psychol. Psychiatry* **34** 1019–30
[33] Kane R L and Kay G G 1992 Computerized assessment in neuropsychology: a review of tests and test batteries *Neuropsychol. Rev.* **3** 1–117
[34] Gualtieri C T and Johnson L 2006 Reliability and validity of a computerized neurocognitive test battery, CNS vital signs *Arch. Clin. Neuropsychol.* **21** 623–43
[35] Achenbach T M, McConaughy S H and Howell C T 1987 Child/adolescent behavioral and emotional problems: implications of cross-informant correlations for situational specificity *Psychol. Bull.* **101** 213–32
[36] Wolraich M L, Lambert E W, Brickman L, Simmons T B S, Doffing M A and Worley K A 2004 Assessing the impact of parent and teacher agreement on diagnosing attention-deficit hyperactivity disorder *J. Dev. Behav. Pediatrics* **25** 41–7

IOP Publishing

Neurological Disorders and Imaging Physics, Volume 4
Application to attention deficit hyperactivity disorder
Ayman El-Baz and Jasjit S Suri

Chapter 5

Resting-state functional magnetic resonance imaging (R-FMRI) as a potential tool for early diagnosis and outcome prediction in attention deficit hyperactivity disorder (ADHD)

Victor Pereira-Sanchez and Pilar de Castro-Manglano

5.1 Introduction

Attention deficit hyperactivity disorder (ADHD) is widely recognized as a neurodevelopmental disorder and counts as the most common psychiatric disorder in childhood, with an estimated prevalence rate of 5%–10% in that population across the world [1]. Its main clinical features include symptoms of inattention and hyperactivity/impulsivity, although it often presents with affective symptoms, learning difficulties and other comorbidities [2]. ADHD symptoms frequently persist into adulthood, with different functional impairments across the lifespan [3].

ADHD diagnosis is based in a clinical interview and observation of patients, supported in third-party reports (in children and adolescents, with the information provided by their caregivers and teachers). Clinicians are required to confirm the presence of enough core symptoms of inattention and/or hyperactivity/impulsivity in different settings, present since childhood, with a functional impairment and not explainable by other disorders [4]. To date, no test or technique is able to reliably confirm the presence of this disorder, and clinical criteria have an inherent degree of subjectivity, with the risks or overdiagnosis, underdiagnosis, late diagnosis and misdiagnosis [5]. Consequently, the need for early and reliable diagnostic biomarkers is compelling.

ADHD treatment involves psychoeducation of the symptoms and consequences for patients and parents, academic support, behavioral interventions and medication, sometimes including a specific psychotherapy [6, 7]. The most common and approved pharmacological treatments are classified in stimulants (methylphenidate and amphetamines) and non-stimulants (atomoxetine and guanfacine). The clinical

doi:10.1088/978-0-7503-1822-8ch5

response to medication is high (70%–80%), especially with stimulant treatments [8], however, each patient responds differently to the available medications, and there is currently no way to individually predict which medication will show the best efficacy and tolerability.

Modern neuroimaging techniques are emerging in the scientific search of biomarkers that could improve our knowledge about this disorder and customize its clinical management [9]. This chapter aims to discuss the rationale for the proposal of resting-state functional magnetic resonance imaging (R-fMRI or rs-fMRI) as a potential neuroimaging tool for the early diagnosis and outcome prediction in patients with ADHD in clinical settings. After discussing the biological basis of ADHD from different research perspectives (section 5.2) and the fundamentals of resting state neuroimaging (section 5.3), a thorough description of how R-fMRI studies are conducted nowadays will be provided (section 5.4). Finally (section 5.5), the potential clinical applications of R-fMRI will be briefly outlined.

5.2 Neurobiology of ADHD and biomarking techniques

The neurobiology of ADHD is a field of growing research, and the theoretical paradigms underneath are continuously evolving under the light of new evidence. The results of research studies with different approaches and techniques (including genetics, biochemical, pharmacological and neuroimaging), taken together, suggest that ADHD is a complex neurodevelopmental disorder in which genetic and environmental factors come together into a series of structural and functional delays and disruptions of the brain development and neurotransmission [10–13]. The consequences are the varying and impairing symptoms seen among the patients.

Some of the most relevant and current challenges to improve the understanding of the neurobiology of ADHD, and most importantly, the care for patients, would be the development of multivariate and multimodal (i.e. combining different approaches and data sources) etiological research [13, 14] and the establishment of reliable and useful clinical biomarkers (this concept will be discussed in section 5.4) for the early diagnosis and outcome prediction [15].

In this section, a general review of current knowledge about the neurobiology of ADHD from different research approaches will be briefly described, excluding the R-fMRI evidence, which will be outlined in section 5.3.

5.2.1 Genetics, epigenetics, omics and biochemistry

Family studies of ADHD demonstrate its high heritability, which ranges between 60%–90%. Genome-wide association studies (GWAS) and other approaches are providing vast amounts of data about genetic alterations in ADHD patients [16]. However, the nature of these alterations is heterogenous and polygenic, and include multiple low-effect common gene variances and a few high-effect rare mutations. Studies have shown a certain genetic overlap of ADHD with autism spectrum disorders and intellectual disabilities, supporting its neurodevelopmental nature [17]. Based on the mechanisms of action of the pharmacological treatments of this disorder, genetic studies have also focused in genes related to neurotransmitters (dopaminergic, noradrenergic, cholinergic, serotoninergic), and in pharmacogenomic research to develop individualized treatments [18]. In addition, other candidate genes (BDNF, SNAP25) have been also analyzed from a neurodevelopmental point of view [19].

Notwithstanding the crucial role of this evidence, there are many molecular processes beyond the DNA with a mediating role between the genes and the environment, constituting with them the biological basis of human behavior. These are also being investigated in ADHD, and comprise the epigenetics (acetylation and methylation mechanisms [20], miRNA [21]), transcriptomics [22], proteomics [23] and metabolomics [24]. Another emergent focus of research is the microbiome, studying the effects on the brain of the genetic material of microorganisms residing in the human body [25].

The final expression of these biological mechanisms and environmental factors results in the presence of proteins and other elements which could be quantified and characterized from different samples. Blood, urine and cerebrospinal fluid (CSF) biomarkers have been traced in patients with ADHD, and the potential role of neurotransmission, nutritional, endocrine, mineral elements has been discussed [19].

Taking all this evidence together, the biological origins of ADHD seem to be based on complex interplays of heritable and acquired mechanisms, with a key role of genetics. However, none of the suggested biomarkers has yet been translated to clinical practice [26].

5.2.2 Neuroimaging

Research on ADHD has taken advantage of most of the current techniques to visualize and analyze the brain structure and function. The current methods can be classified in regards of the modality (and sub-modalities) of imaging (EEG, MRI, nuclear medicine techniques) and the focus on brain anatomy (structural) or activation patterns (functional).

Furthermore, the study designs may report cross-sectional approaches (single observations across different subjects) or longitudinal approaches (repeated observations in the same subjects at different moments); the former compares different individuals at a single moment, whereas the latter allow for the identification and comparison of intra-individual brain changes related to different conditions (time, treatment). Therefore, longitudinal studies have a greater interest in the assessment of brain development or the effects of medications in the brain structure and function.

5.2.2.1 Structural neuroimaging

Structural neuroimaging comprises the anatomical techniques using magnetic resonance imaging (MRI): anatomic MRI, diffusion-tensor imaging (DTI) and spectroscopy. Some nuclear medicine techniques might be classified as structural, but all these will be discussed among the functional modalities. Anatomic MRI has been used to identify differences in the gray matter structure and maturation between patients with ADHD and typically developing controls (TDC). Shaw *et al* studied the development of the brain cortex in a big sample of pediatric patients and controls during years, and described that ADHD is characterized by a delay in the maturation of cortical thickness [12], cortical surface and gyrification [27]. Additionally, those patients with better clinical outcome tended to present a profile of cortical maturation more similar to the healthy controls [28]. Subcortical gray matter has also been extensively studied; in a cross-sectional mega-analysis including more than 3000 subjects across the world within the ENIGMA International Working Group, ADHD patients showed reduced volumes in the bilateral amygdala, accumbens and hippocampus relative to controls, independently of comorbidities and medication [29].

The white matter architecture represents the structural connectivity of the brain, composed by neuronal axons transmitting information among neurons in different regions. The DTI modalities of MRI, tracing the water movement in the brain, allow for a characterization of white matter microstructure [30], and have been explored in children and adults with ADHD. A common DTI index measured across studies is fractional anisotropy (FA), and global brain alterations of this metric have been described in patients [31].

Finally, spectroscopy is an MRI technique to detect and quantify neural metabolites across the brain. It has been less frequently used for ADHD research, but alterations in N-acetylaspartate (NAA), choline and glutamatergic compounds have been reported [32].

Despite the repeated findings of brain structure alterations in patients with ADHD, the mentioned techniques are not yet able to diagnose single patients, nor predict their outcome. Furthermore, the effects of medication in the brain structure are not yet clear [33].

5.2.2.2 Functional neuroimaging

Different methods have been developed during the last decades to map brain function with neuroimaging, both during tasks and in the so-called resting state. Functional neuroimaging provides a dynamic perspective of the brain, sensitive to changes induced by different conditions (tasks, medication). Functional techniques involve those based in radioisotopes (SPECT and PET) and the functional variants of MRI (fMRI).

SPECT and PET involve the intravenous administration of radioactive-marked molecules, which are transported through the blood vessels to different areas of the brain. Some markers are intended to reflect the cerebral blood flow (CBF), which is supposed to increase temporarily in the brain regions activated in the moment of the scan, thus reflecting the relation of that activation with the specific task executed by the patient [34]; whereas other markers target specific brain processes as beta-amyloid deposit [35] or dopamine transmission [36] in different neuropsychiatric disorders. In spite of the great interest these techniques for brain molecular research, the involvement of radiation makes them more challenging for research purposes, especially in pediatric populations. SPECT and PET studies in ADHD [37, 38] have allowed the characterization of CBF in different areas of the brain, repeatedly finding differences in clinical versus control populations. In addition, the study of the dopamine transmission with specific radioligands has provided a unique insight in the understanding of the mechanism of action of methylphenidate, with a strong dopaminergic component.

Functional MRI, developed in the 1990s, has become a popular technique for the study of brain mapping in healthy individuals and in different clinical populations [39]. It comprises the use of specific sequences to track brain activations during the execution of tasks. Most fMRI studies are based in the blood oxygen level dependent (BOLD) approach, an indirect measure of activation which reflects the use of oxygen through hemoglobin in the brain [40], whereas less used techniques with arterial spin labelling (ASL) represent an alternative for a direct measurement of CBF [41].

The performance of ADHD children and adults and the effects of medication in various tasks have been explored with fMRI. Cortese *et al* reported in 2012 a meta-analysis of fMRI studies comparing children, adolescents and adults with ADHD versus healthy controls in inhibition, working memory and vigilance/attention tasks. They adopted a systems neuroscience perspective, interpreting abnormally activated brain regions as dysfunctional nodes in large-scale neural networks (this concept will be described in section 5.3). In children and adolescents with ADHD, they reported consistent hypoactivation in brain areas related to frontoparietal and ventral attention networks, whereas hyperactivation was present in areas related to ventral attention, default and somatomotor networks. In adults with ADHD they found significant hypoactivation in the frontoparietal network, and hyperactivation was described in the dorsal attention, visual and default mode networks. The results were consistent when considering only treatment naïve patients and patients without comorbidities; the findings point to brain areas related to cognitive control, attention and sensory functions, and set a basis for the understanding of the ADHD symptoms from a perspective of a multi-network dysfunction [42]. fMRI studies have also explored the potential effects of ADHD medications in the brain function. Rubia *et al* published in 2014 a meta-analysis of studies involving acute stimulant administration and the performance of stop, working memory and time discrimination tasks. Their results revealed a consistent pattern of activation in areas of cognitive control (bilateral inferior frontal cortex and insula) during inhibition and time discrimination but no effects in working memory networks were found [43]. More recent original studies have also reported results in that direction [44–47].

5.3 Resting-state fMRI (R-fMRI)

Research in task-based brain function with PET and [48] fMRI [49] techniques in the 1990s looking at 'noise signal' led to the discovery of consistent synchronous activity in different regions when subjects where not engaged in particular tasks (i.e. at rest). Actually, these patterns of activity fluctuations in different cerebral regions under non-task conditions reflect not only that the brain is always active, but also that neurons in distant areas are triggered simultaneously. After two decades, R-fMRI has maturated as a powerful set of techniques to capture this resting activity in healthy individuals and patients with different neuropsychiatric disorders.

5.3.1 Functional connectivity and resting-state brain networks

R-fMRI relies on the concept of functional connectivity at rest (intrinsic functional connectivity), which is the temporal correlation of brain signal between distant points of an image. When two or more different areas of the brain show a synchronic pattern of signal, it is assumed that they are somewhat connected (by direct or indirect anatomic/structural connectivity) and probably acting together for the same purpose. In most R-fMRI studies, the characteristics of BOLD low-frequency fluctuations (within the range of 0.01–0.1 Hz) are the phenomenon of interest, although resting-state connectivity can also be captured with ASL techniques [50].

Resting-state functional connectivity is considered a reflect of intrinsic brain functions, which are consistent across diverse populations from all ages (infants, children, adolescents, young adults and elderly populations) and in non-human primates and rodents [51–56], constituting a 'universal functional architecture' or functional connectome.

Systems neuroscience has taken advantage of the R-fMRI techniques to group brain areas into inter-related neural networks whose characteristics can be explored, and whose understanding might overcome the limitations of studying isolated brain regions [57]. Resting-state techniques have described a number of networks which were not apparent in task-studies and have complemented the conventional fMRI into a better understanding on how networks interact during different neuropsychological processes. Yeo *et al* proposed in 2011 a parcellation of the human brain into different networks, the main seven being the visual, somatomotor, dorsal and ventral attention, limbic, frontoparietal and default mode networks [58]; these and other parcellations have become the basic framework for the study of the brain connectome in healthy and disease conditions.

Among the described networks, the default mode (DMN) has raised particular interest. DMN is constituted by a midline core (posterior cingulate cortex and anterior medial prefrontal cortex) with a medial temporal (hyppocampal formation, parahyppocampal cortex, retrosplenial cortex, posterior inferior parietal lobule, ventral medial prefrontal cortex) and dorsal medial (lateral temporal cortex, temporal pole, temporoparietal junction, dorsal medial prefrontal cortex) subsystems structures [59]. The cerebellum, perhaps often overlooked, also plays a role in the DMN. This network, whose activity increases at rest and decreases during tasks (acting as an 'antagonist' of task-focused networks such as the frontoparietal) appears to be related to cognition processes underlying 'mind wandering': self-relevant affective decisions, constructing a mental scene based on memory and social cognition [60]. A graphical representation of the main hubs of the DMN in the three planes of MR imaging (axial, sagittal and coronal) and two surface reconstructions (lateral and medial) is offered in figures 5.1 and 5.2, based in first-level (single individuals) correlation analysis data in the ongoing CUNMET study from the authors of this chapter: medial prefrontal and posterior-cingulate/precuneus areas are highlighted (see figures 5.1 and 5.2).

R-fMRI methods have not only been under intense exploitation as a standard paradigm for human brain mapping (see the 'Human Connectome Project' [61]), but

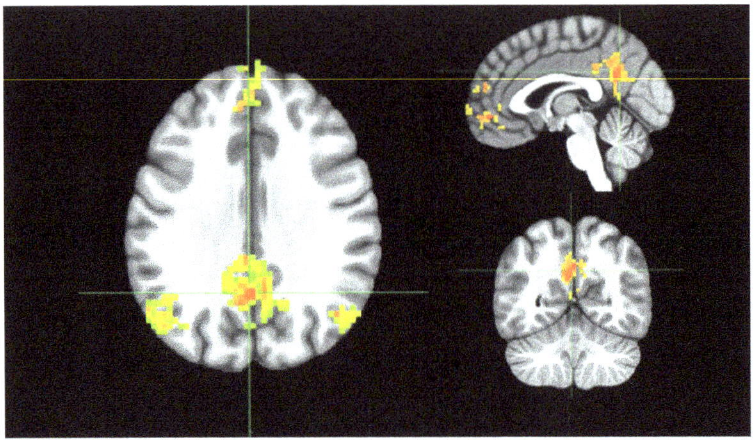

Figure 5.1. Two-dimensional representation of the main nodes of the default mode network in axial (left), sagital (top right) and coronal (bottom right) planes.

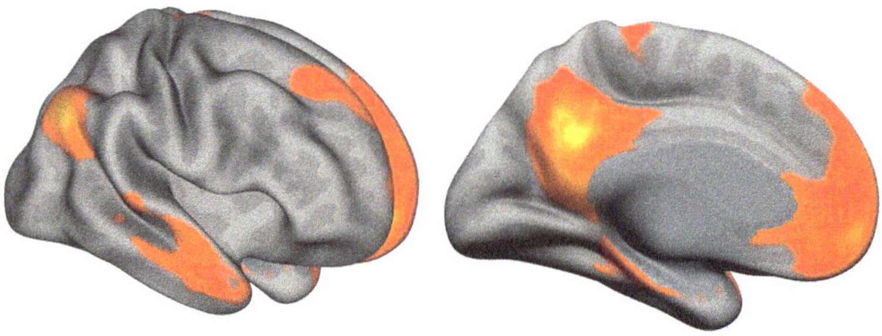

Figure 5.2. Visual representation of the main nodes of the default mode network with a brain surface model.

also as a potential tool for the understanding of brain function in multiple neuropsychiatric conditions, including neurodevelopmental, neurodegenerative and traumatic disorders [62], as well as in psychosis [63]. Discoveries in these areas are supporting the hypotheses of many neurological and mental disorders as, at least in part, brain network impairments.

However, important concerns have been raised on the validity of many findings and conclusions, as R-fMRI is subject to relevant limitations and biases, and the reproducibility of these findings has been questioned. First, the complexity and expensiveness of these studies make them often based on a small number of subjects. Limited sample sizes increase the risk of type II errors (not finding significant differences where they actually exist, so reporting false negatives) due to low statistical power [64]. Second, as resting-state functional connectivity is subject to variation across subjects, technical methods of acquisition and analysis, and even within the same subject at different time points, the test–retest reliability of the resting state metrics and the validation of techniques across different individuals and research teams is crucial [65]. Fortunately, resting-state metrics have shown different ranges of reliability and, although further progress is to be made, these methods

Table 5.1. R-fMRI measures of connectivity.

Functional segregation	Functional integration
Amplitude of low-frequency fluctuations (ALFF and fALFF)	Functional connectivity density (FCD)
Regional homogeneity (ReHo)	Seed-based correlation analysis (SCA)
	Independent component analysis (ICA) dual regression
	Graph theory analysis (GTA): network centrality, node degree, modularity, path length, clustering coefficient

seem to be consistent enough to allow large-scale international research [66]. But even with standardized and reliable methods, the internal and external (i.e. representativity) validity will also rely on the research design and the selection of the populations. An inherent trade off in the designs is the decision to include a homogeneous sample of subjects, balanced with the representativity of that sample regarding the population where they come from. Stringent inclusion and exclusion criteria might enhance the internal validity of the results but compromise their translation to other subjects out of the study. The final but crucial limitation to discuss here is head motion, a known source of bias in neuroimaging, and especially in R-fMRI, as it might induce artificial correlation [67, 68]. Motion is greater in younger children and older adults and is expected to be higher in patients with some neuropsychiatric disorders such as ADHD and dementia. This factor has been somewhat overlooked in many early studies but, as will be discussed later, the degree with which is prevented, recognized, corrected and adjusted during data acquisition and analysis is determinant to ascertain the validity of the R-fMRI reports.

Resting-state functional connectivity is not a univocal concept, as different metrics or indices exist to analyze and describe it, and they show and represent complementary perspectives of a complex phenomenon. Common indices are summarized in table 5.1, and grouped into two categories: metrics of functional segregation and metrics of functional integration [69], although other categorizations have also been reported (local versus global connectivity, voxel-based versus correlation metrics, etc). Importantly, brain mapping approaches are also commonly divided to distinguish those based in previously selected regions of interest (ROI) and those which explore the data without prior hypothesis: hypothesis driven versus data-driven methods (see table 5.1).

Functional segregation refers to the local function of specific brain regions and comprises the amplitude of low-frequency fluctuations (ALFF and fALFF) and the regional homogeneity (ReHo). ALFF measures the power (amplitude) of the BOLD signal fluctuations within the mentioned range of 0.01–0.1 Hz in the brain voxels under study [70]. Fractional ALFF (fALFF) is a refined method resulting in the division of the amplitude of the LFF by the total amplitude of fluctuations in all the detectable range of frequencies [71]. ReHo represents the degree of similarity (Kendall coefficient of concordance) between the BOLD time series of adjacent voxels in the brain [72].

Functional integration metrics describe different insights of the connectivity between distant areas of the brain within network perspectives. They comprise, among others: the functional connectivity density analysis (FCD); the seed-based correlation analysis (SCA); the independent component analysis (ICA) dual regression; graph theory analysis (GTA) approaches and the voxel-mirrored homotopic connectivity (VMHC). Functional connectivity density analyses are a data-driven voxel-based approach to map short-range and long-range correlation of the BOLD timeseries of a given brain area [73]. Seed-based correlation analyses and independent component analysis dual regression, calculate and map the functional connectivity of brain networks with different perspectives [74]. SCA measures the correlation of the BOLD signal a preselected ROI (the seed region) with all other areas of the brain, to determine which are presumably part of its network. ICA are data-driven techniques which explore temporal correlations dividing the brain into independent components, resulting in the main described neural networks. Graph theory analyses are a family of methods (also used in other biomedical and social research areas) which consider brain networks as graphs, consisting of nodes (hubs) interconnected by edges: nodes are brain areas of gray matter, whereas the edges are the direct and indirect connections between these areas [75, 76]. GTA metrics focus on the efficiency of the within-network communication, path lengths among the hubs, degrees of centrality-hubness of the brain areas involved and the hierarchical complex interplay among different networks [77]. Finally, the voxel-mirrored homotopic connectivity provide the inter-hemispheric synchrony patters of geometrically corresponding (homotopic) left and right areas [78], which might reflect hemispheric specialization for certain cognitive functions. Perhaps less commonly, other R-fMRI metrics have been also reported, such as clustering and pattern classification [79], as well as multivariate distance matrix regression (MDMR) [80].

5.3.2 The *restless* ADHD brain

ADHD is a field of neurobiological research which has substantially benefited from the development of the resting-state science, and has furthermore contributed as a pioneer disorder in the study of some of its methods (such as the ALFF) [70]. Early reports conceptualized ADHD as brain network disorder, and the role of DMN has been repeatedly described [81].

Sonuga-Barke and Castellanos proposed in 2007 the DMN ‘interference hypothesis’ of ADHD, in which this network reverts its natural functioning to intrude in the activity of task-focused networks [82]. However, the pathophysiology of ADHD seems to comprise a wide range of resting-state activity alterations in different brain networks/systems [83], as well as the complex and hierarchical interplay between them [84]. Networks studied in ADHD include not only the DMN, but also the frontoparietal, attentional (ventral, dorsal, salience), motor and visual. A great contribution in the global massive-scale study of the functional connectome of patients with ADHD, as compared with typically developing controls was possible thanks to the ADHD-200 consortium, which has made publicly available hundreds of scans and phenotypic data, in an open science effort to accelerate the international research [85]; a number of original studies have used this dataset.

A wide range of R-fMRI techniques and indices have been studied in children, adolescents and adults with ADHD (see also narrative reviews summarizing them in 2014 by Posner *et al* [86], and in 2016 by Castellanos and Aoki [87]), including ALFF [70], fALFF and ReHo [88], SCA [89], ICA-dual regression [90] and GTA [47, 91]. Nevertheless, the resting state functional connectivity in ADHD is still a 'science in construction', as Castellanos and Aoki described in the mentioned review of 2016, acknowledging its achievements and pitfalls [87]. They pointed out some tentative conclusions which might be outlined from the wide heterogeneity of research methods, sample sizes and populations: decreased synchrony between anterior and posterior nodes of the DMN, altered interplay of DMN (including cerebellum) with frontoparietal and attention networks, implication of reward-related circuits (orbitofrontal cortex, ventral prefrontal cortex, ventral striatum) in the hyperactivity/impulsivity symptoms, the role of the amygdala in emotional dysregulation, evidence of delays and alterations in developmental trajectories in the mentioned brain systems, and a repeated report of altered ReHo in medial prefrontal cortex.

The evidence outlined before comes mainly from studies comparing ADHD patients (most treatment-naive) with typically developing controls. However, R-fMRI techniques have also shown its potential in the research for the neural effects of treatment, and its correlation with symptom improvement. The effects of stimulant (methylphenidate, amphetamines) and non-stimulant (atomoxetine) medications have been tested with almost the whole variety of the described methods [80, 92–98]. Interestingly, longitudinal studies have scanned patients before and after acute or chronic treatment administration; however, heterogeneity of research designs and imaging metrics here is high and sample sizes are low. Although sometimes apparently conflicting across studies, results tend to highlight consistent R-fMRI medication-induced changes in the brain. Reports have more frequently included methylphenidate, as it is often the first-line pharmacological treatment in most clinical contexts. The effects of non-pharmacological treatments, like cognitive behavioral therapy (CBT), have also been explored, evidencing a selective modulation of functional connectivity in the frontoparietal network and cerebellum [99] which is similar to that described with pharmacological treatments.

Regarding methodological issues, the named limitations of resting-state fMRI research are also a source of concern in these studies. As research in ADHD often involves young children and/or hyperkinetic individuals, head motion is a critical issue for careful review of the evidence and design and conduction of future studies. In addition, it should be noted that many of the neuroimaging studies with ADHD include homogeneous samples with a limited representation (and often, explicit exclusion) of girls and women, non-right-handed individuals, predominant hyperactive ADHD subtypes/presentations, patients with lower intelligence coefficients and certain comorbidities. Consequently, the results reported in the literature should be interpreted with caution and might not be representative of a wide range of individuals with this disorder.

Current efforts and potential areas for advance include ensuring a better control of head motion [100], longitudinal large and open-access efforts such as the ABCD study [101, 102], and the development of specific analytic methods, such as the PyBASC for corticostriatal parcellation trough bootstrapping techniques [103].

5.3.3 Conducting an R-fMRI study: a stepwise description

An fMRI study involves a series of steps, in which variability might be high depending on the research questions. Basic procedures are depicted in figure 5.3, and involve the study design, subject assessment, image acquisition, data pre-processing, computation of derivatives and group statistical analysis. The following paragraphs describe these steps, whose knowledge is useful both for conducting studies and for a critical reading of the scientific literature.

The COBIDAS report, published by an expert committee of the Organization for Human Brain Mapping (OHBM), provides an excellent guideline on how to conduct, report and assess the steps of fMRI studies to improve their quality and reproducibility, and a checklist is proposed [104].

5.3.3.1 Study design

R-fMRI investigations start with a careful design. A thorough literature review is required to identify the scientific gaps in the area of study, set the targets for the new research and balance the strengths and pitfalls of previous methodologies. Considering the complexity and expensiveness of these techniques, researchers should have enough financial backing and a multidisciplinary team including psychiatrists, psychologists, radiologists, data scientists and engineers, as well as technical and administrative staff. Sample size estimation (power calculation) is recommended; however, the singularity of neuroimaging studies makes it challenging. Some guidelines have been developed to assist in this process [105]. In any case, looking at the sample sizes of previous studies and counting on the, very probable, loss of usable data due to subject motion and other factors is key to avoid finishing with an extremely low number of analyzable subjects. Multi-site international collaborations such as the ADHD-200 consortium are intended to overcome the

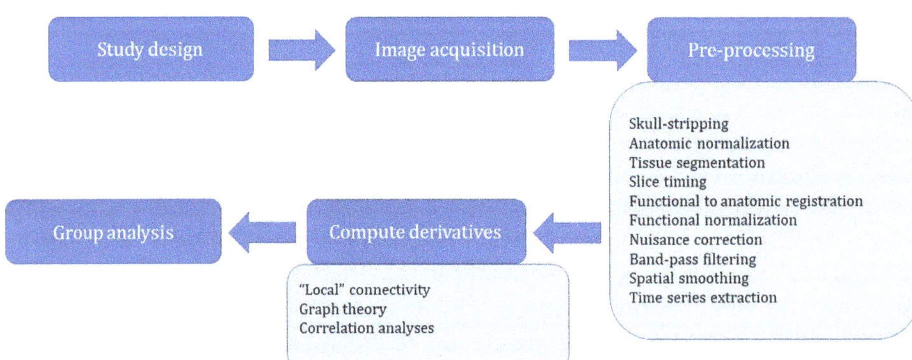

Figure 5.3. Methodological steps in neuroimaging studies.

limitations of a single recruitment center, but heterogeneities in the patient assessment, collection of data and image acquisition, even with very similar scanners, are a potential pitfall of these efforts.

The study design should also very clearly state the inclusion and exclusion criteria, the clinical assessment methods and how to handle and collect the data. These criteria should balance the inclusion of a homogeneous sample with its representativity of the population from which they come. Very often, studies of ADHD exclude female and right-handed patients, as well as those with low intellectual coefficient (IQ) and certain comorbidities: these criteria should acknowledge that an increased homogeneity of the sample results in an underrepresentation of the general population. Other crucial decisions are whether to scan patients once or longitudinally, to include or not healthy controls, and to recruit medication-naïve patients or already medicated ones. Although longitudinal studies with medication-naïve patients and healthy controls are preferred, they are more complex and expensive, and other 'less purist' designs might respond better to certain research questions.

As a reference structural MRI is acquired in these studies, it is important to acknowledge that incidental findings (often non-pathological such as arachnoid cysts, but sometimes life-threatening such as malignant tumors) might arise in the brain anatomy of the subjects, so it is important to establish a procedure for anatomical check of the scans and management of those incidents.

Although R-fMRI analysis techniques are under constant evolution, preprocessing steps and statistical analysis should be planned beforehand as much as possible. Changing the methods during the data analysis poses an important risk of bias. For that reason, it is advisable to preregister in the public domain (for example, in clinicaltrials.gov or in osf.io) the study protocol and stick to it, or justify any deviations. Finally, ethical aspects must be considered. As with any other medical study involving human beings, the international guidelines should be followed, balancing the benefits of the study against their potential risks (see Declaration of Helsinki [106]). An explicit approval by the Institutional Review Board (IRB) or Research Ethics Committee is required, and patients should be informed and give their consent for participation in the study. In the case of children and adolescents with ADHD and typically developing controls, the consent is signed by their parents or caregivers, but the subjects should participate in the decision to the degree they can understand and assent.

5.3.3.2 Subject assessment

Subjects should be assessed by trained staff to confirm they meet the inclusion criteria and have no excluding criteria, and to collect the sociodemographic-general and clinical data (see table 5.2). The diagnostic procedures to confirm or exclude the presence of ADHD and other disorders should be clarified. Structured clinical interviews and international-reliable diagnostic criteria (such as the World Health Organization *International Classification of Diseases ICD-10* or the American Psychiatric Association *Diagnostic and Statistical Manual of Mental Disorders DSM-5*) are preferred. Rating scales are of great value to quantify the presence

Table 5.2. Basic data to collect from subjects.

Type of information	Data to collect
General data	Age (date of birth), sex and gender, handedness, education, socioeconomic and education of parents, weight, height, vital signs
Clinical and psychological	IQ (total, verbal, nonverbal) and other psychometrics (processing speed, working memory), severity of ADHD symptoms (rating scales), age at diagnosis, medication history (including current medication with daily dose), comorbidities, family history, perinatal and developmental history

and severity of the symptoms and have a role in the evaluation of clinical changes in longitudinal studies and in the evaluation of intrinsic functional connectivity correlations.

Assessments should include interviews with subjects and external informers (in the case of children and adolescents, their parents or caregivers). The medication history is key, and in the case of medicated subjects, it is important to register the dosing and the timing of the medication administration in relation to the scanning session: the study design will determine if patients should withdraw the medication previously to the image acquisition or when to take it. Finally, it is important to rule out circumstances that might prevent or artifact the MRI scan such as claustrophobia or wearing paramagnetic objects (such as dental braces).

5.3.3.3 R-fMRI acquisition

Once the subjects have been recruited and the study design has determined the imaging metrics to obtain and compare, and thus the MRI sequences to use, images are acquired. The time of the scan in the day might be important (as resting-state brain connectivity has time fluctuations) and should be registered; ideally, all subjects should be scanned at the same hour of the day.

In contrast with task-based fMRI, resting-state scans do not require patients to perform any specific activity, but instead they are instructed to remain lying, still and awake, without thinking of anything in particular (resting state connectivity in the default mode network has been related to 'mind wandering'). Subjects are placed as comfortable as possible, with headphones to minimize their exposure to the noise of the scanner and with the head immobilized. Controversy and heterogeneity exist on whether subjects should keep their eyes closed or open or, in the latter case, if they should fix their eyes on a particular point or not. No matter the specific instructions, they should be the same for all the subjects in the same study. As remaining still and awake in an unstructured condition might be difficult, especially in long sessions, and for children and ADHD patients, and as head motion is a serious concern regarding the validity of the imaging data, the use of movies or the scanning of sleeping individuals have been discussed, but these conditions probably affect the functional connectivity. Potentially useful additional devices to improve quality include eye trackers, wakefulness detection, real-time head motion monitoring (with feedback to subjects to instate them to remain still) and vital signs (heart and breathing rate) monitoring have been used and proposed [100, 107].

Resting-state fMRI includes a series of anatomical and functional sequences whose parameters are established in advance and required to be constant for all the subjects. For that reason, it is advisable that all the scanners are conducted in the exact same machine. The field strength of the MRI scan is improving: nowadays 3 Tesla are most common. The structural MRI sequence (T1-MPRAGE is common) will be used for a visual check of brain anatomy, ruling out abnormalities, and for normalization of the studied brains within a standard template, as well as for the registration of functional images (with lower spatial resolution) within the anatomical space. Resting-state functional sequences, as stated, are mostly based in BOLD acquisitions, which are weighted in T2* in echo-planar imaging (EPI). However, alternative approaches include spiral techniques [108] and other resting-state sequences with ASL [109]. Different functional sequences may be obtained in the same session, and dual sequences are also possible [110–112]. The duration of the scan is a matter of discussion, as the length of the functional sessions influence their intra-scan and inter-scan reliability [113]. Longer scans could provide a better characterization of the functional connectivity, but have the risk to increase subject boredom, motion and sleeping.

5.3.3.4 Data analysis

From image acquisition to the conclusions, brain images require a series of steps: quality control, pre-processing, extraction of individual resting-state metrics and group statistical analysis. These steps are often grouped in two phases: first level (individual subjects) and second-level (inter-group) analyses. Very often, a first step is to convert the anonymized individual data from the scanner device to standard formats to be read by software tools (e.g. conversion from DICOM to NIfTI format).

Quality control is a step to be conducted before and after pre-process and involves a visual check of the raw images data and the results of the pre-processed images, as well as the assessment of head motion. Anatomical abnormalities and artifacts should be noted, and gross errors in image acquisition should be reported to prevent their repetition in further scans. Head motion can be quantified in six degrees of translation (x, z and y axes) and rotation (roll, pitch and yaw), and condensed in unified metrics such as the framewise displacement (FD) or the spatial root mean of the data after temporal differencing (DVARS) [114], which will be later taken into account in the data pre-processing and group analysis.

Data-preprocessing is an individual-level procedure to clean the brain images from noise, make them comparable across subjects and correlate their space coordinates with the standard anatomy of the brain. It is a delicate step whose results condition the validity of subsequent analysis and their conclusions. However, the heterogeneity here among studies is huge, and no gold standards have been agreed. Furthermore, the different options to be applied are under constant debate and change, and slightly different pre-processing variants might lead to dramatically different results on the same raw data. Nevertheless, the basic pipeline (sequence of pre-processing steps) usually includes: skull stripping (removing non-neural structures around the brain such as skull and soft tissues), anatomic normalization (correlating the structural image with standard brain coordinates of space in the scientific literature, such as the Talairach-Tournoux or Montreal Neurological Institute (MNI) atlases [115]), tissue segmentation (dividing the brain tissue in gray matter, white matter and cerebrospinal fluid), slice timing (adjusting the brain signal by the time of sequence acquisition), functional to anatomic registration and normalization (correlate the functional images with the anatomic ones, and with the standard atlas), nuisance correction (identification and correction of artifactual signal that might be confounded with real brain activation, derived from motion and physiological rhythmic changes due to heart beating and breathing), band-pass filtering (removing oscillatory brain activity out of a frequency range of interest, usually 0.01–0.1 Hz), spatial smoothing (blurring of the signal to improve its strength) and extraction of the time series of the processed data. More detailed information about these steps can be found elsewhere. These steps are sequentially taken in a computerized pipeline whose results should afterwards be checked for quality control.

The pre-processed data is then analyzed at an individual level to extract the resting-state metrics of interest. These could be classified in 'functional segregation' and 'functional integration' indices [69], as described in section 5.3.1 and listed in table 5.1.

Finally, group analyses are conducted to identify statistically significant differences in the functional connectivity metrics between the preestablished groups or conditions of interest. Statistical tests are selected according to the nature of the contrasts (paired tests when the comparison is within the same subjects in different time points, e.g. pre-post medication; and unpaired tests when comparing different subject groups). T-tests, analysis of variance (ANOVA) and regression models can be constructed in the statistical framework of the so-called general linear model (GLM). As these analyses involve a huge number of individual contrasts (due to the large number of voxels in the brain to be compared across subjects), correction methods are required to decrease the chance of finding random false positives (falling into the type I error). The 'surviving' differences are then located in a 3D map of the brain in standard space, and the neurobiological and clinical significance of the differences need to be discussed.

Different software tools have been developed and are available for computerized analysis of R-fMRI data, from the preprocessing steps to the group comparisons. Table 5.3 includes the most common, which are either based on open-source UNIX systems or in Matlab (some using the processing and statistical functionalities of Statistical Parametric Mapping (SPM) software). The UNIX software tools have the advantage of their free availability and their wide flexibility, but are harder to learn, whereas other tools offer more relatively intuitive graphical user interfaces (GUIs) but offer fewer opportunities for customization.

Table 5.3. Software tools for R-fMRI analysis.

Software	Comments
Analysis of Functional NeuroImages (AFNI)	UNIX-based, open access
FSL-MELODIC	UNIX-based, open access
CONN toolbox (SPM based)	SPM/Matlab-based, requires Matlab license
Group ICA of fMRI toolbox (GIFT)	Matlab-based, requires Matlab license
REST toolkit	SPM/Matlab-based, requires Matlab license
Data Processing Assistant for Resting-State fMRI (DPARSF)	SPM/Matlab-based, requires Matlab license

5.3.3.5 Scientific publication and data sharing

The development of the scientific evidence is based in the honest reporting of the results of the studies, acknowledging their methodologies, quality and limitations. A common problem described in the biomedical literature is the publication bias ('file drawer problem'), resulting in the selective publication in journals of 'positive' results (reporting statistical differences) and withholding non-significant results. The so-called 'p-hacking' is a related problem consisting of the continuous analysis and sub-analysis of the data beyond the planned statistics until some significant results show up [116]. These problems result in an inflation of false positive results and seriously challenge the validity and credibility of research; neuroimaging field is not free from this risk [117]. Thus, reporting transparency in the publication of all the results of the planned analyses is especially required for R-fMRI researchers.

Another issue of concern in the neuroimaging studies is the 'reproducibility crisis'. The validity and consistency of scientific results depend, to some extent, on their ability to be potentially replicated by other researchers using the same or similar data and methods. The complexity of neuroimaging studies and the frequent paucity of methodological details reported in the literature make many studies unreproducible, so there is no way to check if they are correct and consistent. Authors and journal editors are increasingly becoming aware of this problem and implementing guidelines and policies to improve transparency and reproducibility of research reports [118].

One way to overcome these problems and to accelerate the pace of scientific discovery though international collaboration is the sharing of neuroimaging datasets in open-access web-based repositories. Anonymized clinical and brain data from subjects is uploaded and any researcher in the world can analyze them. Consequently, simultaneous analysis can be performed in parallel with large populations, collaborative competition is enhanced (see for example the ADHD Global Competition [85]), and the results from the studies could be checked for reproducibility, re-analyzed and integrated in image-based massive meta-analyses [119]. For that reason, researchers are encouraged to take part in this trend with actual and potential high scientific impact [120], providing that research subject's confidentiality is warranted.

5.4 R-fMRI as a potential biomarking tool in ADHD

In this final section, the concept of medical biomarkers will be defined, and the potential role of R-fMRI for clinical diagnostic and prognostic purposes will be evaluated in the light of widespread evidence in neuropsychiatric disorders. Finally, its application to ADHD will be discussed.

5.4.1 Biomarkers and R-fMRI

Biomedical research and, most importantly, clinical care for patients, should ideally require the availability of objective measurements to certainly diagnose a disease or disorder, distinguish it from normality and from other conditions, predict its outcome, customize its treatment and assess its change (stability, improvement, worsening, transformation) over time in response to the interventions taken. Biomarkers, derived from different human diagnostic methods (lab tests of biological samples, imaging, neurophysiology) are meant to serve these purposes.

The need for biomarkers in psychiatry is compelling, as current practice mainly relies on symptom assessment through observation, self-reports and third-person reports of thoughts, emotions and behaviors, with a high degree of subjectivity due to human error, clinical expertise and cultural factors, and there exist notable academic and social controversies.

The development of potential biomarkers starts with good quality research studies, but clinical usefulness of a biomarker goes beyond the statistical significance of the differences found in individual studies, and is based on its validity (accuracy), reliability (precision), sensitivity, specificity and widespread availability. Biomarkers are required to be reliable within and among subjects and reproducible among different sites. Most importantly, the group level statistical differences in research studies should have enough consistency and predictive power to be used in individuals. Here is where the gap between research and clinical practice still compromises the translation and understanding of the experimental evidence.

But even after overcoming these difficulties, the implementation of biomarking techniques will require availability in daily practice, which depends on complexity and cost. Currently, R-fMRI needs expensive devices as well as a multidisciplinary team for image acquisition and analysis, so its use is not within reach for low-income and community settings. On the other hand, image acquisition of R-fMRI does offer interesting advantages over other neuroimaging and non-imaging methods, as it appears to be valid across the whole lifespan and does not require as much collaboration as with fMRI task-based acquisitions. For that reason, it might be useful in the study of young children and people with intellectual disabilities or other cognitive impairments. The optimal duration of an R-fMRI protocol should still be established in research, but a clinical application will need a balance between excellent acquisition and a tolerable length for patients.

Notwithstanding the challenges, R-fMRI is a candidate set of techniques for the development of neuroimage-based biomarkers in different neuropsychiatric disorders. In neurodegenerative disorders it has been proposed as a tool for early diagnosis of cognitive impairment and a predictor of conversion to dementia [121, 122]. In autism spectrum disorders (ASDs), deep learning analysis of resting state data has proven its potential for the distinction of patients from healthy individuals [123]. Non-psychiatric disorders such as multiple sclerosis could also be potentially diagnosed with R-fMRI [124]. The search for neuroimaging biomarkers has integrated machine-learning computerized and statistical approaches such as logistic regression, support vector machine (SVM), decision trees-random forest (RF) algorithms (see [9] for description of these methods) in an effort to convert group findings in individual predictions.

5.4.2 R-fMRI for early diagnosis, outcome prediction and treatment response biomarker in ADHD

Current clinical challenges in the management of ADHD are its accurate early detection and differential diagnosis (separating patients from healthy individuals and distinguishing this disorder from others with similar symptoms) and the election of a customized treatment strategy with the best chance of success. Prognosis of symptomatic and functional short-term and long-term outcomes in affected individuals is still unpredictable and might depend on poorly understood individual differences such as the existence of neurobiologically-based subtypes of ADHD, sociodemographic factors and genetic subtleties.

Therefore, the quest for neuroimaging biomarkers in ADHD is highly relevant but has not yet yielded clinically relevant results [9, 26]. R-fMRI is a candidate tool for this purpose and has proven its consistency in international large datasets, and has been conducted in children, adolescents and adults. However, head motion is and will be an issue to carefully address in these populations. Machine learning neuroimaging analyses have already been studied in ADHD, and could be useful in the future for diagnosis [88], identification of subtypes [125] and prediction of clinical response to medications [92].

To answer the question on whether R-fMRI could be used in the near future as a biomarking tool in ADHD, the challenges cited in the previous subsection should be addressed, and the neuroimaging research in this disorder should be expanded with more longitudinal and inclusive studies, exploring also its capability to detect the disorder before symptoms or their consequences are too impairing (early diagnosis). Furthermore, the neural effects of different medications and interventions, in correlation to their symptomatic and functional outcomes, should be more thoroughly investigated.

Finally, as the brain functioning and the psychopathology are overwhelmingly complex and determined by different bio-psycho-social factors, R-fMRI in isolation will probably never capture the ADHD phenomenon, and its research should be tightly analyzed in the context of sociodemographic and clinical factors, and ideally integrated within multi-modal imaging (task-based fMRI, DTI) and genetic studies (imaging genetics).

5.5 Conclusion

Resting state fMRI techniques are under maturation for standardized, international collaborative mapping of the developing brain in healthy and impaired individuals, and time will tell if the neurobiology of psychiatric disorders can be better understood with them. The enthusiasm with which many fMRI researchers are embracing a collaborative culture of open and reproductible science, as well as the consolidation of large subject datasets, raise the hopes in the potential of neuroimaging research for better understanding of the neurobiology of ADHD.

ADHD is an impairing condition for many individuals from their childhood, but early and optimal interventions can lead to symptom remission or alleviation, prevention of comorbid disorders, improving their quality of life and normalizing their functioning. Although great gaps of knowledge still exist in regard to the neurobiology of ADHD, and its diagnosis and personalized management lack reliable biomarkers, resting-state fMRI is a promising tool whose potential should be further explored.

References

[1] Polanczyk G V, Willcutt E G, Salum G A, Kieling C and Rohde L A 2014 ADHD prevalence estimates across three decades: an updated systematic review and meta-regression analysis *Int. J. Epidemiol.* **43** 434–42

[2] American Psychiatric Association 2013 *Diagnostic and Statistical Manual of Mental Disorders: DSM-5* 5th edn (Arlington, VA: APS)

[3] Franke B *et al* 2018 Live fast, die young? A review on the developmental trajectories of ADHD across the lifespan *Eur. Neuropsychopharmacol.* **28** 1059–88

[4] American Psychiatric Association 2013 Neurodevelopmental disorders *Diagnostic and Statistical Manual of Mental Disorders DSM-V* 5th edn (Arlington, VA: APS)

[5] Ford-Jones P C 2015 Misdiagnosis of attention deficit hyperactivity disorder: 'Normal behaviour' and relative maturity *Paediatr. Child Health* **20** 200–2

[6] Bai G-N, Wang Y-F, Yang L and Niu W-Y 2015 Effectiveness of a focused, brief psychoeducation program for parents of ADHD children: improvement of medication adherence and symptoms *Neuropsychiatr. Dis. Treat.* **11** 2721–35

[7] Rajeh A, Amanullah S, Shivakumar K and Cole J 2017 Interventions in ADHD: a comparative review of stimulant medications and behavioral therapies *Asian J. Psychiatr.* **25** 131–5

[8] Cortese S *et al* 2018 Comparative efficacy and tolerability of medications for attention-deficit hyperactivity disorder in children, adolescents, and adults: a systematic review and network meta-analysis *Lancet Psychiatry* **5** 727–38

[9] Uddin L Q, Dajani D R, Voorhies W, Bednarz H and Kana R K 2017 Progress and roadblocks in the search for brain-based biomarkers of autism and attention-deficit/hyperactivity disorder *Transl. Psychiatry* **7** e1218

[10] Gallo E F and Posner J 2016 Moving towards causality in attention-deficit hyperactivity disorder: overview of neural and genetic mechanisms *Lancet Psychiatry* **3** 555–67

[11] Shaw P, Lalonde F, Lepage C, Rabin C, Eckstrand K, Sharp W, Greenstein D, Evans A, Giedd J N and Rapoport J 2009 Development of cortical asymmetry in typically developing children and its disruption in attention-deficit/hyperactivity disorder *Arch. Gen. Psychiatry* **66** 888–96
[12] Shaw P, Eckstrand K, Sharp W, Blumenthal J, Lerch J P, Greenstein D, Clasen L, Evans A, Giedd J and Rapoport J L 2007 Attention-deficit/hyperactivity disorder is characterized by a delay in cortical maturation *Proc. Natl Acad. Sci. USA* **104** 19649–54
[13] Khadka S, Pearlson G D, Calhoun V D, Liu J, Gelernter J, Bessette K L and Stevens M C 2016 Multivariate imaging genetics study of MRI gray matter volume and SNPs reveals biological pathways correlated with brain structural differences in attention deficit hyperactivity disorder *Front. psychiatry* **7** 128
[14] Moser D A, Doucet G E, Lee W H, Rasgon A, Krinsky H, Leibu E, Ing A, Schumann G, Rasgon N and Frangou S 2018 Multivariate associations among behavioral, clinical, and multimodal imaging phenotypes in patients with psychosis *JAMA Psychiatry* **75** 386
[15] Thome J *et al* 2012 Biomarkers for attention-deficit/hyperactivity disorder (ADHD). A consensus report of the WFSBP task force on biological markers and the World Federation of ADHD *World J. Biol. Psychiatry* **13** 379–400
[16] Demontis D *et al* 2019 Discovery of the first genome-wide significant risk loci for attention deficit/hyperactivity disorder *Nat. Genet.* **51** 63–75
[17] Thapar A 2018 Discoveries on the genetics of ADHD in the 21st century: new findings and their implications *Am. J. Psychiatry* **175** 943–50
[18] Faraone S V and Larsson H 2017 Genetics of attention deficit hyperactivity disorder *Charney & Nestler's Neurobiology of Mental Illness* ed D S Charney, E J Nestler, P Sklar and J D Buxbaum 5th edn (Oxford: Oxford University Press)
[19] Caylak E 2012 Biochemical and genetic analyses of childhood attention deficit/hyperactivity disorder *Am. J. Med. Genet. Part B Neuropsychiatr. Genet* **159B** 613–27
[20] Hamza M, Halayem S, Bourgou S, Daoud M, Charfi F and Belhadj A 2017 Epigenetics and ADHD *J. Atten. Disord.* **23** 655–64
[21] Srivastav S, Walitza S and Grünblatt E 2018 Emerging role of miRNA in attention deficit hyperactivity disorder: a systematic review *ADHD Atten. Deficit Hyperact. Disord.* **10** 49–63
[22] Masuo Y, Shibato J and Rakwal R 2012 ADHD animal model characterization: transcriptomics and proteomics analyses *Methods Mol. Biol. (Clifton, N.J.)* **829** 505–30
[23] Sokolowska I, Ngounou Wetie A G, Wormwood K, Thome J, Darie C C and Woods A G 2015 The potential of biomarkers in psychiatry: focus on proteomics *J. Neural Transm.* **122** 9–18
[24] Bonvicini C, Faraone S V and Scassellati C 2016 Attention-deficit hyperactivity disorder in adults: a systematic review and meta-analysis of genetic, pharmacogenetic and biochemical studies *Mol. Psychiatry* **21** 872–84
[25] Aarts E *et al* 2017 Gut microbiome in ADHD and its relation to neural reward anticipation *PLoS One* **12** e0183509
[26] Thome J *et al* 2012 Biomarkers for attention-deficit/hyperactivity disorder (ADHD). A consensus report of the WFSBP task force on biological markers and the World Federation of ADHD *World J. Biol. Psychiatry* **13** 379–400

[27] Shaw P, Malek M, Watson B, Sharp W, Evans A and Greenstein D 2012 Development of cortical surface area and gyrification in attention-deficit/hyperactivity disorder *Biol. Psychiatry* **72** 191–7
[28] Shaw P, Lerch J, Greenstein D, Sharp W, Clasen L, Evans A, Giedd J, Castellanos F X and Rapoport J 2006 Longitudinal mapping of cortical thickness and clinical outcome in children and adolescents with attention-deficit/hyperactivity disorder *Arch. Gen. Psychiatry* **63** 540–9
[29] Hoogman M *et al* 2017 Subcortical brain volume differences in participants with attention deficit hyperactivity disorder in children and adults: a cross-sectional mega-analysis *Lancet Psychiatry* **4** 310–9
[30] Soares J M, Marques P, Alves V and Sousa N 2013 A Hitchhiker's guide to diffusion tensor imaging *Front. Neurosci.* **7** 31
[31] Aoki Y, Yoncheva Y N, Chen B, Nath T, Sharp D, Lazar M, Velasco P, Milham M P and Di Martino A 2017 Association of white matter structure with autism spectrum disorder and attention-deficit/hyperactivity disorder *JAMA Psychiatry* **74** 1120
[32] Altabella L, Zoratto F, Adriani W and Canese R 2014 MR imaging-detectable metabolic alterations in attention deficit/hyperactivity disorder: from preclinical to clinical studies *AJNR Am. J. Neuroradiol.* **35** S55–63
[33] Spencer T J, Brown A, Seidman L J, Valera E M, Makris N, Lomedico A, Faraone S V and Biederman J 2013 Effect of psychostimulants on brain structure and function in ADHD: a qualitative literature review of magnetic resonance imaging-based neuroimaging studies *J. Clin. Psychiatry* **74** 902–17
[34] Feng C-M, Narayana S, Lancaster J L, Jerabek P A, Arnow T L, Zhu F, Tan L H, Fox P T and Gao J-H 2004 CBF changes during brain activation: fMRI vs. PET *Neuroimage* **22** 443–6
[35] Dupont A-C, Santiago Ribeiro M-J, Guilloteau D and Arlicot N 2017 β-Amyloid PET neuroimaging: a review of radiopharmaceutical development *Méd. Nucl.* **41** 27–35
[36] Ibrahim N, Kusmirek J, Struck A F, Floberg J M, Perlman S B, Gallagher C and Hall L T 2016 The sensitivity and specificity of F-DOPA PET in a movement disorder clinic *Am. J. Nucl. Med. Mol. Imaging* **6** 102–9
[37] Santra A and Kumar R 2014 Brain perfusion single photon emission computed tomography in major psychiatric disorders: from basics to clinical practice *Indian J. Nucl. Med.* **29** 210
[38] Zimmer L 2017 Contribution of clinical neuroimaging to the understanding of the pharmacology of methylphenidate *Trends Pharmacol. Sci.* **38** 608–20
[39] Glover G H 2011 Overview of functional magnetic resonance imaging *Neurosurg. Clin. N. Am.* **22** 133–9 vii
[40] Buxton R B 2013 The physics of functional magnetic resonance imaging (fMRI) *Rep. Prog. Phys.* **76** 096601
[41] Telischak N A, Detre J A and Zaharchuk G 2015 Arterial spin labeling MRI: clinical applications in the brain *J. Magn. Reson. Imaging* **41** 1165–80
[42] Cortese S, Kelly C, Chabernaud C, Proal E, Di Martino A, Milham M P and Castellanos F X 2012 Toward systems neuroscience of ADHD: a meta-analysis of 55 fMRI studies *Am. J. Psychiatry* **169** 1038–55

[43] Rubia K, Alegria A A, Cubillo A I, Smith A B, Brammer M J and Radua J 2014 Effects of stimulants on brain function in attention-deficit/hyperactivity disorder: a systematic review and meta-analysis *Biol. Psychiatry* **76** 616–28
[44] Biehl S C, Merz C J, Dresler T, Heupel J, Reichert S, Jacob C P, Deckert J and Herrmann M J 2016 Increase or decrease of fmri activity in adult attention deficit/hyperactivity disorder: does it depend on task difficulty? *Int. J. Neuropsychopharmacol.* **19**
[45] Schulz K P, Bédard A-C V, Fan J, Hildebrandt T B, Stein M A, Ivanov I, Halperin J M and Newcorn J H 2017 Striatal activation predicts differential therapeutic responses to methylphenidate and atomoxetine *J. Am. Acad. Child Adolesc. Psychiatry* **56** 602–9.e2
[46] Schulz K P, Krone B, Adler L A, Bédard A-C V, Duhoux S, Pedraza J, Mahagabin S and Newcorn J H 2018 Lisdexamfetamine targets amygdala mechanisms that bias cognitive control in attention-deficit/hyperactivity disorder *Biol. Psychiatry Cogn. Neurosci. Neuroimaging* **3** 686–93
[47] Tao J *et al* 2017 Disrupted control-related functional brain networks in drug-naive children with attention-deficit/hyperactivity disorder *Front. Psychiatry* **8** 246
[48] Raichle M E 2015 The brain's default mode network *Annu. Rev. Neurosci.* **38** 433–47
[49] Biswal B B 2012 Resting state fMRI: a personal history *Neuroimage* **62** 938–44
[50] Li Z, Vidorreta M, Katchmar N, Alsop D C, Wolf D H and Detre J A 2018 Effects of resting state condition on reliability, trait specificity, and network connectivity of brain function measured with arterial spin labeled perfusion MRI *Neuroimage* **173** 165–75
[51] Mongerson C R L, Jennings R W, Borsook D, Becerra L and Bajic D 2017 Resting-state functional connectivity in the infant brain: methods, pitfalls, and potentiality *Front. Pediatr.* **5** 159
[52] Wehrle F M, Michels L, Guggenberger R, Huber R, Latal B, O'Gorman R L and Hagmann C F 2018 Altered resting-state functional connectivity in children and adolescents born very preterm short title *NeuroImage Clin.* **20** 1148–56
[53] Solesio-Jofre E, Beets I A M, Woolley D G, Pauwels L, Chalavi S, Mantini D and Swinnen S P 2018 Age-dependent modulations of resting state connectivity following motor practice *Front. Aging Neurosci.* **10** 25
[54] Li G, Rossbach K, Jiang W and Du Y 2018 Resting-state brain activity in Chinese boys with low functioning autism spectrum disorder *Ann. Gen. Psychiatry* **17** 47
[55] Chen L M, Yang P-F, Wang F, Mishra A, Shi Z, Wu R, Wu T-L, Wilson G H, Ding Z and Gore J C 2017 Biophysical and neural basis of resting state functional connectivity: evidence from non-human primates *Magn. Reson. Imaging* **39** 71–81
[56] Bajic D, Craig M M, Mongerson C R L, Borsook D and Becerra L 2017 Identifying rodent resting-state brain networks with independent component analysis *Front. Neurosci.* **11** 685
[57] Kyriazis M 2015 Systems neuroscience in focus: from the human brain to the global brain? *Front. Syst. Neurosci.* **9** 7
[58] Thomas Yeo B T *et al* 2011 The organization of the human cerebral cortex estimated by intrinsic functional connectivity *J. Neurophysiol.* **106** 1125–65
[59] Andrews-Hanna J R, Reidler J S, Sepulcre J, Poulin R and Buckner R L 2010 Functional-anatomic fractionation of the brain's default network *Neuron* **65** 550–62
[60] Poerio G L, Sormaz M, Wang H-T, Margulies D, Jefferies E and Smallwood J 2017 The role of the default mode network in component processes underlying the wandering mind *Soc. Cogn. Affect. Neurosci.* **12** 1047–62

[61] Glasser M F *et al* 2016 The Human Connectome Project's neuroimaging approach *Nat. Neurosci.* **19** 1175–87
[62] Woodward N D and Cascio C J 2015 Resting-state functional connectivity in psychiatric disorders *JAMA Psychiatry* **72** 743–4
[63] Alonso-Solís A *et al* 2012 Altered default network resting state functional connectivity in patients with a first episode of psychosis *Schizophr. Res.* **139** 13–8
[64] Kim H-Y 2015 Statistical notes for clinical researchers: type I and type II errors in statistical decision *Restor. Dent. Endod.* **40** 249–52
[65] Yan C-G, Craddock R C, Zuo X-N, Zang Y-F and Milham M P 2013 Standardizing the intrinsic brain: towards robust measurement of inter-individual variation in 1000 functional connectomes *Neuroimage* **80** 246–62
[66] Zuo X-N, Di Martino A, Kelly C, Shehzad Z E, Gee D G, Klein D F, Castellanos F X, Biswal B B and Milham M P 2010 The oscillating brain: complex and reliable *Neuroimage* **49** 1432–45
[67] Van Dijk K R A, Sabuncu M R and Buckner R L 2012 The influence of head motion on intrinsic functional connectivity MRI *Neuroimage* **59** 431
[68] Power J D, Barnes K A, Snyder A Z, Schlaggar B L and Petersen S E 2012 Spurious but systematic correlations in functional connectivity MRI networks arise from subject motion *Neuroimage* **59** 2142–54
[69] Lv H, Wang Z, Tong E, Williams L M, Zaharchuk G, Zeineh M, Goldstein-Piekarski A N, Ball T M, Liao C and Wintermark M 2018 Resting-state functional MRI: everything that nonexperts have always wanted to know *Am. J. Neuroradiol.* **39** 1390–9
[70] Yu-Feng Z, Yong H, Chao-Zhe Z, Qing-Jiu C, Man-Qiu S, Meng L, Li-Xia T, Tian-Zi J and Yu-Feng W 2007 Altered baseline brain activity in children with ADHD revealed by resting-state functional MRI *Brain Dev.* **29** 83–91
[71] Zou Q-H, Zhu C-Z, Yang Y, Zuo X-N, Long X-Y, Cao Q-J, Wang Y-F and Zang Y-F 2008 An improved approach to detection of amplitude of low-frequency fluctuation (ALFF) for resting-state fMRI: fractional ALFF *J. Neurosci. Methods* **172** 137–41
[72] Zang Y, Jiang T, Lu Y, He Y and Tian L 2004 Regional homogeneity approach to fMRI data analysis *Neuroimage* **22** 394–400
[73] Tomasi D and Volkow N D 2010 Functional connectivity density mapping *Proc. Natl Acad. Sci. USA* **107** 9885–90
[74] Smith D V, Utevsky A V, Bland A R, Clement N, Clithero J A, Harsch A E W, McKell Carter R and Huettel S A 2014 Characterizing individual differences in functional connectivity using dual-regression and seed-based approaches *Neuroimage* **95** 1–12
[75] Zuo X-N, Ehmke R, Mennes M, Imperati D, Castellanos F X, Sporns O and Milham M P 2012 Network centrality in the human functional connectome *Cereb. Cortex* **22** 1862–75
[76] Wang J, Zuo X and He Y 2010 Graph-based network analysis of resting-state functional MRI *Front. Syst. Neurosci.* **4** 16
[77] Sepulcre J, Sabuncu M R, Yeo T B, Liu H and Johnson K A 2012 Stepwise connectivity of the modal cortex reveals the multimodal organization of the human brain *J. Neurosci.* **32** 10649–61
[78] Zuo X-N *et al* 2010 Growing together and growing apart: regional and sex differences in the lifespan developmental trajectories of functional homotopy *J. Neurosci.* **30** 15034–43
[79] Lee M H, Smyser C D and Shimony J S 2013 Resting-state fMRI: a review of methods and clinical applications *Am. J. Neuroradiol.* **34** 1866–72

[80] Yang Z, Kelly C, Castellanos F X, Leon T, Milham M P and Adler L A 2016 Neural correlates of symptom improvement following stimulant treatment in adults with attention-deficit/hyperactivity disorder *J. Child Adolesc. Psychopharmacol.* **26** 0243
[81] Castellanos F X, Kelly C and Milham M P 2009 The restless brain: attention-deficit hyperactivity disorder, resting—state functional connectivity, and intrasubject variability *Can. J. Psychiatry* **54** 665–72
[82] Sonuga-Barke E J S and Castellanos F X 2007 Spontaneous attentional fluctuations in impaired states and pathological conditions: a neurobiological hypothesis *Neurosci. Biobehav. Rev.* **31** 977–86
[83] Castellanos F X and Proal E 2012 Large-scale brain systems in ADHD: beyond the prefrontal-striatal model *Trends Cogn. Sci.* **16** 17–26
[84] Marcos-Vidal L *et al* 2018 Local functional connectivity suggests functional immaturity in children with attention-deficit/hyperactivity disorder *Hum. Brain Mapp.* **39** 2442–54
[85] Brown M R G, Sidhu G S, Greiner R, Asgarian N, Bastani M, Silverstone P H, Greenshaw A J and Dursun S M 2012 ADHD-200 global competition: diagnosing ADHD using personal characteristic data can outperform resting state fMRI measurements *Front. Syst. Neurosci.* **6** 69
[86] Posner J, Park C and Wang Z 2014 Connecting the dots: a review of resting connectivity MRI studies in attention-deficit/hyperactivity disorder *Neuropsychol. Rev.* **24** 3–15
[87] Castellanos F X and Aoki Y 2016 Intrinsic functional connectivity in attention-deficit/ hyperactivity disorder: a science in development *Biol. Psychiatry. Cogn. Neurosci. Neuroimaging* **1** 253–61
[88] Cheng W, Ji X, Zhang J and Feng J 2012 Individual classification of ADHD patients by integrating multiscale neuroimaging markers and advanced pattern recognition techniques *Front. Syst. Neurosci.* **6** 58
[89] Barber A D, Jacobson L A, Wexler J L, Nebel M B, Caffo B S, Pekar J J and Mostofsky S H 2015 Connectivity supporting attention in children with attention deficit hyperactivity disorder *NeuroImage. Clin.* **7** 68–81
[90] Mostert J C, Shumskaya E, Mennes M, Onnink A M H, Hoogman M, Kan C C, Arias Vasquez A, Buitelaar J, Franke B and Norris D G 2016 Characterising resting-state functional connectivity in a large sample of adults with ADHD *Prog. Neuro-Psychopharmacology Biol. Psychiatry* **67** 82–91
[91] Fair D A *et al* 2013 Distinct neural signatures detected for ADHD subtypes after controlling for micro-movements in resting state functional connectivity MRI data *Front. Syst. Neurosci.* **6** 80
[92] Yoo J H, Kim D, Choi J and Jeong B 2018 Treatment effect of methylphenidate on intrinsic functional brain network in medication-naïve ADHD children: a multivariate analysis *Brain Imaging Behav.* **12** 518–31
[93] Battel L, Kieling R R, Kieling C, Anés M, Aurich N K, da Costa J C, Rohde L A and Franco A R 2016 Intrinsic brain connectivity following long-term treatment with methylphenidate in children with attention-deficit/hyperactivity disorder *J. Child Adolesc. Psychopharmacol.* **26** 555–61
[94] Shang C Y, Yan C G, Lin H Y, Tseng W Y, Castellanos F X and Gau S S 2016 Differential effects of methylphenidate and atomoxetine on intrinsic brain activity in children with attention deficit hyperactivity disorder *Psychol. Med.* **46** 3173–85

[95] Marquand A F, O'Daly O G, De Simoni S, Alsop D C, Maguire R P, Williams S C R, Zelaya F O and Mehta M A 2012 Dissociable effects of methylphenidate, atomoxetine and placebo on regional cerebral blood flow in healthy volunteers at rest: a multi-class pattern recognition approach *Neuroimage* **60** 1015–24
[96] Silk T J, Malpas C, Vance A and Bellgrove M A 2016 The effect of single-dose methylphenidate on resting-state network functional connectivity in ADHD *Brain Imaging Behav.* **11** 1422–31
[97] An L, Cao X-H, Cao Q-J, Sun L, Yang L, Zou Q-H, Katya R, Zang Y-F and Wang Y-F 2013 Methylphenidate normalizes resting-state brain dysfunction in boys with attention deficit hyperactivity disorder *Neuropsychopharmacology* **38** 1287–95
[98] Hong S-B, Harrison B J, Fornito A, Sohn C-H, Song I-C and Kim J-W 2015 Functional dysconnectivity of corticostriatal circuitry and differential response to methylphenidate in youth with attention-deficit/hyperactivity disorder *J. Psychiatry Neurosci.* **40** 46–57
[99] Wang X, Cao Q, Wang J, Wu Z, Wang P, Sun L, Cai T and Wang Y 2016 The effects of cognitive-behavioral therapy on intrinsic functional brain networks in adults with attention-deficit/hyperactivity disorder *Behav. Res. Ther.* **76** 32–9
[100] Dosenbach N U F *et al* 2017 Real-time motion analytics during brain MRI improve data quality and reduce costs *Neuroimage* **161** 80–93
[101] Bjork J M, Straub L K, Provost R G and Neale M C 2017 The ABCD study of neurodevelopment: identifying neurocircuit targets for prevention and treatment of adolescent substance abuse *Curr. Treat. Options Psychiatry* **4** 196–209
[102] Casey B J *et al* 2018 The adolescent brain cognitive development (ABCD) study: imaging acquisition across 21 sites *Dev. Cogn. Neurosci.* **32** 43–54
[103] Nikolaidis A, Vogelstein J, Bellec P and Milham M 2018 Improving corticostriatal parcellation through multilevel bagging with PyBASC *NeuroImage* **214** 116678
[104] Nichols T E *et al* 2017 Best practices in data analysis and sharing in neuroimaging using MRI *Nat. Neurosci.* **20** 299–303
[105] Mumford J A 2012 A power calculation guide for fMRI studies *Soc. Cogn. Affect. Neurosci.* **7** 738–42
[106] World Medical Association Declaration of Helsinki 2013 *JAMA* **310** 2191
[107] Wang J, Han J, Nguyen V T, Guo L and Guo C C 2017 Improving the test–retest reliability of resting state fMRI by removing the impact of sleep *Front. Neurosci.* **11** 249
[108] Glover G H 2012 Spiral imaging in fMRI *Neuroimage* **62** 706–12
[109] Haller S, Zaharchuk G, Thomas D L, Lovblad K-O, Barkhof F and Golay X 2016 Arterial spin labeling perfusion of the brain: emerging clinical applications *Radiology* **281** 337–56
[110] Fernández-Seara M A, Rodgers Z B, Englund E K and Wehrli F W 2016 Calibrated bold fMRI with an optimized ASL-BOLD dual-acquisition sequence *Neuroimage* **142** 474–82
[111] Storti S F, Boscolo Galazzo I, Montemezzi S, Menegaz G and Pizzini F B 2017 Dual-echo ASL contributes to decrypting the link between functional connectivity and cerebral blow flow *Hum. Brain Mapp.* **38** 5831–44
[112] Zhang K, Huang D and Shah N J 2018 Comparison of resting-state brain activation detected by bold, blood volume and blood flow *Front. Hum. Neurosci.* **12** 443
[113] Birn R M, Molloy E K, Patriat R, Parker T, Meier T B, Kirk G R, Nair V A, Meyerand M E and Prabhakaran V 2013 The effect of scan length on the reliability of resting-state fMRI connectivity estimates *Neuroimage* **83** 550–8

[114] Goto M, Abe O, Miyati T, Yamasue H, Gomi T and Takeda T 2016 Head motion and correction methods in resting-state functional MRI *Magn. Reson. Med. Sci.* **15** 178–86

[115] Dickie D A, Shenkin S D, Anblagan D, Lee J, Blesa Cabez M, Rodriguez D, Boardman J P, Waldman A, Job D E and Wardlaw J M 2017 Whole brain magnetic resonance image atlases: a systematic review of existing atlases and caveats for use in population imaging *Front. Neuroinform.* **11** 1

[116] Head M L, Holman L, Lanfear R, Kahn A T and Jennions M D 2015 The extent and consequences of P-hacking in science *PLoS Biol.* **13** e1002106

[117] Jennings R G and Horn J D V 2012 Publication bias in neuroimaging research: implications for meta-analyses *Neuroinformatics* **10** 67–80

[118] Gorgolewski K J and Poldrack R A 2016 A practical guide for improving transparency and reproducibility in neuroimaging research *PLoS Biol.* **14** e1002506

[119] Radua J and Mataix-Cols D 2012 Meta-analytic methods for neuroimaging data explained *Biol. Mood Anxiety Disord.* **2** 6

[120] Milham M P *et al* 2018 Assessment of the impact of shared brain imaging data on the scientific literature *Nat. Commun.* **9** 2818

[121] Hojjati S H, Ebrahimzadeh A, Khazaee A, Babajani-Feremi A and Alzheimer's Disease Neuroimaging Initiative 2017 Predicting conversion from MCI to AD using resting-state fMRI, graph theoretical approach and SVM *J. Neurosci. Methods* **282** 69–80

[122] Lin L, Xing G and Han Y 2018 Advances in resting state neuroimaging of mild cognitive impairment *Front. Psychiatry* **9** 671

[123] Heinsfeld A S, Franco A R, Craddock R C, Buchweitz A and Meneguzzi F 2018 Identification of autism spectrum disorder using deep learning and the ABIDE dataset *NeuroImage Clin.* **17** 16–23

[124] Saccà V *et al* 2018 Evaluation of machine learning algorithms performance for the prediction of early multiple sclerosis from resting-state FMRI connectivity data *Brain Imaging Behav.* **13** 1103–14

[125] Kyeong S, Kim J-J and Kim E 2017 Novel subgroups of attention-deficit/hyperactivity disorder identified by topological data analysis and their functional network modular organizations *PLoS One* **12** e0182603

IOP Publishing

Neurological Disorders and Imaging Physics, Volume 4
Application to attention deficit hyperactivity disorder
Ayman El-Baz and Jasjit S Suri

Chapter 6

Brain networks related to automatic and controlled processes in ADHD

Rosa Angela Fabio and Tindara Caprì

6.1 Introduction

Attention deficit hyperactivity disorder (ADHD) represents one of the most common neuropsychiatric disorders in childhood [1–4]. It persists into adolescence and adulthood in 30% to 60% of cases [5]. Worldwide incidence is between 5% and 15% of the school-aged population [6, 7]. ADHD is diagnosed more often in males than females, with female ratios of between 4:1 and 9:1 [8, 9]. The disorder is characterized by the following symptoms: inattention, hyperactivity and impulsivity. According to this symptomatology, ADHD can be classified into three clinical subtypes: predominantly inattentive, predominantly hyperactive, and combined [10].

Decades of research have revealed that ADHD is associated with several executive dsyfunctions [11, 12] such as: set shifting [13], planning [14] working memory (WM) [15], and inhibition [16]. In addition, patients with ADHD also show deficits in autobiographical memory [17], motivational processes [18], decision making [19] and reinforcement learning [20].

Although ADHD is closely linked to executive deficits, it has recently been attributed to procedural learning and automatic processing impairments [21–24]. In particular, it has been found that individuals with ADHD show impaired performance in different automatic or procedural abilities: motor sequence tapping [25–28], serial reaction time [29, 30], probabilistic selection [31], visual category learning [32], artificial grammar learning [33, 34] and verbal fluency [35].

Despite the inextricable relationship between automatic and controlled processes, most works have focused on the executive functions (EF) and only few studies have investigated the role of automatic processes in ADHD. Hence, some questions remain, for example: to what extent can an automatic deficit, associated with executive functioning, explain the core symptoms of ADHD. To answer to this

doi:10.1088/978-0-7503-1822-8ch6

question, we examined the brain networks related to automatic and controlled processes in ADHD, focusing on impaired brain areas in individuals that are affected by ADHD.

In this chapter, we will describe the recent neuropsychological models of ADHD, and we propose to include the role of automatization deficits in ADHD, and the related subcortical activation, to better explain ADHD symptomatology, along with a new theoretical framework, including the cortico-subcortical brain network of cognitive processes.

This chapter is organized into five sections. In the first section, we have introduced the topics of this chapter. In section 6.2, an overview of recent neuropsychological models of ADHD is provided. Section 6.3 provides new evidence on the presence of a deficit in automatic processes in ADHD. In section 6.4, we propose a new theoretical framework of ADHD. In section 6.5, we discuss the new theoretical proposal and suggest future research to validate the automatic hypothesis deficit in ADHD.

6.2 Recent neuropsychological models of ADHD

6.2.1 Cognitive theories

The etiology of ADHD is still unclear, probably because ADHD has a complex background, in which multiple factors contribute to the etiology of this disorder. Several studies have been conducted under the currently prevailing neuropsychiatric paradigm, in which neurobiological conceptualizations of the disorder, genetic parameters and psychosocial factors have been considered to explain the phenotype of ADHD.

The dominating neuropsychological theories of ADHD in the past 25 years have emphasized behavioral and cognitive factors, in particular, the focus has been on executive functions. In this scenario, the most popular and influential theory is Barkley's model [36, 37], which conceptualizes ADHD as a failure of self-control systems. According to this model, the primary deficit in ADHD is the inhibition ability, and, executive deficits are secondary. Precisely, Barkley's theory assumes inhibition (i.e. inhibition of prepotent response, stopping an ongoing response, and interference control) as the core deficit of ADHD symptomatology and associates it with four executive functions: WM, self-regulation of affect-motivation-arousal, internalization of speech, and reconstruction [38]. Barkley [36] states that individuals with ADHD may not lack the skills and knowledge to be successful, but rather, their problems with self-regulation often prevent them from applying their knowledge and skills at the necessary times.

Another prominent neuropsychological theory of ADHD postulates that it arises from an impairment in EF. It is well known that executive deficits can lead to poor attention and planning, difficulties generating and implementing strategies, inability to utilize feedback, and inflexibility of thinking [39]. All these symptoms characterize the phenotype of ADHD. A meta-analysis of 83 studies, which administered EF measures to groups with ADHD (total $N = 3734$) and without ADHD ($N = 2969$), has demonstrated that individuals with ADHD show moderate weaknesses in response inhibition, WM, impulsivity, vigilance, organization, and planning [40], confirming the EF hypothesis.

From the cognitive prospective, another important theory of ADHD is the functional WM model that proposes WM as a core deficit in ADHD [41]. This model changes the level of analysis and assumes that the deficit in inhibition is due to an impairment in WM, as stimuli must gain access to the working memory system before a response can be inhibited [42, 43].

Despite wide literature examining EF in the ADHD population, the identification of a unique core deficit can explain the entire ADHD symptomatology remains elusive [44].

6.2.2 Neurobiological theories

From the neurobiological prospective, some environmental and genetic factors have been identified to contribute to the onset of ADHD. For example, prenatal exposure to alcohol, cigarettes, and illicit drugs have all been associated with an increased risk of ADHD [45]. Low birth weight and adverse life experiences have also demonstrated associations. However, environmental factors are not sufficient to explain the phenotype of ADHD.

Research into the genetic field has focused on candidate genes of ADHD and has identified genes involved in catecholamine (dopamine, noradrenaline) and serotonin transmission as important factors in the etiology of ADHD. The dopamine-deficit theory of ADHD assumes that this disorder is due to a dopamine transfer deficit (DTD). This hypothesis has been confirmed by recent literature, showing: abnormalities in dopamine-modulated frontal-striatal circuits, reflected by size (smaller-than-average components) and function (hypoactivation); agonist effects of stimulant medication on dopaminergic mechanisms at the synaptic and circuit level of analysis; and the most-widely documented ADHD-related neural abnormality in the dopamine system.

6.3 New evidence

As described before, in the explanation of ADHD symptoms, the focus has always been executive deficits, including response inhibition, WM, and general EF. Experts have always seen the ADHD as a disorder of controlled processes, the idea that it can be also due to a deficit in automatic processing has been less investigated. Before illustrating recent studies on automatic processes in ADHD, we briefly explain the construct of automaticity.

6.3.1 Automatic and controlled processes

The first distinction between automatic and controlled processes was introduced by Schneider and Shiffrin [46] and Schneider and Chein [47] with the dual-process theory. This theory suggests that there are two distinctive cognitive processes, namely, controlled and automatic processes (also called controlled cognition and automatic cognition, respectively) that play roles in predicting behavior. Automatic processing is fast, effortless, autonomous, stereotypic, unavailable to conscious awareness and fairly error-free. It can be accomplished simultaneously with other cognitive processes without interference, it is not limited by attentional capacity and it can be unconscious or involuntary [22, 23, 48].

Most commonly, automatic cognitions are depicted as unconscious mental associations between concepts and valences in an associative network or in habitual responses that can generate quick, spontaneous behavioral tendencies without intention [49]. In contrast, controlled processing is effortful, slow, and prone to errors, but at the same time, flexible and useful for dealing with novel situations. Furthermore, in controlled processing, people carry out deliberate behaviors by retrieving information from memory with effort which is particularly important as it supports behaviors that achieve goals and ultimately promote survival [49].

According to classical theories of cognitive control and automaticity, automaticity has been considered as an all-or-none phenomenon, that is, a process is either automatic or controlled. Controlled processes were considered exclusive to the domain of conscious cognition, and automatic processes were thought to be in the domain of unconscious cognition [46, 50, 51]. This classical view implies that a behavioral or neurophysiological effect has to be context-independent to induce a 'truly automatic' process [52].

However, it is difficult to identify processes that actually meet the classical criteria for automaticity as a task frequently demands modulated behavioral and neurophysiological effects [48, 53, 54]. Behavioral studies also suggest a set of phenomena associated with automaticity that indicate a continuous process rather than an all-or-none process: gradual development with practice; concomitant improvements in speed (and a reduction of variance); reduced reliance on, but not complete autonomy from, the effects of attention, the relative nature of interference effects and the interacting influences of stimulus information and attentional allocation on responding.

Unlike classical theories, refined theories of automaticity propose a new view of automatic processing, as a flexible process [55–59]. They argue that automatic processing depends on a configuration of the cognitive system regarding attention and task sets. In particular, it has been suggested that attention, intentions, and task sets are involved in the unconscious processing. For example, Neumann [55] states that unconscious information will only be processed and will influence the action to a target stimulus to the extent that it matches current goals.

Traditionally, it is known that the controlled and automatic processes are two separated processes. This view is partially true. When we perform a task, all our cognitive resources are engaged in the learning of new information. The performance is slow, awkward and prone to errors. After the experience, the task execution requires less vigilance, the number of errors decrease and the performance is faster. This change can be defined as 'automatization' [22].

According to Fabio's model, the individual automatizes learning of the plus sign. As shown in figure 6.1, when we perform a new task, we are positioned in the A level, when the control of attention fulls cognitive load. For example, when a child must learn to read or a young person must learn to drive a car, all cognitive resources are involved in the learning of new abilities.

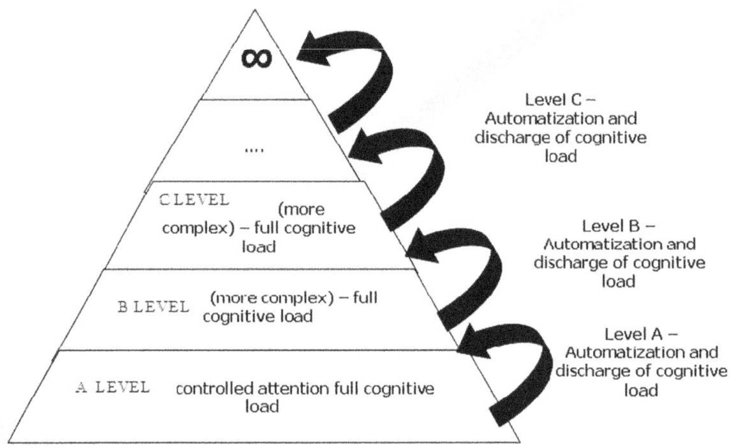

Figure 6.1. Fabio's model (2009).

When the learning is complete, the child has learned to read the words and the young adult has learned to change the gears of a car. Now, the subject can have access to a complex task, for example, reading the full test (B level). This is possible because the A level has become an automatized subroutine [22].

To access to the next level, the controlled processes of attention are needed; other cognitive resources are activated to learn new information. By learning, the initial control of attention becomes automatic. The child is now able to read and repeat the text, the young person can now drive a car in a spontaneous way.

6.3.2 Automatic processes in ADHD

The first studies examining automatic processes in ADHD have postulated that children with ADHD may have difficulties in performing acquired automatic skills [60–62]. Hazell *et al* [63] stated that an individual with ADHD can have problems in both encoding and automatic phase of information processing. Hurks *et al* [64] used a task requiring both automatic and controlled abilities in their study on ADHD. The authors analyzed the semantic category fluency (SCF) versus initial letter fluency (ILF) tasks; word production was recorded for each 15-s time slice on each task. They compared two groups: children with ADHD and typically developing subjects (TD). The results demonstrated that the ADHD group presented difficulties in the automatic skills involved in the abstract verbal information.

Fabio *et al* [24] investigated the automaticity of the auditory vigilance in ADHD and control subjects. They employed two tasks: Merril's [65] procedure with the dual-task interference paradigm and the auditory test with automatic procedure. A deficit in auditory vigilance tests was found when interference is introduced. However, this study provided no definitive support on the role of automatic processes in children with ADHD.

Also, the work of Martino *et al* [23] is in line with previous studies. The authors examined the automatic processing of selective visual attention in two groups (ADHD and TD groups). All participants performed two tasks: a visual information processing task and a clock test. This study also indicated that ADHD groups showed an impairment of automatic processing.

In relation to this weakness in both automatic and controlled processes, in the following we underline the neurological related processes.

6.3.3 Neurological basis of automatic and controlled processes and its relationship to ADHD

Several aspects of brain development, structure, function, and connectivity have been found impaired in the ADHD population [66–72].

Functional MRI (fMRI) studies have indicated total brain volume and total grey matter reduction up to 3%–5% in persons with ADHD compared to TD subjects [67, 73, 74]. These findings have been confirmed by a meta-analysis showing significant volume differences in cerebellar regions, total and right cerebral volume, right caudate, and frontal brain areas in subjects with ADHD [74]. Furthermore, Ellison-Wright *et al* [75], Frodl and Skokauskas [76], Naka *et al* [77], and Norman *et al* [78] conducted four meta-analyses in order to further understand these brain abnormalities, using voxel-based morphometry (VBM) analyses. The results of all the meta-analyses again confirmed grey matter reductions in the ventrolateral prefrontal/insular-striatal regions, such as the right insula, putamen, globus pallidus, and caudate nucleus.

Also, the study of Bralten *et al* [79] identified a reduced grey matter volume in five clusters located in the precentral gyrus, medial and orbital frontal cortex, and (para) cingulate cortices.

Several studies have combined fMRI with cognitive tasks, measuring: inhibition, WM and attention in patients with ADHD and TD subjects. The results have shown a reduced activation of fronto-striatal, fronto-parietal, and ventral attention networks [80–84].

From table 6.1 and figure 6.2, it can be seen that both brain cortical and subcortical areas are impaired in the population with ADHD.

In a meta-analyses of fMRI studies of inhibition and attention, consistent functional abnormalities in two distinct domain-dissociated fronto-basal ganglia networks have been found. These include the inferior frontal cortex, supplementary motor areas, and anteriorcingulate cortex (ACC) for inhibition and the dorsolateral prefrontal cortex (PFC), parietal, and cerebellar areas for attention processes [85].

Other studies on structural and functional neuroimaging have also provided evidence for abnormalities in children and adults with ADHD both in frontostriatal, fronto-parieto-temporal, fronto-cerebellar and fronto-limbic regions and networks [86–90]. Structural fMRI studies have demonstrated that children and adults with ADHD compared to control subjects show reduced white matter connectivity in fronto-striatal, cingulate, as well as fronto-parietal, fronto-cerebellar and parieto-occipital white matter tracts [84, 91–95].

Table 6.1. Reduced brain areas and under activation in population with ADHD.

Authors	Brain areas
Salmi *et al* 2018 [96]	Frontopariental, somato-motor, cerebellar, striatal areas
Rosch *et al* 2018 [97]	Caudate, globus pallidus and thalamus
Nornan *et al* 2018 [98]	Prefrontal cortex, putamen, caudate
Jacboson *et al* 2018 [99]	Pariental lobe, frontal cortex
Ueda *et al* 2018 [100]	Disconnettivity hemispheric
Salavert *et al* 2018 [101]	Medial prefontal cortex
Al-amin *et al* 2018 [102]	Subfields of hyppocampus
Hoogman *et al* 2018 [103]	Hyppocampus
Hoogman *et al* 2017 [104]	Accumbens
Hoogman *et al* 2017 [104]	Amygdala
Hoogman *et al* 2017 [104]	Caudate
Ivanov *et al* 2010 [105]	Thalamus
Narr *et al* 2009 [106]	Cortex
Valera *et al* 2007 [107]	Cerebellum
Pliszka *et al* 2006 [108]	ACC[a]
Durston *et al* 2004 [109]	Occipital lobe
Sowell *et al* 2003 [110]; Castellanos *et al* 2002 [111]	Parietal lobe
Sowell *et al* 2003 [110]; Mostofsky *et al* 2002 [112]	Prefontal cortex

[a] Anterior cingulate cortex.

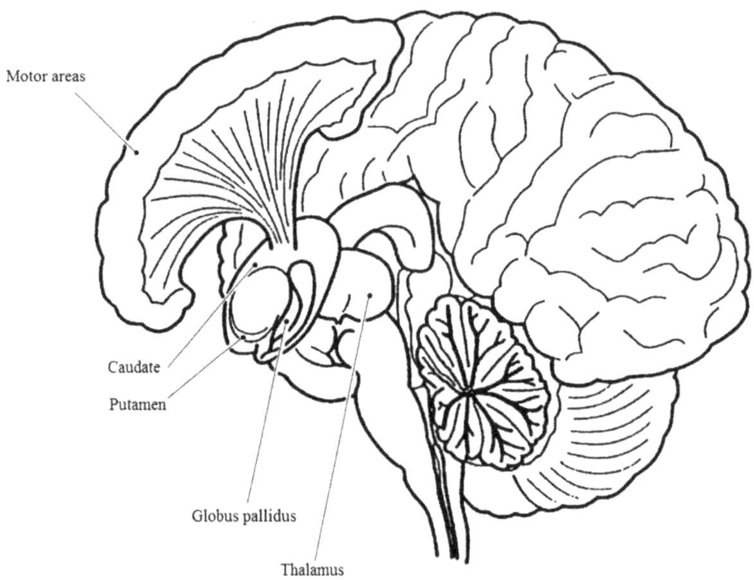

Figure 6.2. Reduced brain areas in the population with ADHD.

In addition, it was found that children with ADHD have shown under activation relative to controls in the DLPFC/IFC, ACC, caudate, supplementary motor area (SMA) as well as in temporo-parietal cortices during motor response inhibition, interference inhibition, vigilant, selective and flexible attention [113–118].

Posner *et al* [119] investigated the cognitive control network, and cortico-striato-thalamo-cortical loops in an ADHD population. He found that the ADHD group has less pronounced or absent correlations in the fronto-striatal circuits [119].

Also, the study by Mostert *et al* [72] demonstrated a lower functional connectivity in the executive control network, and the cerebellum network in a large sample of adults with ADHD compared to TD subjects.

It is well known that the fronto-parietal network mediates goal-directed executive processes, whereas the ventral attention network facilitates reorientation of attention towards salient and behaviorally relevant external stimuli. In addition, it is also recognized that cortico-striato-basal gangli are involved in the automatic processing.

fMRI studies of ADHD have mainly focused on neural circuits implicated in the disorder, especially the default-mode network (DMN), cognitive control network, and cortico-striato-thalamo-cortical loops [119]. But, it is important to note that these brain networks mediate both controlled and automatic processes. Despite this evidence, the automatic deficit in ADHD is not conceptualized as a possible brain phenotype in people with ADHD.

6.4 A new theoretical framework

Considering that an increasing number of studies [80–119] found structural and functional abnormalities in both fronto-cortical and fronto-subcortical networks in children and adults with ADHD, and, considering that these circuits support both controlled and automatic processes [120], it is reasonable to assume that children with ADHD could show both automatic and controlled deficits.

As described before, few previous studies have investigated the procedural deficit hypothesis (PDH) in ADHD. The results have shown an automatic deficit, but new research is needed.

As observed in table 6.1, the cortical and subcortical brain areas are impaired in the ADHD population. At the neural level, neuroimaging studies have demonstrated structural and functional abnormalities in the basal ganglia and cerebellum (core structures of the procedural learning system) and, specifically, deficits in cortical-striatal loops [121–125] (see figure 6.3).

These observations have led some authors to view ADHD as a disorder that arises from a selective disruption in the procedural learning systems [126–132]. However, the PDH has been postulated to explain the specific language impairment (SLI), dyslexia and briefly extended to ADHD.

The PDH of Ullman [126–132] proposes that SLI can be due to a dysfunction of brain network related procedural memory and in particular, portions of frontal/basalganglia circuits and the cerebellum. According to PHD of SLI and dyslexia, these abnormalities can explain the observed deficits of procedural memory, grammar and other functions that depend on these brain structures.

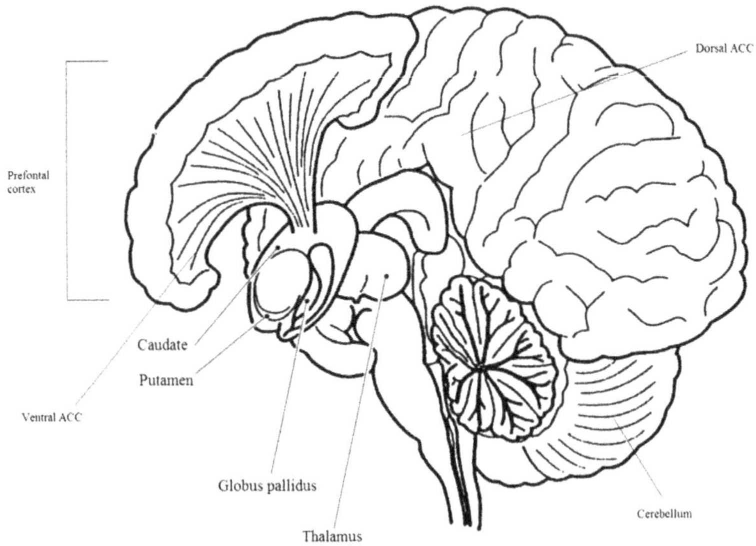

Figure 6.3. Cortical and subcortical brain areas.

In this chapter, we represent the PDH and the Cumulative and Emergent Automatic Deficit model of Fabio [22] (CEAD model) and propose a new theoretical framework of ADHD.

The underlying logic of the CEAD is that if basic processes are not well automatized, they will engage in a high cognitive load. Consequently, automatic deficits can lead to a deficit in controlled processes [22]. This could explain the ADHD symptoms.

Here, we propose that ADHD may be considered a disorder affecting the brain structures of the procedural system, in particular frontal/basal-ganglia circuits (especially the caudate), and therefore, a disorder overlapping but partially distinguished by cognitive functions.

In other words, we suggest that abnormalities of brain structures underlying procedural memory, largely documented in the ADHD population, can explain the core deficit of this disorder. In particular, we propose that abnormalities in the frontal/basal-ganglia circuits and the cerebellum can justify both controlled and automatic deficit in ADHD, because these networks rule both processes.

In addition to the executive dysfunctions [133–139], children and adults with ADHD can have procedural learning impairments, as shown by some previous studies. Also, there was found to be an automatic deficit in other disorders and disabilities, for example Rett Syndrome and autism [140–166].

In light of all the observations argued in this chapter, we suggest that brain abnormalities in the fronto-cerebellum network can lead to an impairment in the ability to 'automatize' behaviors, resulting in increased demands on attentional resources. This is manifested in the ADHD phenotype, in which individuals fail to resist interference or distractions, have need to excessive cognitive resources to perform a task. The abnormalities of brain structures subserving the procedural memory system can lead to difficulties with executive functioning ruled in this system, as well as problems with other functions that depend on these brain structures (fronto-cerebellum circuit).

In conclusion, given that the control of attention involves networks in cerebro-cortical and subcortical brain structures and these areas are impaired in ADHD, we state that ADHD is a disorder involving both executive and procedural impairments.

6.5 Discussion

In this chapter, we described the brain networks related to automatic and controlled processes and its relationship to ADHD. We presented a new theoretical framework for this disorder. Recent evidence from functional connectivity fMRI studies have demonstrated that functional abnormalities in ADHD not only affect isolated brain regions, but also the functional interregional interconnectivity between fronto-striatal, cingulate, fronto-parietal, temporoparietal and fronto-cerebellar networks [167].

As described in this chapter, these brain networks modulate both automatic and controlled processing, but in neuropsychological literature the hypothesis that children with ADHD fail to develop automatic processing is less consolidated.

Some studies [60–64] have shown that children with ADHD have deficits both in automatic and controlled processes.

In accordance with neuroimaging studies on the ADHD population [60–125], we suggest that abnormalities of fronto-striatal and fronto-cerebellar networks can be explained by automatic deficits in children with ADHD. Since these brain circuits modulate both automatic and controlled processes, these abnormalities may be one of the causes of the core deficits of ADHD, which in turn explains the controlled and automatic problems associated with this disorder. However, further research should be conducted to validate PDH in ADHD.

In light of the observations described in this chapter, conceptualizing EF as the sole account for the diverse range of deficits observed in ADHD may represent a partial prospective to view and study a complex disorder, such as ADHD.

6.6 Conclusion

In the present chapter, we propose that brain structures underlying procedural memory, a system that is critical for learning automatized skills, may apply to ADHD. This hypothesis is similar to the PHD of Ullman [126–132], but we add other factors.

First, in accordance with Ullman [127–132], since ADHD is comorbid with dyslexia and possibly SLI, these disorders may share etiological mechanisms. Second, like developmental disorders of reading and language, ADHD is also neurodevelopmental and thus a brain-based account could have substantial explanatory power. Third, in accordance with CEAD, if basic processes are not well automatized, subjects with ADHD should thus show deficits following aberrations to automatic processing. Finally, the ADHD population shows abnormalities in the fronto-cerebellum circuit, a brain network underlying both controlled and automatic processes.

In conclusion, we propose that automatic and controlled deficits in ADHD may be largely explained by abnormalities of brain structures underlying these processes, in particular, the frontal/cerebellum circuit. However, there is a need for more research to support this proposal.

In particular, future research on automatic deficits in ADHD is needed to improve understanding of the nature of the underlying impairments of ADHD. From a theoretical and clinical point of view, it is important to obtain a clearer picture on deficits in early bottom-up (automatic) and top-down (controlled) attention processes in ADHD.

References

[1] Greenhill L L, Posner K, Vaughan B S and Kratochvil C J 2008 Attention deficit hyperactivity disorder in preschool children *Child Adolesc. Psychiatr. Clin. N. Am.* **17** 347–66

[2] Kieling R and Rohde L A 2012 ADHD in children and adults: diagnosis and prognosis *Curr. Top. Behav. Neurosci.* **9** 1–16

[3] Thomas R, Sanders S, Doust J, Beller E and Glasziou P 2015 Prevalence of attention-deficit/hyperactivity disorder: a systematic review and meta-analysis *Pediatrics* **135** 994–1001

[4] Faraone S V, Asherson P, Banaschewski T, Biederman J, Buitelaar J K, Ramos-Quiroga J A, Rohde L A, Sonuga-Barke E J S, Tannock R and Franke B 2015 Attention-deficit/hyperactivity disorder *Nat. Rev. Dis. Prim.* **1** 150

[5] Biederman J *et al* 2006 Young adult outcome of attention deficit hyperactivity disorder: a controlled 10-year follow-up study *Psychol. Med.* **6** 167–79

[6] Asherson P, Buitelaar J, Faraone S V and Rohde L A 2016 Adult attention-deficit hyperactivity disorder: key conceptual issues *Lancet Psychiatry* **3** 568–78

[7] Faraone S V, Biederman J and Mick E 2006 The age-dependent decline of attention deficit hyperactivity disorder: a meta-analysis of follow-up studies *Psychol. Med.* **36** 159–65

[8] Biederman J, Mick E and Faraone S V *et al* 2002 Influence of gender on attention deficit hyperactivity disorder in children referred to a psychiatric clinic *Am. J. Psychiatry* **159** 36–42

[9] Cuffe S P, Moore C G and McKeown R E 2005 Prevalence and correlates of ADHD symptoms in the national health interview survey *J. Atten. Disord.* **9** 392–401

[10] American Psychiatric Association 2013 *Diagnostic and Statistical Manual of Mental Disorders* 5th ed (Arlington, VA: American Psychiatric Association)

[11] Willcutt E G, Doyle A E, Nigg J T, Faraone S V and Pennington B F 2005 Validity of the executive function theory of attention-deficit/hyperactivity disorder: a meta-analytic review *Biol. Psychiatry* **57** 1336–46

[12] Fabio R A and Caprì T 2017 The executive functions in a sample of Italian adults with ADHD: attention, response inhibition and planning/organization *Mediterr. J. Clin. Psychol.* **5** 1–17

[13] Boonstra A M, Kooij J, Oosterlaan J, Sergeant J A and Buitelaar J K 2010 To act or not to act, that's the problem: primarily inhibition difficulties in adult ADHD *Neuropsychology* **24** 209

[14] Kofman O, Larson J G and Mostofsky S H 2008 A novel task for examining strategic planning: evidence for impairment in children with ADHD *J. Clin. Exp. Neuropsychol.* **30** 261–71
[15] Schweitzer J B, Faber T L, Grafton S T, Tune L E, Hoffman J M and Kilts C D 2000 Alterations in the functional anatomy of working memory in adult attention deficit hyperactivity disorder *Am. J. Psychiat.* **157** 278–80
[16] Barkley R A 1997 Behavioral inhibition, sustained attention, and executive functions: constructing a unifying theory of ADHD *Psychol. Bull.* **121** 65
[17] Fabio R A and Caprì T 2015 Autobiographical memory in ADHD subtypes *J. Intellect. Dev. Disabil.* **40** 26–36
[18] Stark R, Bauer E, Merz C, Zimmermann M, Reuter M, Plichta M M and Vaitl D 2011 ADHD related behaviors are associated with brain activation in the reward system *Neuropsychologia* **49** 426–34
[19] Sonuga-Barke E J S and Fairchild G 2012 Neuroeconomics of attention-deficit/hyperactivity disorder: differential influences of medial, dorsal, and ventral prefrontal brain networks on suboptimal decision making? *Biol. Psychiatry* **72** 126–33
[20] Nigg J T 2013 Attention-deficit/hyperactivity disorder and adverse health outcomes *Clin. Psychol. Rev.* **33** 215–28
[21] Mohammadhasani N, Fardanesh H, Hatami J, Mozayani N and Fabio R A 2018 The pedagogical agent enhances mathematics learning in ADHD students *ITLT* **23** 2299–308
[22] Fabio R A 2017 The study of automatic and controlled processes in ADHD: a reread and a new proposal *Mediterr. J. Clin. Psychol.* **5** 1–8
[23] Martino G, Caprì T, Castriciano C and Fabio R A 2017 Automatic Deficits can lead to executive deficits in ADHD *Mediterr. J. Clin. Psychol.* **5** 1–32
[24] Fabio R A, Castriciano C and Rondanini A 2015 ADHD: auditory and visual stimuli in automatic and controlled processes *J. Atten. Disord.* **19** 771–8
[25] Adi-Japha E, Fox O and Karni A 2011 Atypical acquisition and atypical expression of memory consolidation gains in a motor skill in young female adults with ADHD *Res. Dev. Disabil.* **32** 1011–20
[26] Fox O, Adi-Japha E and Karni A 2014 The effect of a skipped dose (placebo) of methylphenidate on the learning and retention of a motor skill in adolescents with Attention Deficit Hyperactivity Disorder *Eur. Neuropsychopharmacol.* **24** 391–6
[27] Fox O, Adi-Japha E and Karni A 2016 Motor memory consolidation processes in young female adults with ADHD may be less susceptible to interference *Neurosci. Lett.* **637** 91–5
[28] Fox O, Karni A and Adi-Japha E 2016 The consolidation of a motor skill in young adults with ADHD: shorter practice can be better *Res. Dev. Disabil.* **51** 135–44
[29] Barnes K A, Howard J H, Howard D V, Kenealy L and Vaidya C J 2010 Two forms of implicit learning in childhood ADHD *Dev. Neuropsychol.* **35** 494–505
[30] Prehn-Kristensen A, Molzow I, Munz M, Wilhelm I, Müller K, Freytag D and Baving L 2011 Sleep restores daytime deficits in procedural memory in children with attention deficit/hyperactivity disorder *Res. Dev. Disabil.* **32** 2480–8
[31] Frank M J, Santamaria A, O'Reilly R C and Willcutt E 2007 Testing computational models of dopamine and noradrenaline dysfunction in attention deficit/hyperactivity disorder *Neuropsychopharmacol.* **32** 1583–99

[32] Huang-Pollock C L, Maddox W T and Tam H 2014 Rule-based and informationintegration perceptual category learning in children with attention-deficit/ hyperactivity disorder *Neuropsychology* **28** 594
[33] Laasonen M, Väre J, Oksanen-Hennah H, Leppämäki S, Tani P, Harno H and Cleeremans A 2014 Project DyAdd: implicit learning in adult dyslexia and ADHD *Ann. Dyslexia* **64** 1–33
[34] Rosas R, Ceric F, Tenorio M, Mourgues C, Thibaut C, Hurtado E and Aravena M T 2010 ADHD children outperform normal children in an artificial grammar implicit learning task: ERP and RT evidence *Conscious Cogn.* **19** 341–51
[35] Hurks P P M, Hendriksen J S H and Vles A C *et al* 2004 Verbal fluency over time as a measure of automatic and controlled processing in children with ADHD *Brain Cogn.* **55** 535–44
[36] Barkley R A 2002 International consensus statement on ADHD. Clinical child and family *Psychol. Rev.* **5** 89–111
[37] Barkley R A, Murphy K R and Fischer M 2008 Identifying new symptoms of ADHD in adulthood ed R A Barkley, K R Murphy and M Fischer *ADHD in Adults* pp 170–204 (New York: Guilford Press)
[38] Arnsten A F 2009 Toward a new understanding of attention-deficit hyperactivity disorder pathophysiology: an important role for prefrontal cortex dysfunction *CNS Drugs.* **23** 33–41
[39] Willcutt E G, Pennington B F, Boada R, Ogline J S, Tunick R A, Chhabildas N A and Olson R K 2001 A comparison of the cognitive deficits in reading disability and attention-deficit/hyperactivity disorder *J. Abnorm. Psychol.* **110** 157–72
[40] Kofler M J, Rapport M D, Bolden J and Altro T A 2008 Working memory as a core deficit in ADHD: preliminary findings and implications *ADHD Rep.* **16** 8–14
[41] Rapport M D, Chung K M, Shore G and Isaacs P 2001 A conceptual model of child psychopathology: implications for understanding attention-deficit/hyperactivity disorder (ADHD) and treatment efficacy *J. Clin. Child Psychol.* **30** 48–58
[42] Schreiber J E, Possin K L, Girard J M and Rey-Casserly R 2014 Executive function in children with attention deficit/hyperactivity disorder: the NIH examiner battery *J. Int. Neuropsychol. Soc.* **20** 41–51
[43] Doyle A E 2006 Executive functions in attention-deficit/hyperactivity disorder *J. Clin. Psychiat.* **67** 21–6
[44] Sagvolden T, Johansen E B, Aase H and Russell V A 2005 A dynamic developmental theory of attention-deficit/hyperactivity disorder (ADHD) predominantly *Behav. Brain Sci.* **28** 397–419
[45] Ziegler S *et al* 2016 Etiologic subtypes of attention-deficit/hyperactivity disorder: brain imaging, molecular genetic and environmental factors and the dopamine hypothesis *Neurosci. Biobehav. Rev.* **71** 633–56
[46] Shiffrin R M and Schneider W 1977 Controlled and automatic human information processing: II. Perceptual learning, automatic attending, and a general theory *Psychol. Rev.* **84** 1–66
[47] Schneider W and Chein J M 2003 Controlled & automatic processing: behavior, theory, and biological mechanisms *Cogn. Sci.* **27** 525–59
[48] Moors A and De Houwer J 2006 Automaticity: a theoretical and conceptual analysis *Psychol. Bull.* **132** 297–326

[49] Xu Y, Li Y, Ding W and Lu F 2014 Controlled versus automatic processes which is dominant to safety the moderating effect of inhibitory control *PLoS One* **9** 1–9
[50] Fabio R A 2009 *Relationship between automatic and controlled processes of attention and leading to complex thinking* (New York: Nova Science)
[51] Posner M I and Snyder C R R 1975 Attention and cognitive control ed R L Solso *Information Processing and Cognition: The Loyola Symposium* pp 55–85 (Hillsdale, NJ: Erlbaum)
[52] Pessoa L, Kastner S and Ungerleider L G 2003 Neuroimaging studies of attention: from modulation of sensory processing to top-down control *J. Neurosci.* **23** 3990–8
[53] Kiefer M 2012 Executive control over unconscious cognition: attentional sensitization of unconscious information processing *Front. Hum. Neurosci.* **6** 1–12
[54] Kiefer M 2007 Top down modulation of unconscious 'automatic' processes: a gating framework *Adv. Cogn. Psychol.* **3** 289–306
[55] Neumann O 1990 Direct parameter specification and the concept of perception *Psychol. Res.* **52** 207–15
[56] Naccache L, Blandin E and Dehaene S 2002 Unconscious masked priming depends on temporal attention *Psychol. Sci.* **13** 416–24
[57] Kiefer M and Martens U 2010 Attentional sensitization of unconscious cognition: task sets modulate subsequent masked semantic priming *J. Exp. Psychol. Gen.* **139** 464–89
[58] Fabio R A and Towey G E 2018 Long-term meditation: the relationship between cognitive processes, thinking styles and mindfulness *Cogn. Process* **19** 73–85
[59] Dehaene S and Naccache L 2001 Towards a cognitive neuroscience of consciousness: basic evidence and a workspace framework *Cognition* **79** 1–37
[60] Ackerman P T, Anhalt J M, Holcomb P J and Dykman R A 1986 Presumably innate and acquired automatic processes reading problems *J. Child Psychol. Psychiatry* **27** 513–29
[61] Borcherding B, Thompson K, Kruesi M, Bartko J J, Rapoport J and Weingartener H 1988 Automatic and effortful processing in attention deficit/hyperactivity disorder *J. Abnorm. Child Psychol.* **16** 333–45
[62] Ott D A and Lyman R D 1993 Automatic and effortful memory in children exhibiting attention-deficit hyperactivity disorder *J. Clin. Child Psychol.* **22** 420–7
[63] Hazell P L, Carr V J, Lewin T J, Dewis S A M, Heathcote D M and Brucki B M 1999 Effortful and automatic information processing in boys with ADHD and specific learning disorders *J. Child Psychol. Psychiatry* **2** 275–86
[64] Hurks P P M, Hendriksen J G M, Vles J S H, Kalff A C, Feron F J M, Kroes M and Jolles J 2004 Verbal fluency over time as a measure of automatic and controlled processing in children with ADHD *Brain Cogn.* **55** 535–44
[65] Merril E D 1992 Attentional resource demands of stimulus encoding for persons with and without mental retardation *Am. J. Ment. Retard.* **97** 87–98
[66] Cortese S, Kelly C, Chabernaud C, Proal E, Di Martino A, Milham M P and Castellanos F X 2012 Toward systems neuroscience of ADHD: a meta-analysis of 55 fMRI studies *Am. J. Psychiatry* **169** 1038–55
[67] Greven C U *et al* 2015 Developmentally stable whole-brain volume reductions and developmentally sensitive caudate and putamen volume alterations in those with attention-deficit/hyperactivity disorder and their unaffected siblings *J. Am. Psychiatry* **72** 490–9
[68] Onnink A M, Zwiers M P and Hoogman M 2015 Deviant white matter structure in adults with attention-deficit/hyperactivity disorder points to aberrant myelination and affects neuropsychological performance *Prog. Neuropsychopharmacol. Biol. Psychiatry* **63** 14–22

[69] Shaw P, Malek M, Watson B, Sharp W, Evans E and Greenstein D 2012 Development of cortical surface area and gyrification in attention-deficit/hyperactivity disorder *Biol. Psychiatry* **72** 191–7
[70] van Ewijk H, Heslenfeld D J, Zwiers M P, Buitelaar J K and Oosterlaan J 2012 Diffusion tensor imaging in attention deficit/hyperactivity disorder: a systematic review and meta-analysis *Neurosci. Biobehav. Rev.* **36** 1093–106
[71] van Ewijk H, Heslenfeld D J, Zwiers M P, Faraone S V, Luman M, Hartman C A, Hoekstra P J, Franke B, Buitelaar J K and Oosterlaan J 2014 Different mechanisms of white matter abnormalities in attention-deficit/hyperactivity disorder: a diffusion tensor imaging study *J. Am. Acad. Child Adolesc. Psychiatry* **53** 790–9
[72] Mostert J C *et al* 2016 Characterising resting-state functional connectivity in a large sample of adults with ADHD *Prog. Neuropsychopharmacol. Biol. Psychiatry* **67** 82–91
[73] Castellanos F X *et al* 2002 Developmental trajectories of brain volume abnormalities in children and adolescents with attention-deficit/hyperactivity disorder *JAMA* **288** 1740–8
[74] Valera E M, Faraone S V, Murray K E and Seidman L J 2007 Meta-analysis of structural imaging findings in attention-deficit/hyperactivity disorder *Biol. Psychiatry* **61** 1361–9
[75] Ellison-Wright I, Ellison-Wright Z and Bullmore E 2008 Structural brain change in Attention Deficit Hyperactivity Disorder identified by meta-analysis *BMC Psychiatry* **8** 51
[76] Frodl T and Skokauskas N 2012 Meta-analysis of structural MRI studies in children and adults with attention deficit hyperactivity disorder indicates treatment effects *Acta Psychiatr. Scand.* **125** 114–26
[77] Nakao T, Radua J, Rubia K and Mataix-Cols D 2011 Gray matter volume abnormalities in ADHD: voxel-based meta-analysis exploring the effects of age and stimulant medication *Am. J. Psychiatry* **168** 1154–63
[78] Norman L J, Carlisi C, Lukito S, Hart H, Mataix-Cols D, Radua J and Rubia K 2016 Structural and functional brain abnormalities in attention-deficit/hyperactivity disorder and obsessive-compulsive disorder: a comparative meta-analysis *JAMA Psychiatry* **73** 815–25
[79] Bralten J *et al* 2015 Voxel-basedmorphometry analysis reveals frontal brain differences in participants withADHD and their unaffected siblings *J. Psychiatry Neurosci.* **4** 140–377
[80] Castellanos F X *et al* 2008 Cingulate-precuneus interactions: a new locus of dysfunction in adult attention-deficit/hyperactivity disorder *Biol. Psychiatry* **63** 332–7
[81] Cubillo A, Halari R, Giampietro V, Taylor E and Rubia K 2011 Fronto-striatal under-activation during interference inhibition and attention allocation in grown up children with attention deficit/hyperactivity disorder and persistent symptoms *Psychiatry Res.* **30** 17–27
[82] Dickstein S G, Bannon K, Castellanos F X and Milham M P 2006 The neural correlates of attention deficit hyperactivity disorder: an ALE meta-analysis *J. Child Psychol. Psychiatry* **47** 1051–62
[83] Karch S, Voelker J M, Thalmeier T, Ertl M, Leicht G, Pogarell O and Mulert C 2014 Deficits during voluntary selection in adult patients with ADHD: new insights from single-trial coupling of simultaneous EEG/fMRI *Front. Psychiatry* **22** 41
[84] Hoogman M *et al* 2017 Subcortical brain volume differences in participants with attention deficit hyperactivity disorder in children and adults: a cross-sectional mega-analysis *Lancet Psychiatry* **4** 310–9
[85] Hart H, Radua J, Nakao T, Mataix-Cols D and Rubia K 2013 Meta-analysis of functional magnetic resonance imaging studies of inhibition and attention in attention-deficit/

hyperactivity disorder: exploring task-specific, stimulant medication, and age effects *JAMA Psychiatry* **70** 185–98

[86] Batty M J, Liddle E B, Pitiot A, Toro R, Groom M J, Scerif G, Liotti M, Liddle P F, Paus T and Hollis C 2010 Cortical gray matter in attention-deficit/hyperactivity disorder: a structural magnetic resonance imaging study *J. Am. Acad. Child Adolesc. Psychiatry* **49** 229–38

[87] Cao Q J, Zang Y F, Sun L, Sui M, Long X, Zou Q and Wang Y 2006 Abnormal neural activity in children with attention deficit hyperactivity disorder: a resting-state functional magnetic resonance imaging study *Neuro Report* **17** 1033–6

[88] Cao X, Cao Q, Long X, Sun L, Sui M, Zhu C, Zuo X, Zang Y and Wang Y 2009 Abnormal restingstate functional connectivity patterns of the putamen in medication-naive children with attention deficit hyperactivity disorder *Brain Res.* **1303** 195–206

[89] Carmona S *et al* 2005 Global and regional gray matter reductions in ADHD: a voxel-based morphometric study *Neurosci. Lett.* **389** 88–93

[90] Carmona S *et al* 2009 Ventro-striatal reductions underpin symptoms of hyperactivity and impulsivity in attention-deficit/hyperactivity disorder *Biol. Psychiatry* **66** 972–7

[91] Davenport N D, Karatekin C, White T and Lim K O 2010 Differential fractional anisotropy abnormalities in adolescents with ADHD or schizophrenia *Psychiatry Res.* **181** 193–8

[92] Konrad A, Dielentheis T F, El Masri D, Bayerl M, Fehr C, Gesierich T, Vucurevic G, Stoeter P and Winterer G 2010 Disturbed structural connectivity is related to inattention and impulsivity in adult attention deficit hyperactivity disorder *Eur. J. Neurosci.* **31** 912–9

[93] Konrad K, Neufang S, Hanisch C, Fink G R and Herpertz Dahlmann B 2006 Dysfunctional attentional networks in children with attention deficit/hyperactivity disorder: evidence from an event-related functional magnetic resonance imaging study *Biol. Psychiatry* **59** 643–51

[94] Konrad K and Eickhoff S B 2010 Is the ADHD brain wired differently? A review on structural and functional connectivity in attention deficit hyperactivity disorder *Hum. Brain Mapping* **31** 904–16

[95] Krain A L and Castellanos F X 2006 Brain development and ADHD *Clin. Psychol. Rev.* **26** 433–44

[96] Salmi J, Salmela V, Salo E, Mikkola K, Leppämäki S, Tani P, Hokkanen L, Laasonen M, Numminen J and Alho K 2018 Out of focus—Brain attention control deficits in adult ADHD *Brain Res.* **1692** 12–22

[97] Rosch K S, Crocetti D, Hirabayashi K, Denckla M B, Mostofsky S H and Mahone E M 2018 Reduced subcortical volumes among preschool-age girls and boys with ADHD Psychiatry *Res. Neuroimaging* **271** 67–74

[98] Norman L *et al* 2018 Fronto-striatal dysfunction during decision-making in attention-deficit/hyperactivity disorder and obsessive-compulsive disorder *Biol. Psychiatry Cogn. Neurosci. Neuroimaging* **3** 694–703

[99] Jacobson L A, Crocetti D, Dirlikov B, Slifer K, Denckla M B, Mostofsky S H and Mahone E M 2018 Anomalous brain development is evident in preschoolers with attention-deficit/hyperactivity disorder *J. Int. Neuropsychol. Soc.* **24** 531–9

[100] Ueda S, Ota T, Iida J, Yamamuro K, Yoshino H, Kishimoto N and Kishimoto T 2018 Reduced prefrontal hemodynamic response in adult attention-deficit hyperactivity disorder as measured by near-infrared spectroscopy *Psychiatry Clin. Neurosci.* **72** 380–90

[101] Salavert J *et al* 2018 Functional Imaging Changes in the Medial Prefrontal Cortex in Adult ADHD *J. Atten. Disord.* **22** 679–93

[102] Al-Amin M, Artyom Z and Thomas G 2018 Hippocampal subfield volume changes in subtypes of attention deficit hyperactivity disorder *Brain Res.* **1685** 1–8

[103] Douglas P K *et al* 2018 Hemispheric brain asymmetry differences in youths with attention-deficit/hyperactivity disorder *Neuroimage Clin.* **24** 744–52

[104] Hoogman M *et al* 2017 Subcortical brain volume differences in participants with attention deficit hyperactivity disorder in children and adults: a cross-sectional mega-analysis *Lancet Psychiatry* **4** 310–19

[105] Ivanov I *et al* 2010 Morphological abnormalities of the thalamus in youths with attention deficit hyperactivity disorder *Am. J. Psychiatry* **167** 397–408

[106] Narr K L, Woods R P, Lin J, Kim J, Phillips O R, Del'Homme M, Caplan R, Toga A W, McCracken J T and Levitt J G 2009 Widespread cortical thinning is a robust anatomical marker for attention-deficit/hyperactivity disorder *J. Am. Acad. Child. Adolesc. Psychiatry* **48** 1014–22

[107] Valera E M, Faraone S V, Murray K E and Seidman L J 2007 Meta-analysis of structural imaging findings in attention-deficit/hyperactivity disorder *Biol. Psychiatry* **61** 1361–9

[108] Pliszka S R, Glahn D C, Semrud-Clikeman M, Franklin C, Perez R, Xiong J and Liotti M 2006 Neuroimaging of inhibitory control areas in children with attention deficit hyperactivity disorder who were treatment naive or in long-term treatment *Am. J. Psychiatry* **163** 1052–60

[109] Durston S, Hulshoff Pol H E, Schnack H G, Buitelaar J K, Steenhuis M P, Minderaa R B, Kahn R S and van Engeland H 2004 Magnetic resonance imaging of boys with attention-deficit/hyperactivity disorder and their unaffected siblings *J. Am. Acad. Child Adolesc. Psychiatry* **43** 332–40

[110] Sowell E R, Thompson P M, Welcome S E, Henkenius A L, Toga A W and Peterson B S 2003 Cortical abnormalities in children and adolescents with attention-deficit hyperactivity disorder *Lancet* **362** 1699–707

[111] Castellanos F X *et al* 2002 Developmental trajectories of brain volume abnormalities in children and adolescents with attention-deficit/hyperactivity disorder *JAMA* **288** 1740–8

[112] Mostofsky S H, Cooper K L, Kates W R, Denckla M B and Kaufmann W E 2002 Smaller prefrontal and premotor volumes in boys with attention-deficit/hyperactivity disorder *Biol. Psychiatry* **52** 785–94

[113] Dibbets P, Evers L, Hurks P, Marchetta N and Jolles J 2009 Differences in feedback- and inhibition-related neural activity in adult ADHD *Brain Cogn.* **70** 73–83

[114] Dibbets P, Evers E A, Hurks P P, Bakker K and Jolles J 2010 Differential brain activation patterns in adult attention-deficit hyperactivity disorder (ADHD) associated with task switching *Neuropsychology* **24** 413–23

[115] Frodl T *et al* 2009 Amygdala reduction in patients with ADHD compared with major depression and healthy volunteers *Acta Psychiatr. Scand.* **121** 111–8

[116] Rubia K, Halari R, Christakou A and Taylor E 2009a Impulsiveness as a timing disturbance: neurocognitive abnormalities in attention-deficit hyperactivity disorder during temporal processes and normalization with methylphenidate *Philos. Trans. R. Soc. Lond. B Biol. Sci.* **364** 1919–31

[117] Rubia K, Halari R, Smith A, Mohammad M, Scott S and Brammer M 2009b Shared and disorder-specific prefrontal abnormalities in boys with pure attention-deficit/hyperactivity

disorder compared to boys with pure CD during interference inhibition and attention allocation *J. Child Psychol. Psychiatry* **50** 669–78
[118] Rubia K, Smith A, Halari R, Matsukura F, Mohammad M, Taylor E and Brammer M J 2009c Disorder-specific dissociation of orbitofrontal dysfunction in boys with pure conduct disorder during reward and ventrolateral prefrontal dysfunction in boys with pure attention-deficit/hyperactivity disorder during sustained attention *Am. J. Psychiatry* **166** 83–94
[119] Posner J, Park C and Wang Z 2014 Connecting the dots: a review of resting connectivity MRI studies in attention-deficit/hyperactivity disorder *Neuropsychol. Rev.* **24** 3–15
[120] Salmi J, Rinne T, Koistinen S, Salonen O and Alho K 2009 Brain networks ofbottom-up triggered and top-down controlled shifting of auditory attention *Brain Res.* **1286** 155–64
[121] Salmi J, Salmela V, Salo E, Mikkola K, Leppamaki S, Tani P, Hokkanen L, Laasonen M, Numminen J and Alho K 2018 Out of focus – brain attention control deficits in adults ADHD *Brain Res.* **1692** 12–22
[122] Cao M, Shu N, Cao Q, Wang Y and He Y 2014 Imaging functional and structuralbrain connectomics in attention-deficit/hyperactivity disorder *Mol. Neurobiol.* **50** 1111–23
[123] Castellanos F X and Proal E 2012 Large-scale brain systems in ADHD: beyond the prefrontal-striatal model *Trends Cogn. Sci.* **16** 17–26
[124] Rubia K, Alegria A A and Brinson H 2014 Brain abnormalities in attention-deficit hyperactivity disorder: a review *Rev. Neurol.* **58** S3–16
[125] Salmela V, Salo E, Salmi J and Alho K 2018 Spatiotemporal dynamics of attention networks as revealed by representational similarity analysis of EEG and fMRI data *Cereb. Cortex* **28** 549–60
[126] Nicolson R I and Fawcett A J 2007 Procedural learning difficulties: reuniting the developmental disorders? *Trends Neurosci.* **30** 135–41
[127] Ullman M 2016 The declarative/procedural model: a neurobiological model of language learning, knowledge, and use *Neurobiology of Language* ed G Hickok and G A Small (Amsterdam: Elsevier) 953–68
[128] Ullman M T 2004 Contributions of memory circuits to language: the declarative/procedural model *Cognition* **92** 231–70
[129] Ullman M T 2015 The declarative/procedural model: a neurobiologically motivated theory of first and second language *Theories in Second Language Acquisition* ed B Van Patten and J Williams (London: Routledge) 135–58
[130] Ullman M T and Pierpont E I 2005 Specific language impairment is not specific to language: the procedural deficit hypothesis *Cortex* **41** 399–433
[131] Ullman M T and Pullman M Y 2015 A compensatory role for declarative memory in neurodevelopmental disorders *Neurosci. Biobehav. Rev.* **51** 205–22
[132] Ullman M T, Pullman M, Lovelett J T, Pierpont E I and Turkeltaub P E 2017 The neuroanatomy of specific language impairment *Annu. Rev. Psychol.*
[133] Fabio R A, Caprì T, Mohammadhasani N, Gangemi A, Gagliano A and Martino G 2018 Frequency bands in seeing and remembering: comparing ADHD and typically developing children *Neuropsychol Trends* **24** 97–116
[134] Mohammadhasani N, Fabio R A, Fardanesh H and Hatami J 2015 The link between visual attention and memory in ADHD and normally developing students: seeing is remembering? *Reti, Saperi e Linguaggi Ita J. Cogn. Sci.* **1** 89–102
[135] Sempio O L, Fabio R A, Tiezzi P and Cedro C 2016 Parental and teachers attachment in children at risk of ADHD and with ADHD *Life Span Disabil.* **19** 57–77

[136] Fabio R A and Urso M 2014 The analysis of attention network in ADHD, attention problems and typically developing subjects *Life Span Disabil.* **17** 199–221

[137] Fabio R A and Antonietti A 2012 Effects of hypermedia instruction on declarative, conditional and procedural knowledge in ADHD students *Res. Dev. Disabil.* **33** 2028–39

[138] Antonietti A, Monnier A S, Gatti E and Fabio R A 2010 Emotional and relational processes in pre-adolescents with attentional deficits: an attempt to test some psychodynamic hypotheses *Psicol. Clin. dello Svilupp* **14** 359–78

[139] Fabio R A, Piran S G and Antonietti A 2005 Vigilanza uditiva nei soggetti normali e con deficit di attenzione *Psicol. Clin. dello Svilupp.* **9** 151–7

[140] Fabio R A, Gangemi A, Capri T, Budden S and Falzone A 2018 Neurophysiological and cognitive effects of Transcranial Direct Current Stimulation in three girls with Rett Syndrome with chronic language impairments *Res. Dev. Disabil.* **76** 76–87

[141] Fabio R A, Caprì T, Lotan M, Towey G E and Martino G 2018 Motor abilities are related to the specific genotype in Rett Syndrome ed K V Urbano *Advances in Genetics Research* vol 18 (New York: Nova Science)

[142] Fabio R A, Magaudda C, Caprì T, Towey G E and Martino G 2018 Choice behavior in Rett Syndrome: the consistency parameter *Life Span Disabil.* **21** 47–62

[143] Gangemi A, Caprì T, Fabio R A, Puggioni P, Falzone A M and Martino G 2018 Transcranial Direct Current Stimulation (tDCS) and Cognitive Empowerment for the functional recovery of diseases with chronic impairment and genetic etiopathogenesis ed K V Urbano *Advances in Research* vol 18 (New York: Nova Science)

[144] Fabio R A, Billeci L, Crifaci G, Troise E, Tortorella G and Pioggia G 2016 Cognitive training modifies frequency EEG bands and neuropsychological measures in Rett syndrome *Res. Dev. Disabil.* **54** 73–85

[145] Fabio R A, Gullà I and Errante R 2015 Emotions and eye movements: eye tracker and mnestic parameters *Memory Consolidation* 235–58

[146] Falzone A, Gangemi G and Fabio R A 2015 Genotype-phenotype relationships in language processes in rett syndrome ed K V Urbano *Advances in Research* vol 14 pp 153–70 (New York: Nova Science)

[147] Fabio R A, Colombo B, Russo S, Cogliati F, Masciadri M, Foglia S, Antonietti A and Tavian D 2014 Recent insights into genotype-phenotype relationships in patients with Rett syndrome using a fine grain scale *Res. Dev. Disabilities* **35** 2976–86

[148] Fabio R A, Castelli I, Marchetti A and Antonietti A 2013 Training communication abilities in Rett syndrome through reading and writing *Front. Psychol.* **4** 9–11

[149] Castelli I, Antonietti A, Fabio R A, Lucchini B and Marchetti A 2013 Do Rett syndrome persons possess theory of mind? Some evidence from not-treated girls *Life Span Disabil.* **16** 157–68

[150] Fabio R A, Giannatiempo S, Oliva P and Murdaca A M 2011 The increase of attention in Rett syndrome: a pre-test/post-test research design *J. Dev. Physic. Disabil.* **23** 99–111

[151] Vignoli A, Fabio R A, La Briola F, Giannatiempo S, Antonietti A, Maggiolini S and Canevini M P 2010 Correlations between neurophysiological, behavioral, and cognitive function in Rett syndrome *Epilepsy Behav.* **17** 489–96

[152] Fabio R A, Antonietti A, Castelli I and Marchetti A 2009 Attention and communication in Rett Syndrome *Res. Autism Spectr. Disord.* **3** 329–35

[153] Fabio R A, Giannatiempo S, Antonietti A and Budden S 2009 The role of stereotypies in overselectivity process in Rett syndrome *Res. Dev. Disabil.* **30** 136–45

[154] Ciccocioppi L and Fabio R A 2013 Improvement of cognitive processes through yoga practice *Psychot. Psychos.* **82** 19–20

[155] Brivitello U, Nucera S, Fabio R A and Plebe A 2016 The sweet smell of altruism. Correlations between smells and prosocial behavior. A short review *Reti, Saperi e Linguaggi Ita J. Cogn. Sci.* **3** 301–16

[156] Fabio R A 2012 Cognitive skills enhancement in intellectual disability *Intel. Disabil. Manag. Caus. Social Percep.* 147–66

[157] Fabio R A 2012 Emerging trends of research on new technologies on cognitive skills enhancement in intellectual disability *Intel. Disabil. Manag. Caus. Social Percep.* 167–70

[158] Fabio R A, Oliva P and Murdaca A M 2011 Systematic and emotional contents in over selectivity processes in autism *Res. Autism Spectr. Disord.* **5** 575–83

[159] Martino G, Catalano A, Bellone F, Sardella A, Lasco C, Capri T, Langher V, Caputo A, Fabio R A and Morabito N 2018 Vitamin D status is associated with anxiety levels in postmenopausal women evaluated for osteoporosis *Mediterr. J. Clin. Psychol.* **6** 1–16

[160] Fabio R A and Towey G E 2018 Cognitive and personality factors in the regular practice of martial arts *J. Sports Med. Phys. Fitness* **58** 933–43

[161] Fabio R A, Caprì T, Campana R and Buzzai C 2018 The construction and validation of an Italian Dsyfunctional Beliefs Questionnaire *Curr. Psychol.* **1** 1–10

[162] Fabio R A 2007 New directions in psychological intelligence tests: the dynamic measures *Psychological Tests and Testing Research Trends* ed P M Goldfarb (New York: Nova Science) pp 1–5

[163] Fabio R A 2007 Gifted with dynamic intelligence test measures and normal with static intelligence test measures: what does it mean? *Psychological Tests and Testing Research Trends* ed P M Goldfarb (New York: Nova Science) pp 83–111

[164] Fabio R A 2005 Dynamic assessment of intelligence is a better reply to adaptive behavior and cognitive plasticity *J. Gen. Psychol.* **132** 41–66

[165] Fabio R A, Martinazzoli C and Antonietti A 2005 Development and standardization of the 'R.A.R.S.' (Rett Assessment Rating Scale) *Life Span Disab.* **8** 257–81

[166] Fabio R A, Caprì T, Nucita A, Iannizzotto G and Mohammadhasani N 2018 Eye gaze digital games to improve motivational and attentional ability in Rett Syndrome *J. Spe. Educ. Rehab.* **19** 105–26

[167] Cocchi L, Bramati I E, Zalesky A, Furukawa E, Fontenelle L F, Moll J, Tripp G and Mattos P 2012 Altered functional brain connectivity in a non-clinical sample of young adults with attention-deficit/hyperactivity disorder *J. Neurosci.* **32** 17753–61

IOP Publishing

Neurological Disorders and Imaging Physics, Volume 4
Application to attention deficit hyperactivity disorder
Ayman El-Baz and Jasjit S Suri

Chapter 7

Attention deficit and hyperactivity disorder (ADHD) and criminal behavior: a criminological viewpoint

Marc Ruffinengo and Anthony Walsh

7.1 Introduction

Attention deficit and hyperactivity disorder (ADHD) is one of the most well-known as well as the most frequently diagnosed mental and behavioral issues that is found in children from a young age through adolescence [1]. Although children have been known to be rambunctious for some time, it was not until the second half of the 20th century that academia began to pay attention to the details of the symptoms and behaviors of children who seemed to be more energetic and inattentive than what is considered normal for a youth or adolescent. Until the 1980s these constellations of symptoms that we now know as ADHD were often referred to as hyperactivity or hyperkinesis. Nevertheless, according to Curatolo *et al* [2] there is evidence of attempts characterize the grouping of symptoms of what we now know as ADHD in children over 100 years ago, meaning that awareness of the condition has existed for some time. These terms are a description of one of the more well-known symptoms of ADHD, which is restless, but not involuntary, movements [3]. However, the symptoms of the disorder are not completely static as restless movements often diminish as a child progresses through adolescence. Some other features of disorder, such as a diminished capacity to complete longitudinal tasks, often persist throughout the life-course for up to 50% of patients, however [4].

ADHD can manifest in a variety of ways along a spectrum of severity. Although children are often hyperactive and inattentive, ADHD is typically considered when these behaviors are present and more severe than what would be considered normal for individuals at a similar age or developmental step. The most recent conceptions of the disorder according to the *Diagnostic and Statistical Manual of Mental Disorders* (DSM-V) describe the disorder as one that begins in childhood but often persists into adulthood. Those afflicted have behavioral issues that can cause

doi:10.1088/978-0-7503-1822-8ch7

difficulty at work, school, and in social settings. There are two broad categories of symptoms from which those 17 and over must present with five, and those under 17 must present with six symptoms from the two categories. The categories are inattentiveness and hyperactivity/impulsivity [5].

Although the prevalence of ADHD is not completely known, the most widely cited estimates place the prevalence at 10% or less of the population of children. According to the DSM-V the prevalence of ADHD in children is around 5% [5]. The prevalence of the disorder varies widely across nations with the United States showing a higher diagnosed prevalence than European nations. Within the United States there are regional variations in distribution as well, with prevalence lower in the western United States than in other parts of the country. Furthermore, prevalence appears to be on the increase since the 1990s. The 5% figure in the DSM-V is typically on the low-end of various estimates of prevalence. Some estimates place the prevalence over 10% [6]. Others place the estimate at between 5%–10% [7]. Regardless, the disorder is commonly diagnosed in children and adolescents worldwide. Variations in the severity of the disorder as well as inconsistencies in diagnostic criteria across medical practitioners may contribute to the variations in prevalence [3].

ADHD is also one of the most highly heritable behavioral disorders as well with most heritability estimates falling above 0.70. Furthermore, there is typically high concordance between monozygotic twins as opposed to dizygotic twins [8, 9]. This would indicate that genetics play a crucial role in ADHD although the specific etiology is not well understood. More near causes of specific ADHD behaviors are linked to specific neurotransmitters, in particular dopamine, norepinephrine, and serotonin, but it is the underlying relationship between genes and neurotransmitter functioning that is of particular interest going forward [1]. However, the role of the environment in shaping ADHD should not be minimized or underestimated as even with high heritability this leaves room for significant variation that is explained by environmental conditions.

Treatment for ADHD has been largely pharmacological over the years. Early treatments involved methylphenidate-based stimulants that increase available dopamine via reuptake inhibition. Atomoxetine, which increases norepinephrine via reuptake inhibition also has been available for some time as well. Promising physical interventions such as repetitive transcranial magnetic stimulation (rTMS), which involves the use of magnetic fields in a noninvasive manner to promote alterations in cortical functioning, are now available as well. Pharmacological interventions remain the standard treatment for ADHD, however [10].

Despite the uncertainty about the exact etiology, precise prevalence, as well as diagnostic inconsistency, the disorder has long been linked to criminal behavior as well as other detrimental life outcomes. In fact, ADHD is one of the most durable correlates of antisocial and criminal behavior. A wide array of the extant literature using wildly inconsistent methodologies have found positive relationships between ADHD, as well as various symptoms of ADHD prior to the disorder being more consistently classified starting in the 1980s, and various measures of offending. It has been linked to antisocial behavior in late adolescence and adulthood [11]. It has also been linked to delinquency in teenagers in a follow up study of children who were diagnosed as being hyperactive [12]. There were also early recognized positive associations with recidivism as well [13]. Findings such as these have remained consistent in the literature over the subsequent decades [14].

7.2 Definitions, presentation, and co-morbidity

As mentioned previously, ADHD can vary widely in the quantity and severity of symptoms and many children and adolescents exhibit symptoms without qualifying for a diagnosis of ADHD. According to the DSM-V, symptoms generally fall into two broad categories of inattentiveness related symptoms and hyperactivity and impulsivity related symptoms. Based on the observed constellation of symptoms in each individual case the presentation of the disorder is described as falling into one of three-categories: *Predominantly inattentive, predominantly hyperactive and impulsive, and combined* [5]. Furthermore, ADHD is often co-morbid with other disorders such as oppositional defiant disorder (ODD) and conduct disorder (CD). These associations are of particular interest in criminology as there is strong evidence that ADHD that is co-morbid with other disorders is more strongly linked with various delinquency and offending measures than ADHD alone [15, 16].

7.2.1 Definitions

The DSM-V [5] describes the symptoms (paraphrased here) of ADHD as oriented on inattention:

1. Often fails to give attention to detail and makes mistakes.
2. Has trouble focusing on one task for a significant period of time.
3. Has trouble listening.
4. Does not follow instructions or fails to complete tasks.
5. Has issues with organization.
6. Does not seem interested in tasks that involve a long period of time.
7. Frequently misplaces important items.
8. Frequently and easily distracted.
9. Frequently forgetful.

And oriented on hyperactivity and impulsivity:

1. Frequently moves hands or feet or cannot sit still.
2. Frequently moves around or leaves seat.
3. Runs or climbs in inappropriate situations.
4. Has trouble participating in activities quietly.
5. Described as frequently ‘on the go’ with excessive energy.
6. Talks excessively.
7. Blurts out answers to incomplete questions.
8. Difficulty waiting for one’s turn.
9. Interrupts or intrudes on others.

Children up to 16 must have six symptoms from each category, while adolescents and adults 17 and up must have five symptoms. It is possible to have the requisite number of symptoms from one category but not the other. This would describe whether the presentation is *Predominantly inattentive, predominantly hyperactive and impulsive, or combined* [5]. Additionally, as ADHD is considered a childhood disorder that persists into adulthood, it is also required that at least some symptoms were present prior to age 12. The symptoms should also be present in multiple settings such as work/school and home. Lastly, the symptoms should clearly interfere with normal functioning and should not be indicative of or explained more thoroughly by any other mental disorder [5].

7.2.2 Presentation

The distribution of symptoms in an individual will also typically place ADHD into one of the three aforementioned categories. The majority of diagnosed cases fall into the combined presentation of the disorder indicating that most individuals display some inattentiveness as well as hyperactivity/impulsivity [1]. While many, if not most, children will display one or several of these symptoms in varying intensity over the course of their childhood and even into adulthood, it is the polysymptomatic and persistent nature of the disorder that differentiates those presenting with the disorder from children who are occasionally inattentive, hyperactive and/or impulsive. In popular discourse it is not uncommon to come across the perception that the symptoms are rather similar to what is considered common and thus appropriate childhood behavior. There is evidence that children who do not fully meet the ADHD diagnostic criteria are treated with stimulants nevertheless, potentially being enumerated as having the disorder. Furthermore, there is evidence that the condition is overdiagnosed generally, but it is less clear what the implications of this are [17].

7.2.3 Co-morbidity

While ADHD can be co-morbid with a variety of other disorders, it is of particular interest in criminology when ADHD is co-morbid with oppositional defiant disorder (ODD) and conduct disorder (CD). As mentioned previously, there is evidence that the presentation of ADHD and co-morbidity with either ODD or CD increases the risk of antisocial behavior [1, 16].

7.2.3.1 Oppositional defiant disorder (ODD)

The DSM-V [5] describes ODD as a pattern of excessive anger, irritability, vindictiveness, and argumentative behavior. While children, again, frequently display these behaviors to some degree during normal developmental processes, the differences lie in the intensity, distribution across settings, and duration of the behaviors. The spectrum of severity ranges from mild to severe and is determined by whether symptoms manifest in one or several settings such as home, work, school, peer groups, and the like [5]. According to Loeber and Burke [18] ADHD is often co-morbid with ODD. ODD is also frequently co-morbid with CD and often precedes that disorder [19]. The linkage between ODD and CD is strong although the majority of children with ODD will not progress into CD [20]. Nevertheless, youths with CD are much more likely to either have or have had ODD. A suggested developmental pathway has ADHD leading to ODD and subsequently to CD and antisocial personality disorder [18]. It should be stressed however, that such a progression is probabilistic as many children will have been diagnosed as having ADHD or ODD/CD but not progress along that pathway.

7.2.3.2 Conduct disorder (CD)

CD is described by the DSM-V [5] as repetitive and persistent behaviors in which the rights of others and various norms, laws, or rules are violated. A diagnosis is made when an individual exhibits at least three of 15 behaviors over the previous 12 months. The behaviors fall into categories of: aggression to people and/or animals, lying and/or theft, destruction of property, and serious rule violations. Furthermore, the behaviors should cause significant impairment in regular social/occupational/academic functioning. Like ODD, the severity occurs across a spectrum [5].

CD and ODD are related in that ODD typically manifests earlier, and individuals with CD often have ODD. This overlap occurs in as much as 60%–96% of cases of CD [21, 22]. While some have speculated that ODD may actually be an earlier, milder, or age-specific manifestation of CD [23], others point out that despite the similarities and the fact that genetic associations indicate a related origin, there is insufficient evidence to show that they are in fact age-specific manifestations of the same disorder or that one is merely a less severe form of the other [24]. Nevertheless, there is no dispute that these disorders are related even if specific mechanisms are not completely understood.

Of particular interest in criminology is the co-morbidity of ADHD and CD. Lynam's [25, p 209] statement that the presentation of ADHD and CD is 'fledgling psychopathy' has received further attention as this intersection of disorders is recognized as particularly problematic in criminology. Psychopathic personality traits are more common in individuals presenting with ADHD and CD when compared to individuals with either of those conditions by themselves. Moffitt [26] labeled these individuals as life-course persistent offenders, terminology that is well-known in criminology without specifically referring to ADHD or CD. Thrill-seeking and impulsiveness were found to be the factors that were most associated with overall delinquency and violent behavior [27].

There is also evidence that ADHD and CD may have a compounding effect on behavior in the sense that ADHD works through a behavioral inhibition system (BIS) that underfunctions and CD works via a hypersensitive behavioral approach system (BAS). The implication is that individuals that are co-morbid for these two disorders will seek higher levels of stimulation to alleviate their hypersensitive BAS and that the underperforming BIS decreases the probability that they will be able to stop the stimulating activity once it has started [1, 28, 29].

The broad relationship between impulsivity, ADHD and other co-morbid disorders highlights another important facet of ADHD and criminology which is the precise role of impulsivity, or low-self-control as conceptualized by Gottfredson and Hirschi [30] and its relationship to delinquency. This conception of impulsivity has emerged in recent decades as one of the most well-known predictors of delinquent behavior [31]. While it is clear that impulsivity or low-self-control has a strong association with delinquency, it is less clear what the precise etiology of low-self-control is. Unnever *et al* [32] speculate that the underlying etiology of ADHD and low-self-control may be similar. DeLisi [33, p 103] famously labeled low-self-control the 'Tyrannosaurus Rex of criminology' with the implication being that other criminological theories took a back seat to the supposed alpha predator that is the theory of low-self-control. As the association between ADHD and impulsivity as a symptom of that disorder have caught the attention of criminologists more and more, coupled with the wide prevalence of ADHD, led Eme [34, p 446] to further posit that 'If the brain-based disorder of low-self-control is the T-Rex of criminology, then ADHD is the T-Rex of the brain-based disorder of low-self-control'.

7.3 ADHD neuroscience, reinforcement sensitivity theory, genetics, and environment

ADHD has long been considered an arousal disorder, in that individuals are less likely to be aroused by relatively average stimuli [35]. This underarousal often leads to sensation seeking behavior that can correct this under-arousal. Sensation seeking often leads individuals into riskier, and more dangerous activities in order to reach a similar level of arousal that other people have in the face of more mundane stimuli [16]. Early success with pharmacological interventions for ADHD led to the recognition that certain neurotransmitters are implicated in ADHD. Specifically, success with methylphenidate-based stimulants, including the widely known Ritalin, implicated dopamine as these classes of drugs are dopamine reuptake inhibitors which increase available dopamine. More recent findings show that ADHD sufferers also exhibit low levels of an important dopamine metabolite, homovanillic acid, in their cerebral spinal fluid further implicating a dearth of dopamine activity in the disorder [36]. Atomoxetine-class drugs are norepinephrine reuptake inhibitors and also dopamine function facilitators implicating the former neurotransmitter as well [10]. Serotonin is also known to play a large role via its role as an inhibitory neurotransmitter that regulates other inhibitory and excitatory neurotransmitters. Current pharmacological interventions for ADHD, however, do not specifically target this neurotransmitter [37]. When successful these drugs allow sufferers of ADHD to achieve normal levels of arousal in response to environmental stimuli. While these neurotransmitters are definitively indicated as a proximate cause of ADHD, the ultimate, and largely genetic due to high heritability, causes of ADHD are less clear as mentioned previously.

7.3.1 ADHD neuroscience

For some time, many neuroscience models of ADHD have zeroed in on some aspect of frontal lobe connectivity, specifically with other subcortical structures as the basis for understanding the symptomatic manifestations of ADHD [38]. The role of the prefrontal cortex in ADHD cannot be overlooked, and in fact as Goldberg [39] noted this portion of the brain may contribute the most to what makes us 'human'.

While ADHD may have ultimate genetic causes, brain plasticity may temper the impact of ADHD as those afflicted transition into adulthood. According to Sudre *et al* [40], reduction in ADHD symptoms may be indicative of recovery of function that partially compensates for ADHD symptoms. There have been many imaging studies, addressed significantly in other parts of this book, that isolate ADHD in specific parts of the neural anatomy. Functional magnetic resonance imaging and positron emission tomography show that ADHD frequently manifests as dysfunction in the prefrontal cortex, basal ganglion, corpus callosum, temporal lobe and cerebellum. Much of the interest centers around the frontal lobe and cortex, however, as other functional magnetic resonance imaging has zeroed in on the right dorsolateral prefrontal cortex as showing significant differences in ADHD sufferers when contrasted with non-ADHD controls [10].

The prefrontal cortex has been recognized as one of the most important parts of the brain that frequently shows functional deficits in populations with higher propensities for aggression and antisocial behavior [41]. Other brain structures have been implicated in ADHD as well, largely via imaging studies. According to Gallo and Posner [42] there are three main neural circuit networks that are suspects in ADHD. These are frontoparietal circuits that play a role in attention alerting and how an individual orients their available capacity for attention to a specific stimulus. The dorsal frontostriatal circuitry is critical for regulating inhibitions and selecting various responses to a variety of stimuli. Lastly, mesocorticolimbic circuit pathways which include the nucleus accumbens, ventral tegmental area, orbitofrontal cortex, hippocampus, and ventral striatum are implicated as well. Several of these structures, in particular the ventral striatum and the orbitofrontal cortex have been heavily implicated in ADHD via their management of reward calculations, which is an issue for ADHD sufferers. Increased reward signals and inefficient/less effective connectivity between the ventral striatum and motor control areas have also been noted in ADHD sufferers implying that their responsiveness to rewards is abnormal [43]. Additionally, these circuits are also related to the management of emotions, motivation, focus, and inhibition [42].

The prefrontal cortex is also late to myelinate compared with other parts of the brain. Myelin is a high lipid substance that serves as a form of electrical insulation to facilitate transmission of electric signals down the axon of a given neuron. As myelination occurs, neuronal function becomes more efficient along developed neuronal pathways. Typically, the prefrontal cortex fully myelinates in late adolescence and early adulthood which coincides with an improvement in ADHD symptoms, in particular impulsiveness which has known links to criminal behavior. A high percentage of ADHD individuals display symptoms into adulthood but the intensity of the symptoms is reduced [44, 45]. As further evidence of the complexity of neural anatomy and ADHD is the finding of Nagel *et al* [46], that even in very young children the distribution and connectivity of white matter (mostly myelinated axons) was atypical. Further, the atypicality was associated with areas of the white matter with known relationships to behaviors and symptoms of ADHD. These findings are important as they stress that ADHD is a complicated disorder that involves impaired brain connectivity in the white matter but also variations in the specific structures that are a part of that connected neural network. Furthermore, cognitive improvement that is associated with brain development in normal and abnormal individuals is to some degree dependent on white matter integrity [47]. Successful improvements in cognition that are reliant to some degree on white matter development may be impaired in individuals with ADHD and their atypical white matter connectivity.

Gray matter development is also implicated, as Shaw *et al* [48] found that gray matter peak development was achieved about three years later in sufferers of ADHD than in controls. In fact, abnormalities in the volume of various structures are a consistent finding in sufferers of ADHD. Several analyses have found significant reductions in the prefrontal cortex, cerebellum, parietal and temporal lobes, and also total brain volume [49]. In particular, volume loss, when contrasted with controls, of the basal ganglia is considered the most reproducible structural abnormality associated with ADHD. The caudate nucleus, which is part of the dorsal striatum in primates, and the lentiform nucleus which together largely make up the striatum, are shown to be reduced in volume in ADHD sufferers [50]. However, there is evidence, as mentioned previously, that ADHD symptomology improves with age. The decreased volume tends to normalize with age in those ADHD sufferers who show symptom improvement. Pharmacological treatments for ADHD are also implicated in a normalization of brain volume with age. However, when symptoms of ADHD persist despite aging, these individuals are associated with less of a normalization in brain volume, suggesting that decreased brain volume in critical areas is strongly associated with symptoms of ADHD [49, 50].

7.3.1.1 Neurotransmitters

Much of what is known about the neurochemistry of ADHD stems from neuropharmacological work on ADHD treatment [51]. The norepinephrine and dopamine systems have been implicated [52]. Most pharmacological interventions for ADHD are directed towards increasing the availability of dopamine and norepinephrine in the synaptic cleft. This is accomplished by either increasing the neuronal release of these transmitters or by blocking their reuptake, thus increasing the duration of the time that they spend in the synaptic cleft. Some pharmacological interventions accomplish both [2]. As a disorder that is highlighted by difficulty in regulating responses to stimuli the serotonergic system is implicated as well. In fact, while most pharmacological interventions attempt to address a dearth of dopamine and norepinephrine, genetic studies and the role of serotonin in regulating a host of neural functions means that this neurotransmitter plays a role as well [36]. There is also recent work that indicates that gamma-aminobutyric acid (GABA), an inhibitory neurotransmitter, is present in significantly lower quantities in ADHD sufferers. Glutamate, an excitatory neurotransmitter, is present in abnormally high quantities in ADHD sufferers as well [53].

7.3.2 Reinforcement sensitivity theory

Criminology, as a discipline, has been interested in some of the most basic conceptions of risk/reward calculation for some time. Many early theories of crime that constituted the classical school of criminology dealt with these issues specifically. The work of Cesare Beccaria, an 18th century Italian economist emphasized that offenders should be assumed to have weighed the risk/reward of their crime. Jeremy Bentham, an English contemporary of Cesare Beccaria, also argued that crime is simply a risk/reward assessment by potential offenders, something that he called the hedonistic calculus. These early conceptions of human behavior as it pertains to crime understandably lacked the wealth of knowledge about cortical function that has been accumulated in the intervening centuries. Deterrence was the obvious policy implication of the belief that behavior, in particular criminal behavior, was based on a calculation of possible risks and rewards. However, Beccaria and most contemporaries assumed that the risk/reward assessments worked the same in offenders and non-offenders. As time went on this view became inadequate [16].

Reinforcement sensitivity theory is as close as criminology can get to a scientific theory of 18th century risk and reward conceptions [54]. Reinforcement sensitivity theory was first conceptualized in the 1970s [55]. The basic concept has individuals varying in their sensitivity to reward and punishment cues. If humans are to function in a society, they must have societally appropriate responses to incentives and disincentives. If incentives are typically perceived as stronger and disincentives as weaker, the end result is usually anti-social, and possibly criminal, behavior [16]. Reinforcement sensitivity theory basically proposes that three interacting systems facilitate the normal social functioning of humans. These systems are the behavioral approach system (BAS), the behavioral inhibition system (BIS) and the fight/flee/freeze system. These systems are part of the limbic system and the autonomic nervous system [1]. A crude analogy can be drawn between these systems and Sigmund Freud's id, ego, and superego but with more significant supporting evidence and a specific neuroanatomical and genetic foundation. Some early work was supportive of Gray's contentions, indicating that a stronger behavioral approach system (BAS) is predictive of antisocial behavior in boys [56].

The behavioral approach system (BAS) is critical in pleasure-seeking behavior. Reproduction, nutrition, social bonding, and other critical life activities have a reward system that promotes these behaviors, which are obviously important in the success of most organisms. This system is sensitive to both conditioned stimuli such as drugs but also unconditioned stimuli such as food or reproduction [57]. The system depends on dopamine and the neural anatomy that responds to dopamine [58]. Considering what is known about dopamine and ADHD, the connection of the behavioral approach system (BAS) with ADHD is apparent. A lack of dopamine means an underperforming behavioral approach system (BAS), which would then require higher levels of stimulation. While individuals with a normally functioning behavioral approach system (BAS) are adequately rewarded by normal stimuli, those with ADHD must seek more and more intense stimuli to elicit the same response.

The behavioral inhibition system (BIS) evolved because humans are predominantly social beings and an unregulated seeking of pleasure would lead to excessive conflict. The desire and necessity to function in large social groups required some method of regulating pleasure-seeking behavior so that it did not conflict with the normal social functioning of the group [59]. Like the behavioral approach system (BAS), the behavioral inhibition system (BIS) responds to conditioned (incarceration/law breaking) an unconditioned (fire, dangerous animals, heights, etc) threats of danger or punishment [57]. The behavioral inhibition system (BIS) is linked with the serotonergic system [54, 60].

Organisms frequently experience unanticipated or surprising stimuli (such as an attack by a predator or, in the case of humans, an attack by another human or other unexpected situation). In these situations, the early warning system that is the fight/flee/freeze system of the autonomic nervous system comes into play. This system, once activated, releases norepinephrine and epinephrine in order to facilitate the appropriate behavior (fighting, fleeing, or freezing). According to Corr [61] the behavioral inhibition system (BIS) and the fight/flee/freeze system may actually be part of a larger behavioral inhibition system (BIS) that deals with conditioned and unconditioned threats in slightly different ways.

All three of these systems work in concert to produce behavior in the presence of certain stimuli. Certainly, potential rewards and threats of danger frequently coexist in routine situations (meaning that perceived probabilities of reward and punishment can be similar). The behavioral inhibition system (BIS), when functioning normally, inhibits behavior until the behavioral activating system (BAS) or the fight/flee/freeze system activate to determine appropriate responses from available options. Criminals may have issues making appropriate calculations when rewards, punishments, and social expectations are in disharmony. An overly potent behavioral approach system (BAS) coupled with weaker than normal behavioral inhibition system (BIS) and fight/flee/freeze system may make it more difficult for criminals to say no to certain stimuli even when the social costs of doing so are high. The frequent result is elevated social and legal trouble [62].

The role of the serotonergic and dopaminergic systems as well as the role of epinephrine and norepinephrine is important here due to the links that these neurotransmitters have with ADHD via pharmacology and genetics but to behavior in general. Any dysfunction in these systems in the form of hypo and/or hyperactivity is relevant in a wide array of behavioral and cognitive problems that should interest criminologists [1].

7.3.3 Genetics and environment

7.3.3.1 Genetics

As mentioned earlier, ADHD is a disorder that has very high heritability. Most estimates are above 0.70, with some approaching 0.90 and above [63]. Faraone and Larsson [9] examined 37 twin studies as far back as the 1970s and found a mean heritability of 0.74. Very few of the examined studies showed a heritability of less than 0.6. One issue with such comparisons is the inevitable methodological and operational variations across studies. ADHD is not measured consistently across studies as it is treated as a spectrum disorder by some but as a clustering of specific symptoms by others. Nevertheless, despite methodological variation there is consistency and clustering in disparate heritability estimates [64]. Heritability is much lower in twin studies of adults, near half of the heritability for ADHD generally, but this may be due to the self-rating of symptoms and other issues with interrater reliability [63].

One issue that has become clear over time is that ADHD is a highly polygenic disorder [65]. No single polymorphism is implicated in the disorder and the polygenic nature of ADHD may explain why the presentation and intensity of the disorder vary so widely. While public discourse of genetics tends to focus on the role of single genes, such a discussion is not possible with ADHD. In fact, the single nucleotide polymorphism heritability for ADHD is 0.22, which is considerably lower than the heritability of the disorder in general which is indicative of large impacts being the additive result of many polymorphisms [9]. Much research in the genetics of ADHD attempts to link genetic variations to specific diagnosable criteria of the disorder. Genetic variance often predicts traits that resemble symptoms of the disorder in those who were never diagnosed [66]. According to Gallo and Posner [42] this is problematic, however, as diagnostic criteria and presentations of the disorder can vary. Also, the fact that ADHD is frequently co-morbid with other disorders as well can complicate attempts to pinpoint genetic etiology. They propose that further examination of endophenotypes, or quantifiable biological traits, may actually be more instructive. Reaction time, during attention-based tasks, variance within individuals has been identified as a robust endophenotype of ADHD. Other candidate endophenotypes have been identified as well, such as working memory and discontinuing possibly undesirable responses to certain stimuli.

While there are numerous candidate genes for ADHD and genome wide association studies have revealed a number of potential genetic suspects, many have not replicated or done so inconsistently. Unsurprisingly, as ADHD is fundamentally a regulation disorder, genes involving dopamine and serotonin are implicated and have replicated [1, 42]. Replicability of the involvement of certain genes has centered around a dopamine receptor gene (DRD4), a dopamine transporter gene (DAT1) and a serotonin transporter (5-HTT). Disharmony in the balance between dopamine and serotonin plays a large role in resource sensitivity theory and in managing responses to stimuli, something that ADHD sufferers obviously struggle with.

DRD4 has been implicated in ADHD for some time [67, 68]. DRD4 is a gene that repeats between two and 11 times with longer repeats being associated with less responsivity to dopamine [69]. Of particular interest is the seven-repeat allele of this gene which is associated with less than optimal arousal that may be experienced as boredom. Individuals with shorter repeats are either over stimulated or adequately stimulated by stimuli that would underarouse those with the seven-repeat allele.

The DAT1 gene is a dopamine transporter gene that plays a role in determining how much dopamine is available in the synaptic spaces via reuptake effectiveness. This gene does not have as many repeat alleles as the DRD4 gene, but the most common variants are associated with greater dopamine reuptake [70]. If reuptake is more efficient, dopamine does not persist in the synaptic spaces diminishing sensations of pleasure from various stimuli. This could potentially lead to more sensation seeking, which has the potential to run afoul of social norms. The ten-repeat allele of DAT1 has been associated with a greater number of sexual partners as well as antisocial behavior, which is obviously a risk factor for a variety negative outcomes [71, 72].

The 5-HTT gene is a transporter gene that plays a role similar to DAT1 but for serotonin. One particular polymorphism produces long and short variants. The short variant is associated with less efficient reuptake of serotonin, allowing persistence in the synaptic spaces, which can serve as an inhibiting factor. The long variant is associated with ADHD via its much more efficient reuptake of serotonin which means that there is potentially less of it for behavioral inhibition [36, 37, 73].

7.3.3.2 Environment

Despite the high heritability of ADHD, even a coefficient above .80 leaves room for environmental variables to explain significant variation in the disorder. However, a wide array of potential environmental influences, including pre-natal ones, makes it difficult to control for environments in research. Because individuals are constantly creating and responding to environments through gene–environment-correlations and gene–environment-interactions these processes can be difficult to discriminate from each other. Individuals impact differential exposure to environments based on their genes through gene–environment-correlation. They also will have differential susceptibility to environments because of their genes through gene–environment-interactions.

Studies have established a link between exposure to alcohol and tobacco during pregnancy and an increased risk of ADHD. Alcohol use during pregnancy increased the risk of ADHD by over 1.5-fold in offspring while prenatal tobacco exposure, which has been linked to low-self-control, a key criminological variable, increases the risk of ADHD by over 2.6-fold [74–76]. Also of interest is the role that maternal disease during pregnancy can play as well. Conditions that produce inflammatory responses, such as rheumatoid arthritis and hypothyroidism were associated with a higher risk of ADHD in offspring [77]. Low birth weight, prematurity at delivery, toxin exposure, and cocaine use have come up as significant in some studies as well [78]. Head trauma has been implicated also [51]. While environment is not the ultimate cause of ADHD it can make symptoms substantially worse and environment may play a role in the co-morbidity with other disorders. Environmental toxins such as lead have been linked with a variety of symptoms and behaviors associated with ADHD such as impulsivity and low-self-control [79]. Greater proximity to certain hazardous wastes have been associated with a heightened risk of many disorders and deleterious symptoms, including ADHD [80]. Furthermore, the behavior of children with ADHD can lead to negative reactions, erratic responses, and coercive parenting techniques from parents, teachers, and others that, via evocative gene–environment-correlations, makes problems that the child has worse [25, 81].

As ADHD is a common disorder and because so many genes have been implicated in the disorder, it is likely that some ADHD behaviors and their corresponding genes granted an evolutionary advantage at some level. According to Hartmann [82], ADHD behaviors may have been an evolutionary advantage when most humans lived in nomadic hunter–gatherer type societies. As a hunter, impulsivity and sensation seeking(due to low arousal) may have made for a more effective hunter in that one would be more likely to seek out novel stimuli (which may improve hunting opportunities). Additionally, impulsivity in hunting may lead to greater payoffs than meticulous planning and detail orientation through flexible hunting strategies and the ability to change course quickly. This could conceivably lead to greater reproductive success via the ability to secure more resources (food) necessary for survival. Today these 'hunter' traits are a disadvantage in the form of being easily distracted or impulsive, which can inhibit long-term success. The 'farmer' traits of skillful long-term planning and lowered impulsivity were more beneficial in an agricultural environment that has only been around for about 12 000 years [83].

The DRD4 seven-repeat allele has been around for about 40 000 years indicating that it has been around both before the advent of agriculture (in hunter–gather type societies) and that it has been selected for as well [84]. Others have posited that there is an evolutionary model of ADHD that fits with the history of human social development. Williams and Taylor [85], found that unpredictable behavior by some produces overall benefits for groups using simulations centered around the seven-repeat allele of the DRD4 gene. The willingness to explore and take risks was a benefit when you were not growing your own food.

Hartmann's theory was tested when, conveniently, the Ariaal peoples of Kenya split into two groups in the middle of the 20th century. A traditionally nomadic ethnic group, some members preferred to maintain that lifestyle while others preferred a more modern and sedentary agricultural life. Genetic information was gathered from both groups and the seven-repeat allele of DRD 4 was found in about 20% of each group. Health outcomes for those carrying the allele differed depending on the environment that carriers were in. In the nomadic group carriers were generally healthier, while in the agricultural population having the allele was associated with poorer health outcomes. In this context, the gene–environment-interaction of the seven-repeat allele produced an advantage in one environment and a disadvantage in another. This is consistent with Hartmann's hunter/farmer conception of ADHD [86]. As human environments today are more variable it is perhaps not surprising that the rate of genome variation has increased significantly in the Holocene when compared to the Pleistocene [87].

7.4 ADHD treatment

Considering that the proximate causes of ADHD are neurotransmitter dysfunction, interventions have typically attempted to address these issues. In fact, as mentioned previously, success with pharmacological interventions was helpful in identifying specific neurotransmitters that play a role in the disorder [51, 88]. Stimulants have been the main treatment for ADHD for some time. Methylphenidate and amphetamine-based stimulants, which are available under a variety of well-known brand names, are some of the most frequently prescribed medicines period [89]. Methylphenidates and amphetamines both block the reuptake of dopamine and norepinephrine, increasing its availability, while amphetamines additionally further increase the release of dopamine and norepinephrine working on both sides of the availability equation. Increased availability of dopamine and norepinephrine bring less than optimally aroused individuals up to more normal levels of arousal [90]. Methylphenidate-based stimulants have been proven effective when measured against a variety of outcomes such as a reduction in certain bone fractures (suggestive of less involvement high-risk activities where bones are often broken) [91].

Atomoxetine is a less well known, but widely used, non-stimulant drug that increases the availability of both dopamine and norepinephrine by acting on the norepinephrine transporter (which is involved in the reuptake of dopamine as well) [88]. Certain alpha-2 norepinephrine agonists are used as non-stimulant treatments as well [92].

The distinction between stimulant and non-stimulant pharmacological interventions is of relevance to criminologists as the use of stimulants in jail and prison populations is controversial. According to Burns [93], stimulants should never be used in correctional settings due to widespread substance-abuse issues among inmates, frequent misuse of stimulants prescribed for ADHD, as well as the frequent taking and misuse of drugs from weaker inmates by stronger ones. Non-stimulant drugs, such as atomoxetine, clonidine, and guanfacine may be more appropriate for prison populations despite slightly less efficacy than stimulant drugs [92].

Regardless of setting (correctional versus non-correctional), inconsistent use of prescribed medications is problematic in ADHD. Also problematic are increases in heart rate and blood pressure with certain stimulants and atomoxetine that make them inappropriate for some cases. It has also been argued that the misdiagnosis and treatment of ADHD with drugs that often produce serious side effects is seriously problematic [94]. A promising new treatment is repetitive transcranial magnetic stimulation (rTMS) which is a non-invasive, non-pharmacological intervention that uses magnetic stimulation on cranial locations determined by imaging. Stimulation sends magnetic pulses that depolarize neurons and rearrange neural pathways. While the precise mechanism of function is not entirely understood, it possibly acts through plasticity, recovery of function, as well as dopamine release which has obvious implications for ADHD given the goal of pharmacological treatments [95]. It has been shown to have therapeutic impacts in treating depression, anxiety, and other disorders [96, 97]. It has also been shown to be effective in the treatment of ADHD as well. Niederhoffer [98] found significant improvement when compared to non-treatment controls. Others found improvement in attention measures compared to controls [99]. Of particular interest to criminologists may be the finding that when repetitive transcranial magnetic stimulation (rTMS) is combined with atomoxetine it produces significant improvement in ADHD symptoms and executive function beyond what is achieved with either treatment alone. Given the aforementioned issues with the use of stimulant drugs in correctional settings, these findings may have implications for the treatment of incarcerated ADHD sufferers [10].

7.5 ADHD and crime

ADHD, symptoms of ADHD, and disorders that ADHD is co-morbid with have all been linked to various measures of offending for quite some time. While variances in methodology, as well as measures, make comparisons difficult, it should be stressed that findings in general show a positive association. In fact, Ellis *et al* [3] reviewed dozens of studies dating back to the early 1970s and found positive associations between ADHD and violent offenses, drug offenses, alcoholism, antisocial behavior, recidivism and general offending. They noted a pair of studies that found no significant relationship between ADHD and illegal drug use only out of the dozens reviewed. Clearly the weight of the extant literature on ADHD and crime is indicative of a strong association. It is worth noting that early work on subjects such as susceptibility to boredom was likely tapping into ADHD without or being only peripherally aware of it [100]. It is also worth noting that while the link between ADHD and crime is robust, ADHD is also indicated in many undesirable behaviors and pathologies that are not explicitly criminal yet may be problematic such as alcoholism and antisocial behavior in general [3].

7.5.1 Co-morbid conditions and crime

While ADHD is more worrisome when it presents as co-morbid with ODD and CD in particular, these conditions alone have been linked to a variety of offending measures just by themselves. Also, there was early recognition that a variety of similar 'behavioral' disorders would cluster within individuals and that among children the behavioral problems were exacerbated when more than one diagnosis was noted [101]. These authors made a connection between ODD and antisocial behavior. Such a connection has ongoing support in the literature [102]. It is also worth noting that arbitrary diagnostic criteria until the DSM-IV prevented CD and ODD from being diagnosed together, so that researchers could not consider the possibility of distinct pathways from ODD to CD, despite the fact that it was known that these conditions are co-morbid. Longitudinal work showing ODD as a risk factor for CD was needed [24]. Despite the association, they are considered separate disorders and criminologists have treated them as such for much of the early extant work on the subject [103]. It is also worth noting that ODD has also been linked to adult criminality later in life in a sample of Pittsburgh adolescents followed up to the age of 25 [104]. Needless to say, the findings in the literature that associate ODD with criminal and delinquent behavior are robust and with consistent findings in a positive direction [3].

Perhaps of more interest to criminologists, at least as evidenced by the volume of research, is the intersection between ADHD and CD. In addition to Lynam's [25, p 209] aforementioned observation that ADHD and CD represent a form of 'fledgling psychopathy' others have put forth the idea that criminologists should be especially interested in this relationship. Comings [105] posited that because ADHD is often co-morbid with CD, it may actually be ADHD and CD that produce the most deleterious outcomes as opposed to ADHD alone. The argument is that ADHD and co-morbid CD are actually driving adolescent and adult delinquency rather than ADHD alone. Due to diagnostic inconsistency and the similarities between outward symptoms of the disorder, early links between ADHD and crime may have been indicative of undiagnosed CD that was co-morbid with ADHD. It is important that future research examines this intersection more closely as it could have profound impacts on how such disorders are approached in the real world [16]. Also interesting to note is the association of CD and other deleterious outcomes or conditions. CD is associated with a higher risk of post-traumatic stress disorder, which according to some may be due to the increased likelihood of those with CD being in situations where traumatic outcomes are more likely [106]. Furthermore, CD is strongly and consistently associated with a greater likelihood of antisocial personality disorder and psychopathy, which themselves have known links to criminal behavior and delinquency. In fact, criminologists have examined the impact of not just the specific disorders mentioned in this chapter on criminal activity, but individual symptoms and characteristics of the disorders as well. Consistent links in a positive direction have also been found for behaviors that could easily be considered ADHD, CD, or ODD symptoms such as boredom and novelty seeking among others [3]. It is also worth noting however that a 30-year longitudinal study of Norwegian youth found a strong link between childhood CD and adult offending, but no such association for ADHD alone [107].

7.5.2 ADHD

It is important to note the obvious connections between ADHD characteristics and one of the pillar independent variables of the discipline of criminology which is the robust link between various conceptions of low-self-control and crime. As mentioned earlier, the role of low-self-control in criminology has been compared to an extinct cretaceous super-predator [33]. While this may be an over-the-top comparison, it captures the influence of low-self-control in the discipline, which has been robustly supported as being linked to offending since the early 1990s [30, 31]. Despite the empirical necessity to disentangle the precise nature of the relationship between ADHD and criminological constructs of low-self-control, both factors have been strongly linked with crime when examined by themselves. This suggests that regardless of how future scholars should treat ADHD and low-self-control (as having a similar etiology or being diverse measures of the same underlying condition), that the links to offending will be present regardless. According to Schoepfer *et al* [108], low-self-control and ADHD are predictive of delinquency in a similar manner, which has been a consistent finding for some time. However, the exact nature of the relationship between low-self-control and ADHD is not entirely clear currently.

Over the decades ADHD has been linked to both self-reported and criminal justice system detected offenses, with the vast majority of links being in a positive direction. Most of the extant literature has focused on offenses other than serious violent crimes, which suggests that such an area is worthy of deeper exploration, as public discourse of criminal activity often centers on serious violent felonies rather than things such as self-reported drug use [3]. While the body of literature is consistent in finding links between ADHD and offending, it is worth noting that criminology as a discipline has had problems with consistency of measures. Measures such as antisocial behavior have been frequently used in the criminological literature over the decades as dependent variables and have been measured in a wide variety of ways. As a purely social construct antisocial behavior is often subjective (although there is some consistency in what people consider antisocial in certain situations) and also may not be criminal at all, weakening the generalizability of much of the older criminological literature [16]. It is easy to see this in older work that linked ADHD and aggression such as that by Hinshaw [109]. ADHD as an independent variable is also problematic as well, due to wide inconsistencies in how it has been conceptualized over the years but also overdiagnosis has probably led many individuals who did not meet rigid diagnostic criteria for having ADHD being included in studies as ADHD sufferers, further muddying the picture [17].

One area where ADHD sufferers are overrepresented however is among incarcerated individuals, suggesting that ADHD sufferers frequently run foul of conventional norms. One study reviewed nine other studies examining ADHD and prisoners and found that the prevalence among inmates was between 24% and 67%. Needless to say, this is far above all of the estimates of the prevalence of ADHD for the general population [110]. Another study found that almost half of inmates had some presentation of ADHD but also that over 85% of ADHD sufferers were comorbid for some form of substance-abuse and nearly a third of those with ADHD were also showing indications of antisocial personality disorder [111]. More recently, one study additionally found that ADHD sufferers were again overrepresented as inmates but also that there was an association between psychopathy and psychopathic traits. This is further evidence that ADHD has complex co-morbidities with other disorders [112]. Buitelaar *et al* [113], reviewed several studies that showed a link between ADHD and future domestic or intimate partner violence. According to Eme [114], about a third of the entrants into the juvenile justice system have diagnosed ADHD and that this is probably a conservative statistic. Berryessa [115], also notes that individuals with ADHD also have difficulties extricating themselves from the criminal justice system due to the inability to meet the conditions of release and probation, as they represent long-term tasks. Furthermore, impulsivity may contribute to a longer period of incarceration as ADHD sufferers are more likely to accumulate infractions and be involved in altercations with both correctional officers and other inmates.

ADHD also represents a significant cost to society as well. Fletcher and Wolfe [116] find that ADHD symptoms during childhood are strongly predictive of adolescent offending and that this relationship is present regardless of whether they present with *predominantly inattentive, predominantly hyperactive and impulsive, or combined* presentation of the disorder. Perhaps more interesting though is that they attempt to measure the cost to both victims and society of crimes committed by individuals with ADHD. Using disorder prevalence data, the likelihood of individuals with ADHD offending and the mean costs of various types of victimization they conclude that ADHD costs victims alone between 58 and 170 million dollars annually. Furthermore, ADHD is estimated to cost society as a whole between 1.8 and 4.1 billion dollars annually as well. This is clearly a massive social cost in crime alone for just one disorder.

7.6 Conclusion

There is little doubt that there are strong links between ADHD, criminal behavior but also non-criminal undesirable behavior. Decades of extant literature on this topic that have been summarized here demonstrate that thoroughly. Criminologists have been saying that ADHD has been neglected by the discipline for quite some time [32]. However, only somewhat more attention has been recently directed towards this disorder since that observation was made in the early 2000s. Due to the wealth of knowledge about this disorder from many other disciplines, criminologists might want to reconsider the role of ADHD within the discipline. Biologically informed perspectives are making a larger contribution to the discipline and have much to contribute argue Wright and Boisvert [117]. Despite this, criticism is a common feature that has been associated with attempts to integrate biological and criminological perspectives [118]. It is worth exploring ADHD as a disorder from a biological and criminological perspective because of the association between ADHD and the criminological super-variable that are the various conceptions of low-self-control. Understanding the relationship further could have significant implications in both the treatment, management, and societal approach to the disorder but also policy ramifications for the criminal justice system as well. If ADHD is truly as important as the relationship between it and crime would suggest, then it is possible that many future criminal justice, and other, interventions could be directed towards mitigating some of the worst outcomes of ADHD. There are many areas that are implicated for future research and the more that we understand about this very common disorder, the more successful we might be in addressing it in the criminal justice system but also in society as a whole.

References

[1] Walsh A 2019 *Reinforcement Sensitivity Theory: A Metatheory for Biosocial Criminology.* (New York: Routledge)

[2] Curatolo P, Dagati E and Moavero R 2010 The neurobiological basis of ADHD *Ital. J. Pediatr.* **36** 79

[3] Ellis L, Beaver K and Wright J 2009 *Handbook of Crime Correlates.* (Amsterdam: Academic)

[4] Roskell N S, Setyawan J, Zimovetz E A and Hodgkins P 2014 Systematic evidence synthesis of treatments for ADHD in children and adolescents: indirect treatment comparisons of lisdexamfetamine with methylphenidate and atomoxetine *Curr. Med. Res. Opin.* **30** 1673–85
[5] American Psychiatric Association 2013 *Diagnostic and Statistical Manual of Mental Disorders* 5th ed. (Arlington, VA: American Psychiatric Publishing)
[6] Xu G, Strathearn L, Liu B, Yang B and Bao W 2018 Twenty-year trends in diagnosed attention-deficit/hyperactivity disorder among U.S. children and adolescents, 1997–2016 *JAMA Network Open* **1** e181471
[7] Danielson M L, Bitsko R H, Ghandour R M, Holbrook J R, Kogan M D and Blumberg S J 2018 Prevalence of parent-reported ADHD diagnosis and associated treatment among U.S. children and adolescents, 2016 *J. Clin. Child Adolesc. Psychol.* **47** 199–212
[8] Langner I, Garbe E, Banaschewski T and Mikolajczyk R T 2013 Twin and sibling studies using health insurance data: the example of attention deficit/hyperactivity disorder (ADHD) *PLoS One* **8** e62177
[9] Faraone S V and Larsson H 2018 Genetics of attention deficit hyperactivity disorder *Mol. Psychiatry* **24** 562–75
[10] Cao P, Xing J, Cao Y, Cheng Q, Sun X, Kang Q, Dai L, Zhou X and Song Z 2018 Clinical effects of repetitive transcranial magnetic stimulation combined with atomoxetine in the treatment of attention-deficit hyperactivity disorder *Neuropsychiatr. Dis. Treat.* **14** 3231–40
[11] Hare R D 1970 *Psychopathy: Theory and Research: Theory and Research.* (New York: Wiley)
[12] Mendelson W, Johnson N and Stewart M A 1971 Hyperactive children as teenagers: a follow-up study *J. Nerv. Ment. Dis.* **153** 273–9
[13] Knight B J and West D J 1975 Temporary and continuing delinquency *Br. J. Criminol.* **15** 43–50
[14] Watts S J 2018 ADHD symptomatology and criminal behavior during adolescence: exploring the mediating role of school factors *Int. J. Offender Ther. Comp. Criminol.* **62** 3–23
[15] Schilling C M, Walsh A and Yun I 2011 ADHD and criminality: a primer on the genetic, neurobiological, evolutionary and treatment literature for criminologists *J. Crim. Justice* **39** 3–11
[16] Lilly J R, Cullen F T and Ball R A 2019 *Criminological Theory: Context and Consequences.* (Thousand Oaks, CA: Sage)
[17] Merten E C, Cwik J C, Margraf J and Schneider S 2017 Overdiagnosis of mental disorders in children and adolescents (in developed countries) *Child Adolesc. Psychiatry Ment. Health* **11** 5
[18] Loeber R and Burke J D 2011 Developmental pathways in juvenile externalizing and internalizing problems *J. Res. Adolesc.* **21** 34–46
[19] Nock M K, Kazdin A E, Hiripi E and Kessler R C 2007 Lifetime prevalence, correlates, and persistence of oppositional defiant disorder: results from the national comorbidity survey replication *J. Child Psychol. Psychiatry* **48** 703–13
[20] Burke J D, Loeber R and Birmaher B 2002 Oppositional defiant disorder and conduct disorder: a review of the past 10 years, part II *J. Am. Acad. Child Adolesc. Psychiatry* **41** 1275–93

[21] Maughan B, Rowe R, Messer J, Goodman R and Meltzer H 2004 Conduct disorder and oppositional defiant disorder in a national sample: developmental epidemiology *J. Child Psychol. Psychiatry* **45** 609–21
[22] Frick P J, Lahey B B, Loeber R, Stouthamer-Loeber M, Christ M A G and Hanson K 1992 Familial risk factors to oppositional defiant disorder and conduct disorder: parental psychopathology and maternal parenting *J. Consult. Clin. Psychol.* **60** 49–55
[23] Lahey B B, Waldman I D and Mcburnett K 1999 Annotation: the development of antisocial behavior: an integrative causal model *J. Child Psychol. Psychiatry* **40** 669–82
[24] Rowe R, Costello E J, Angold A, Copeland W E and Maughan B 2010 Developmental pathways in oppositional defiant disorder and conduct disorder *J. Abnormal Psychol.* **119** 726–38
[25] Lynam D R 1996 Early identification of chronic offenders: who is the fledgling psychopath? *Psychol. Bull.* **120** 209–34
[26] Moffitt T E 1993 Adolescence-limited and life-course-persistent antisocial behavior: a developmental taxonomy *Psychol. Rev.* **100** 674–701
[27] DeLisi M, Peters D J, Dansby T, Vaughn M G, Shook J J and Hochstetler A 2014 Dynamics of psychopathy and moral disengagement in the etiology of crime *Youth Violence Juv. Justice* **12** 295–314
[28] Quay H C 1997 Inhibition and attention deficit hyperactivity disorder *J. Abnormal Child Psychol.* **25** 7–13
[29] Levy F 2004 Synaptic gating and ADHD: a biological theory of comorbidity of ADHD and anxiety *Neuropsychopharmacology* **29** 1589–96
[30] Gottfredson M and Hirschi T 1990 *A General Theory of Crime.* (Stanford, CA: Stanford University Press)
[31] Pratt T C and Cullen F T 2000 The empirical status of Gottfredson and Hirschi's general theory of crime: a meta-analysis *Criminology* **38** 931–64
[32] Unnever J D, Cullen F T and Pratt T C 2003 Parental management, ADHD, and delinquent involvement: reassessing Gottfredson and Hirschis general theory *Justice Q.* **20** 471–500
[33] DeLisi M 2011 Self-control theory: the *Tyrannosaurus rex* of criminology is poised to devour criminal justice *J. Crim. Justice* **39** 103–5
[34] Eme R 2015 Beauchaine ontogenic process model of externalizing psychopathology a biosocial theory of crime and delinquency *J. Crim. Justice* **43** 443–9
[35] James S-N, Cheung C H M, Rommel A-S, Mcloughlin G, Brandeis D, Banaschewski T, Asherson P and Kuntsi J 2017 Peripheral hypoarousal but not preparation-vigilance impairment endures in ADHD remission *J. Atten. Disord.* **31**
[36] Dalley J W and Roiser J P 2012 Dopamine, serotonin and impulsivity *Neuroscience* **215** 42–58
[37] Oades R 2008 Dopamine–serotonin interactions in attention-deficit hyperactivity disorder (ADHD) *Prog. Brain Res.* **172** 543–65
[38] Rosch K S, Crocetti D, Hirabayashi K, Denckla M B, Mostofsky S H and Mahone E M 2018 Reduced subcortical volumes among preschool-age girls and boys with ADHD *Psychiatry Res.: Neuroimaging* **271** 67–74
[39] Goldberg E 2001 *The Executive Brain: Frontal Lobes and the Civilized Mind.* (Oxford: Oxford University Press)

[40] Sudre G, Mangalmurti A and Shaw P 2018 Growing out of attention deficit hyperactivity disorder: insights from the 'remitted' brain *Neurosci. Biobehav. Rev.* **94** 198–209

[41] Yang Y and Raine A 2009 Prefrontal structural and functional brain imaging findings in antisocial, violent, and psychopathic individuals: a meta-analysis *Psychiatry Res. Neuroimaging* **174** 81–8

[42] Gallo E F and Posner J 2016 Moving towards causality in attention-deficit hyperactivity disorder: overview of neural and genetic mechanisms *Lancet Psychiatry* **3** 555–67

[43] Ma I, Holstein M V, Mies G W, Mennes M, Buitelaar J, Cools R, Cillessen A H, Krebs R M and Scheres A 2016 Ventral striatal hyperconnectivity during rewarded interference control in adolescents with ADHD *Cortex* **82** 225–36

[44] Willoughby M T 2003 Developmental course of ADHD symptomatology during the transition from childhood to adolescence: a review with recommendations *J. Child Psychol. Psychiatry* **44** 88–106

[45] Sowell E R, Thompson P M and Toga A W 2004 Mapping changes in the human cortex throughout the span of life *Neuroscientist* **10** 372–92

[46] Nagel B J, Bathula D, Herting M, Schmitt C, Kroenke C D, Fair D and Nigg J T 2011 Altered white matter microstructure in children with attention-deficit/hyperactivity disorder *J. Am. Acad. Child Adolesc. Psychiatry* **50** 283–92

[47] Stevens M C, Skudlarski P, Pearlson G D and Calhoun V D 2009 Age-related cognitive gains are mediated by the effects of white matter development on brain network integration *NeuroImage* **48** 738–46

[48] Shaw P, Lerch J, Greenstein D, Sharp W, Clasen L, Evans A, Giedd J, Castellanos F X and Rapoport J 2006 Longitudinal mapping of cortical thickness and clinical outcome in children and adolescents with attention-deficit/hyperactivity disorder *Arch. General Psychiatry* **63** 540–49

[49] Friedman L A and Rapoport J L 2015 Brain development in ADHD *Curr. Opin. Neurobiol.* **30** 106–11

[50] Nakao T, Radua J, Rubia K and Mataix-Cols D 2011 Gray matter volume abnormalities in ADHD: voxel-based meta-analysis exploring the effects of age and stimulant medication *Am. J. Psychiatry* **168** 1154–63

[51] Durston S 2003 A review of the biological bases of ADHD: what have we learned from imaging studies? *Ment. Retard. Dev. Disabil. Res. Rev.* **9** 184–95

[52] Pliszka S R 2005 The neuropsychopharmacology of attention-deficit/hyperactivity disorder *Biol. Psychiatry* **57** 1385–90

[53] Purkayastha P, Malapati A, Yogeeswari P and Sriram D 2015 A review on GABA/glutamate pathway for therapeutic intervention of ASD and ADHD *Curr. Med. Chem.* **22** 1850–59

[54] Hughes K A, Moore R A, Morris P H and Corr P J 2012 Throwing light on the dark side of personality: reinforcement sensitivity theory and primary/secondary psychopathy in a student population *Pers. Individ. Differ.* **52** 532–36

[55] Gray J A 1970 The psychophysiological basis of introversion–extraversion *Behav. Res. Therapy* **8** 249–66

[56] Walker J L, Lahey B B, Russo M F, Frick P J, Christ M A G, Mcburnett K, Loeber R, Stouthamer-Loeber M and Green S M 1991 Anxiety, inhibition, and conduct disorder in children: I. Relations to social impairment *J. Am. Acad. Child Adolesc. Psychiatry* **30** 187–91

[57] Corr P J 2004 Reinforcement sensitivity theory and personality *Neurosci. Biobehav. Rev.* **28** 317–32

[58] Day J J and Carelli R M 2007 The nucleus accumbens and Pavlovian reward learning *Neuroscientist* **13** 148–59

[59] Dunbar R I M and Shultz S 2007 Evolution in the social brain *Science* **317** 1344–47

[60] Rogers R D 2011 The roles of dopamine and serotonin in decision making: evidence from pharmacological experiments in humans *Neuropsychopharmacology* **36** 114–32

[61] Corr P J 2013 Approach and avoidance behaviour: multiple systems and their interactions *Emotion Rev.* **5** 285–90

[62] Walsh A, Johnson H and Bolen J D 2012 Drugs, crime, and the epigenetics of hedonic allostasis *J. Contemp. Crim. Justice* **28** 314–28

[63] Larsson H, Chang Z, Donofrio B M and Lichtenstein P 2013 The heritability of clinically diagnosed attention deficit hyperactivity disorder across the lifespan *Psychol. Med.* **44** 2223–29

[64] Faraone S V and Mick E 2010 Molecular genetics of attention deficit hyperactivity disorder *Psychiatric Clin. N. Am.* **33** 159–80

[65] Coings D, Chen T, Blum K, Mengucci J, Blum S and Meshkin B 2005 Neurogenetic interactions and aberrant behavioral co-morbidity of attention deficit hyperactivity disorder (ADHD): dispelling myths *Theor. Biol. Med. Modell.* **2** 50

[66] Martin J, ODonovan M C, Thapar A, Langley K and Williams N 2015 The relative contribution of common and rare genetic variants to ADHD *Transl. Psychiatry* **5** e506

[67] Bobb A J, Castellanos F X, Addington A M and Rapoport J L 2006 Molecular genetic studies of ADHD: 1991 to 2004 *Am. J. Med. Genetics Part B* **141B** 551–65

[68] Shaw P *et al* 2007 Polymorphisms of the dopamine D4 receptor, clinical outcome, and cortical structure in attention-deficit/hyperactivity disorder *Arch. Gen. Psychiatry* **64** 921–31

[69] Ding Y-C *et al* 2002 Evidence of positive selection acting at the human dopamine receptor D4 gene locus *Proc. Natl. Acad. Sci.* **99** 309–14

[70] Miller-Butterworth C M, Kaplan J R, Shaffer J, Devlin B, Manuck S B and Ferrell R E 2007 Sequence variation in the primate dopamine transporter gene and its relationship to social dominance *Mol. Biol. Evol.* **25** 18–28

[71] Guo G, Tong Y, Xie C-W and Lange L A 2007 Dopamine transporter, gender and number of sexual partners among young adults *Eur. J. Human Genetics* **15** 279–87

[72] Beaver K M, Wright J P and Walsh A 2008 A gene-based evolutionary explanation for the association between criminal involvement and number of sex partners *Biodemography Social Biol.* **54** 47–55

[73] Nikolas M, Friderici K, Waldman I, Jernigan K and Nigg J T 2010 Gene × environment interactions for ADHD: synergistic effect of 5HTTLPR genotype and youth appraisals of inter-parental conflict *Behav. Brain Functions* **6** 1–15

[74] Coghill D and Banaschewski T 2009 The genetics of attention-deficit/hyperactivity disorder *Expert Rev. Neurother.* **9** 1547–65

[75] Wright J P and Beaver K M 2013 Parenting and crime *The Oxford Handbook of Criminological Theory* (Oxford: Oxford University Press) pp 40–65

[76] Han J-Y, Kwon H-J, Ha M, Paik K-C, Lim M-H, Lee S G, Yoo S-J and Kim E-J 2015 The effects of prenatal exposure to alcohol and environmental tobacco smoke on risk for ADHD: a large population-based study *Psychiatry Res.* **225** 164–8

[77] Instanes J T, Halmøy A, Engeland A, Haavik J, Furu K and Klungsøyr K 2017 Attention-deficit/hyperactivity disorder in offspring of mothers with inflammatory and immune system diseases *Biol. Psychiatry* **81** 452–9
[78] Millichap J G 2008 Etiologic classification of attention-deficit/hyperactivity disorder *Pediatrics* **121** 358–65
[79] Muller C, Sampson R J and Winter A S 2018 Environmental inequality: the social causes and consequences of lead exposure *Annu. Rev. Sociol* **44** 263–82
[80] Lynch M, Schwendinger H and Schwendinger J 2008 The state of empirical research in radical criminology *Taking Stock: The Status of Criminological Theory* 15 (New Brunswick, NJ: Transaction) 191–215
[81] Ficks C A and Waldman I D 2009 Gene–environment interactions in attention-deficit/hyperactivity disorder *Curr. Psychiatr. Rep.* **11** 387–92
[82] Hartmann T 2000 *Thom Hartmanns Complete Guide to ADHD: Help for Your Family at Home, School and Work* (Nevada City, CA: Underwood)
[83] Fuller D Q, Denham T, Arroyo-Kalin M, Lucas L, Stevens C J, Qin L, Allaby R G and Purugganan M D 2014 Convergent evolution and parallelism in plant domestication revealed by an expanding archaeological record *Proc. Natl Acad. Sci.* **111** 6147–52
[84] Arcos-Burgos M and Acosta M T 2007 Tuning major gene variants conditioning human behavior: the anachronism of ADHD *Curr. Opin. Genetics Dev.* **17** 234–38
[85] Williams J and Taylor E 2006 The evolution of hyperactivity, impulsivity and cognitive diversity *J. R. Soc. Interface* **3** 399–413
[86] Eisenberg D T, Campbell B, Gray P B and Sorenson M D 2008 Dopamine receptor genetic polymorphisms and body composition in undernourished pastoralists: an exploration of nutrition indices among nomadic and recently settled Ariaal men of northern Kenya *BMC Evol. Biol.* **8** 6–12
[87] Hawks J, Wang E T, Cochran G M, Harpending H C and Moyzis R K 2007 Recent acceleration of human adaptive evolution *Proc. Natl Acad. Sci.* **104** 20753–8
[88] Cortese S 2012 The neurobiology and genetics of attention-deficit/hyperactivity disorder (ADHD): what every clinician should know *Eur. J. Paediatr. Neurol.* **16** 422–33
[89] Gilbert D L, Ridel K R, Sallee F R, Zhang J, Lipps T D and Wassermann E M 2006 Comparison of the inhibitory and excitatory effects of ADHD medications methylphenidate and atomoxetine on motor cortex *Neuropsychopharmacology* **31** 442–9
[90] Purper-Ouakil D, Ramoz N, Lepagnol-Bestel A-M, Gorwood P and Simonneau M 2011 Neurobiology of attention deficit/hyperactivity disorder *Pediatr. Res.* **69** 69r–76r
[91] Schermann H, Ankory R, Shlaifer A, Dolkart O, Rotman D, Yoffe V, Karakis I and Chechik O 2019 Lower risk of stress fractures in young adults with ADHD under chronic treatment with methylphenidate *Bone* **120** 20–4
[92] Mattes J A Treating ADHD in prison: focus on alpha-2 agonists (clonidine and guanfacine) *J. Am. Acad. Psychiatry Law* **44** 151–7
[93] Burns K A Commentary: the top ten reasons to limit prescription of controlled substances in prisons *J. Am. Acad. Psychiatry Law* **37** 50–2
[94] August G J, Realmuto G M, Macdonald A W, Nugent S M and Crosby R 1996 Prevalence of ADHD and comorbid disorders among elementary school children screened for disruptive behavior *J. Abnorm. Child Psychol.* **24** 571–95

[95] Theiner P, Ustohal L, Skront T, Bares M and Kasparek T 2015 Repetitive transcranial magnetic stimulation in ADHD *ADHD – New Directions in Diagnosis and Treatment* (Rijeka: InTech) 331–50
[96] Balconi M and Ferrari C 2013 Left DLPFC rTMS stimulation reduced the anxiety bias effect or how to restore the positive memory processing in high-anxiety subjects *Psychiatry Res.* **209** 554–9
[97] Fox M D, Liu H and Pascual-Leone A 2013 Identification of reproducible individualized targets for treatment of depression with TMS based on intrinsic connectivity *NeuroImage* **66** 151–60
[98] Niederhofer H 2008 Effectiveness of the repetitive transcranical magnetic stimulation (rTMS) of 1 Hz for attention-deficit hyperactivity disorder (ADHD) *Psychiat. Danub.* **20** 91–2
[99] Bloch Y, Harel E, Aviram S, Govezensky J, Ratzoni G and Levkovitz Y 2010 Positive effects of repetitive transcranial magnetic stimulation on attention in ADHD subjects: a randomized controlled pilot study *World J. Biol. Psychiatry* **11** 755–8
[100] Wasson A S 1981 Susceptibility to boredom and deviant behavior at school *Psychol. Rep.* **48** 901–2
[101] Anderson J C, Williams S, McGee R and Silva P A 1987 DSM-III disorders in preadolescent children. Prevalence in a large sample from the general population *Arch. Gen. Psychiatry* **44** 69–76
[102] Langbehn D R, Cadoret R J, Yates W R, Troughton E P and Stewart M A 1998 Distinct contributions of conduct and oppositional defiant symptoms to adult antisocial behavior: evidence from an adoption study *Arch. Gen. Psychiatry* **55** 821–9
[103] Ghosh A, Ray A and Basu A 2017 Oppositional defiant disorder: current insight *Psychol. Res. Behav. Manag.* **10** 353–67
[104] Hirschfield P, Maschi T, White H R, Traub L G and Loeber R 2006 Mental health and juvenile arrests: criminality, criminalization, or compassion? *Criminology* **44** 593–630
[105] Comings D E Conduct disorder: a genetic orbitofrontal lobe disorder and the major predictor of adult antisocial behavior *Biosocial Criminology: Challenging Environmentalisms Supremacy* (Hauppauge, NY: Nova Science) 145–64
[106] Sareen J, Stein M B, Cox B J and Hassard S T 2004 Understanding comorbidity of anxiety disorders with antisocial behavior: findings from two large community surveys *J. Nerv. Ment. Dis.* **192** 178–86
[107] Mordre M, Groholt B, Kjelsberg E, Sandstad B and Myhre A M 2011 The impact of ADHD and conduct disorder in childhood on adult delinquency: a 30 years follow-up study using official crime records *BMC Psychiatry* **11** 57
[108] Schoepfer A, Reitzel J D and Norris A 2018 Low self-control and ADHD: similar yet different concepts in the study of crime *J. Crim. Justice* 1–12
[109] Hinshaw S P 1992 Academic underachievement, attention deficits, and aggression: comorbidity and implications for intervention *J. Consult. Clin. Psychol.* **60** 893–903
[110] Gudjonsson G H, Sigurdsson J F, Young S, Newton A K and Peersen M 2009 Attention deficit hyperactivity disorder (ADHD). How do ADHD symptoms relate to personality among prisoners? *Pers. Individ. Differ.* **47** 64–8
[111] Rösler M *et al* 2004 Prevalence of attention deficit/hyperactivity disorder (ADHD) and comorbid disorders in young male prison inmates *Eur. Arch. Psychiatry Clin. Neurosci.* **254** 365–71

[112] Machado A, Rafaela D, Silva T, Veigas T and Cerejeira J 2017 ADHD among offenders: prevalence and relationship with psychopathic traits *J. Atten. Disord* **24** 2020
[113] Buitelaar N J L, Posthumus J A and Buitelaar J K 2015 ADHD in childhood and/or adulthood as a risk factor for domestic violence or intimate partner violence *J. Attent. Disord* **24** 1203–14
[114] Eme R Attention deficit hyperactivity disorder and males in the juvenile justice system *Contemporary Trends in ADHD Research* (New York: InTech) 183–96
[115] Berryessa C M 2016 Attention, reward, and inhibition: symptomatic features of ADHD and issues for offenders in the criminal justice system *ADHD Attent. Deficit Hyperactivity Disord.* **9** 5–10
[116] Fletcher J M and Wolfe B L 2009 Long-term consequences of childhood ADHD on criminal activities *J. Ment. Health Policy Econ.* **12** 119–38
[117] Wright J P and Boisvert D 2009 What biosocial criminology offers criminology *Crim. Justice Behav.* **36** 1228–40
[118] Heylen B, Pauwels L, Beaver K and Ruffinengo M 2015 Defending biosocial criminology: on the discursive style of our critics, the separation of ideology and science, and a biologically informed defense of fundamental values *J. Theor. Philos. Criminol.* **7** 83–96

IOP Publishing

Neurological Disorders and Imaging Physics, Volume 4
Application to attention deficit hyperactivity disorder
Ayman El-Baz and Jasjit S Suri

Chapter 8

Supporting academic activities of children with developmental disorders and off-task behavior through technological aids and cognitive-behavioral strategies: a selective overview

Fabrizio Stasolla and Alessandro O Caffò

8.1 Introduction

Students with developmental disabilities (DD) and off-task behavior may experience significant learning problems. Thus, the may be affected by attention deficit hyperactivity disorders (ADHD), which may have negative outcomes in their daily academic life [1, 2]. A basic feature of ADHD is a delay in executive functions, which reflects in the inability to adequately manage cognitive processes, emotional responses, and actions [3]. Furthermore, ADHD may have deleterious outcomes on the individual's academic performance and on-task behavior in the classroom [4]. Thus, it may significantly hamper the child's social image, desirability and status [5]. Additionally, these difficulties may impact the individual's capacities for regulating time, managing everyday life activities, monitoring tasks, behavior, and frustration tolerance or emotional regulation [6]. Different contributions emphasize that attention and cognitive fluency, and executive functions in students with ADHD are relevantly compromised [7–10]. Typically, both medical/pharmacological and/or psychological approaches are considered [11, 12]. Behavioral strategies are commonly embedded [13]. Recently, a novel and unexplored option such as exercise has been investigated [14]. Few studies considered the use of assistive technology (AT) to promote self-determination and independence, most of which rely on conference papers [15–18]. Fewer deal with the effects of cognitive-behavioral treatments on ADHD and academic performance, while none is available on the on-task behavior, at least by searching on Scopus database using ADHD, cognitive-behavioral interventions and on-task behavior as keywords [19, 20].

doi:10.1088/978-0-7503-1822-8ch8

The medical approach mostly depends on the use of stimulants (e.g., amphetamine, and methylphenidate), which may have intolerable side effects and many families are concerned about overmedicating the child with negative outcomes in both the short-term (e.g., headache, nausea, and/or lack of appetite), or long-term (e.g., reduced growth progression) side consequences of stimulants [21]. Moreover, a certain number of patients do not adequately respond to the pharmacological intervention [22]. Behavioral and psychological strategies may be considered bulky and hard to follow based on patient and family reports [23]. Symptoms of ADHD may re-emerge with the interruption of medical or psychological therapies [24]. Physical exercise is revealed to have beneficial and long-term effects on cognitive functions, blood pressure and flow, enhanced brain plasticity, attention and information processing [25]. However, none of the aforementioned approaches promotes the child's positive participation and independent behavioral responses. To tackle the latter issue, one should rely on cognitive-behavioral and/or AT-based intervention, aimed at pursuing the above indicated rehabilitative goals [26, 27].

Cognitive-behavioral strategies support the progressive awareness of the participant's own behavior, based on learning processes (i.e., causal relation between participant's response and rewarding events). An illustrative example is provided by the self-monitoring technique. That is, during a self-monitoring intervention phase, the child is equipped with a 2-columns grid representing the attention and inattention behaviors, respectively and irregular instruction cues automatically delivered by the teacher, the caregiver, and/or a suitable technological system. The child, who is preliminarily informed about the operant definitions of both the on/off task behaviors and the coding systems (i.e., a total interval coding system is usually adopted for the on task behavior while a partial interval coding system is commonly used for the off-task behavior) is requested to monitor his/her own behavior contingently to the instruction cues for each observed interval. Thus, the child is gradually expected to acquire the awareness of his/her on/off task behaviors and regulate both accordingly [28].

AT includes all equipment, pieces, instruments, and systems finalized at fostering the inclusion and the positive occupation of an individual with ADHD, learning difficulties, and/or developmental disabilities. That is, the AT-based intervention will fill the existing gap between the personal capacities and the environmental requests. Once the participant exhibits a behavioral response will be enabled with independence, positive occupation, and constructive engagement [29, 30]. For instance, a child with ADHD may be enabled to achieve the academic tasks in the classroom through the implementation of an AT-based solution with verbal or pictorial prompts [31].

In light of the above, the first goal of this chapter will be to present a selective review of the newest empirical studies available in the literature on the implementation of both cognitive-behavioral programs and AT-based interventions to reduce the off-task behavior and improve the academic life of students with DD during classroom. Second, the effects of the aforementioned trainings on the indices of constructive engagement as an index of the participants' satisfaction will be emphasized whenever available. Additionally, data concerning the social validation assessments to emphasize the effectiveness will be reported. Third, strengths and weaknesses of the reviewed studies will be critically discussed as well as practical features of the findings. Fourth, the limitations of the current selective overview will be pointed out. Finally, relevant directions for future perspectives on this specific topic will be highlighted.

8.2 Method

An electronic search was completed in Scopus database. ADHD, learning difficulties, developmental disabilities, on-task behavior, academic performance, classroom, cognitive-behavioral interventions, AT-based programs, self-determination, independence, social validation, positive participation, constructive engagement, and quality of life were merged in Scopus as keywords. A supplementary manual search was added. The eligibility criteria included (a) an empirical contribution (i.e., review papers and/or theoretical articles were preliminarily excluded), (b) the implementation of an AT-based intervention and/or a cognitive-behavioral program, (c) publication time interval comprised between 2010 and 2019, (d) English language of the retained study, and (e) at least a participant who was diagnosed with ADHD and who was aged between 6 and 19 years (i.e., we were focused on childhood and adolescence).

Accordingly, five basic categories of studies were selected, specifically (a) the executive functions, (b) the neuropsychological features, (c) emotional control, (d) time management, and (e) brain–computer interfaces. Overall, 24 studies were retained with 2617 participants involved. Along the following paragraphs, we present a concise description of the selected studies, with the objectives of the contributions, the recruited participants, the adopted procedures, and the main findings. A synoptic table with the implemented interventions, the AT devices used, and outcomes will be added as completion (table 8.1).

8.3 Literature overview

8.3.1 Executive functions

Executive functions are significantly impaired among individuals with ADHD. Notably, children with ADHD may experience relevant delays in cognitive processes. Thus, they are sensitive to time variance [32]. For example, approximately 30% of children with ADHD emphasize working memory abnormalities. That is, the capacities of encoding, storing, and manipulating information are negatively affected. Accordingly, on-task behavior and academic performance may be frequently compromised. AT-based programs and cognitive-behavioral interventions are commonly focused on promoting the inclusion and task achievements in school settings. Four contributions were reviewed within this section with 135 participants recruited (see table 8.1) [33–36].

Ackermann *et al* [33] randomly assigned sixty participants who were aged between 11 and 15 years to cognitive working memory training, whereas medication (i.e., pharmacological treatment) was either pursued or not included because any randomization was considered. Data showed positive outcomes of the cognitive training on the various elements of the executive functions. Specifically, the training

Table 8.1. Reviewed studies grouped according their category and arranged in alphabetic order.

Authors	Participants	Ages	Group	Strategy	Outcomes
Abikoff *et al* [56]	158	8–10	TM	Behavioral intervention	Eight negative
Ackermann *et al* [33]	60	11–15	EF	Cognitive training	Three negative
Bikic *et al* [34]	70	6–13	EF	Clinical trial	All positive
Brunstein-Klomek *et al* [47]	18	10–17	TM	Psychotherapy	All positive
Bul *et al* [54]	170	7–10	TM	Clinical trial	Two negative
Chcko *et al* [40]	85	7–11	NF	Neurological treatment	Five negative
Davis *et al* [41]	40	8–10	NF	Digital intervention	All positive
Eyouboglu & Eyouboglu [55]	83	6–12	TM	Questionnaire	Three negative
Fabio *et al* [37]	23	9–10	NF	Neurological treatment	All positive
Fabio and Urso [38]	280	7–10	NF	Neurological treatment	All positive
Geissler *et al* [53]	1160	12–17	TM	Randomized study	Ten negative
Lim *et al* [60]	172	6–12	BCI	Training program	Two negative
Lim *et al* [62]	20	6–12	BCI	Training program	All positive
Lynch *et al* [42]	10	8–12	NF	Parents interviews	Two negative
Miranda *et al* [49]	172	7–11	EC	Theory of mind	Two negative
Park *et al* [59]	5	7.8	BCI	Game training	All positive
Pezzica *et al* [52]	46	6–9	TM	Pictorial cues	Six negative
Qian *et al* [61]	66	9–10	BCI	Training program	All positive
Smith *et al* [50]	80	14–18	EC	Longitudinal study	All positive
Stasolla *et al* [36]	3	8–10	EF	Self-monitoring	All positive
Tsai *et al* [51]	61	6–16	EC	Questionnaire	One negative
Veenman *et al* [46]	114	8–10	EC	Behavioral program	Four negative
Wei *et al* [48]	20	10	EC	Experimental training	All positive
Zuckerman *et al* [35]	2	6–7	EF	Assistive technology	All positive

Note: EF = executive functions; nf = neuropsychological features; ec = emotional control; tm = time management; bci = brain–computer interface.

enabled the participants with ADHD to achieve their academic tasks similarly to the control group. With regard to the central executive control, the contingent effect of the cognitive training and the pharmacological assumption outlined an improved performance of the participants with ADHD, comparable to the performance of the typically-developed children. No transfer was either detected or recorded to other cognitive processes. Nevertheless, the pharmacological assumption by participants with ADHD demonstrated that the cognitive training successfully decreased both hyperactivity and impulsivity manifestations at two-month follow-up.

Bikic *et al* [34] carried out a clinical trial, which evaluated the effects of a computerized intervention focused on multiple cognitive functions. Seventy participants who were aged between 6 and 13 years were enrolled and assigned to intervention or control group. The experimental group was exposed to an eight-week training and both groups were treated as usual and were examined with respect to cognitive processes, symptoms, behavioral and functional outcomes measures after 8, 12, and 24 weeks. No relevant effects emerged either on the basic outcome variable (i.e., sustained attention) or on the secondary outcome measure (i.e., parent and teacher-rated ADHD).

Zuckerman *et al* [35] developed a prototype tangible assistive technology aimed at enhancing executive functions during daily activities. It was planned on the following features: (a) programmed techniques suggested by experts, (b) decreased conflicts with caregivers, (c) avoidance of intrusion, (d) improved flexibility and independence. These features were included in a prototype encompassing six tangible items, each representing an activity that needed to be concluded during a child's morning activity, and a tablet application for programmed tasks and matching them with items. An initial assessment of the prototype with two case-studies evidenced an improved organization and time management, enhanced fulfillment, and fewer conflicts with the family during morning activities.

Stasolla *et al* [36] exposed three children with cerebral palsy and symptoms of ADHD (i.e., off-task behaviors and limited capacities of executive functions), who were aged between 8 and 10 years old, to a systematic comparison between a DRA, that is a differential reinforcement of an alternative behavior and a self-monitoring procedure to achieve academic activities in the classroom (i.e., focused on promoting the on-task and reducing the off-task behaviors). Besides the academic performance, the participants' positive mood was considered. Participants' preference checks on both strategies were additionally considered. Finally, a social rating with 24 external support teachers was evaluated. The study was conducted following an alternating treatments design embedded in a non-concurrent multiple baseline design across participants. A three-month maintenance phase was implemented. Results demonstrated the effectiveness of both strategies. All the participants assessed the self-monitoring during the preference checks as more preferable. Social experts considered the self-monitoring as preferable as well, if compared to the DRA.

8.3.2 Neuropsychological features

Besides the executive functions, the neuropsychological correlates represent a critical feature of children with ADHD. Thus, the literature commonly emphasizes that individuals with ADHD usually have multiple neuropsychological deficits, with some of them displaying a single deficit, while others have multiple deficits and/or any other deficit. Therefore, considering the neuropsychological features in the ADHD population seems to be crucial. Essentially, the reaction time variability and lack of emotional regulation have been largely reported in school-aged children. Both (i.e., time variability and lack of emotional regulation) are associated with ADHD but considered independently of deficits in executive functions. Consequently, this section examines the neuropsychological aspects separately from the executive functions as a result from the literature available. Five studies were reviewed with 183 participants recruited (see table 8.1) [37, 38, 40–42].

For example, Fabio *et al* [37] assessed whether visual working memory phases such as encoding and recall were impaired in children with ADHD. Second, the electroencephalogram (EEG) measures as neuropsychological correlated were recorded with regard to both effective and ineffective encoding. The EEG measures were evaluated before, during and after the working memory task. That is, encoding and recall were examined. Twenty-three children between 9 and 10 years old and a diagnosis of ADHD were compared to twenty-three typically developed children (i.e., control group). The encoding phase was recorded through eye-tracker and the recall phase through the free recall span measure. Results emphasized lower eye-tracker measurements and free span recall in the experimental group (i.e., children with ADHD). Furthermore, lower levels of EEG alpha, beta, and theta bands were evidenced in children with ADHD, except for the effective encoding, where beta bands for both groups were comparable.

Fabio and Urso [38] analyzed the attention network comparing three different groups, namely (a) children with a typical development, (b) children with low attention, and (c) children affected by ADHD. Fifteen participants were enrolled for both groups (a) and (b), and 14 children were recruited for the group of ADHD (c). The study was conducted according to the *Attention Network Theory* [39]. Data demonstrated that children with ADHD had low scores of accuracy, and high measures of reaction time. No deficits were evidenced for orienting and vigilance among children with ADHD. Conversely, systematic delays in the effectiveness of executive network were outlined if compared to typically-developed children and participants with low levels of attention.

Chacko *et al* [40] evaluated the potential of combining a neuro-cognitive treatment with behavioral parent training (BPT) to enhance cognitive functions, decrease psychiatric symptoms, and different indices of functional delay in school-age children who were aged between 7 and 11 years and received a diagnosis of ADHD by their neurologist. Eighty-five participants were randomly included to either *Cognitive Working Memory Training* (CWMT) linked with an empirically supported manual-based BPT program or to a placebo version of the CWMT, associated with an identical BPT intervention. Executive functions consolidation (i.e., attention control/short-long term memory), working memory processing and manipulation, ADHD and symptoms oppositional defiant disorder (ODD) symptoms, impairments in parent–child dynamics, familial impairments, and overall functional compromise were examined as dependent variables. Data suggested significant outcomes of the combined program (i.e., CWMT and BPT) on the improvement of executive functions. However, no relevant effects on ADHD, ODD symptoms and functional outcomes emerged. Hence, the data did not corroborate the efficacy of the combined sequence of the aforementioned interventions for helping children with neurodevelopmental disorders and ADHD.

Davis *et al* [41] conducted an empirical investigation aimed at assessing the suitability and examined dependent measures for a novel digital intervention, which targeted executive functions involved in ADHD. Forty participants with ADHD and forty participants without ADHD were enrolled. Following psychiatric assessment, ADHD evaluations, and neuropsychological measures, participants were exposed to 28-days of at-home treatment. Neuropsychological evaluation was retested at end-of-study along with treatment satisfaction variables. Eighty-four percent of intervention sessions were successfully completed. Relevant enhancements were found on a computerized attention activity for the ADHD group and significantly compromised ADHD High Severity subgroup. Any variation was observed for the control group. Spatial working memory was additionally enhanced for both ADHD group and High Severity subgroup.

Lynch *et al* [42] examined the manifestation of hoarding disorder among students with an age included between 8 and 12 years old and a diagnosis of ADHD through parents' perception. Ten parents responded to a semi-structured interview. Data were assessed using an Interpretative Phenomenological Perspective. Six different themes were considered, namely (a) emotional distress, (b) parental avoidance and accommodating behaviors, (c) family impacts of hoarding, (d) excessive acquisition and saving, (e) executive functions, and (f) parental insight and intervention. Conversely to other findings, data suggested that emotional distress was closely linked to hoarding disorder and constituted its core. Accordingly, practitioners, psychologists, clinicians, and neurologists may analyze conceptualizing, evaluating, and evaluating hoarding disorder in children with ADHD, through cognitive-behavioral programs.

8.3.3 Emotional control

One of the most compromised features among children with ADHD is undoubtedly their emotional control. Children with ADHD and developmental disorders frequently fail to profitably manage their emotional responses due to impulsivity and frontal lobe disorders matched to limbic region damage. In fact, they may experience tantrum behaviors if combined with autism spectrum disorders. Additionally, emotional regulation may be significantly lacking, with negative outcomes on social interactions with peers and teachers or caregivers. Moreover, academic performance and the on-task behaviors may be commonly poor accordingly [43, 44]. To tackle this issue, one may use AT-based interventions and cognitive-behavioral approaches aimed at adequately calibrating emotional control itself [45]. Six contributions were retained along the current section with 419 students recruited (see table 8.1) [46–51].

Veenman *et al* [46] evaluated the suitability of the positive and rules program (PR program), a behavioral teacher treatment focused on ADHD disorders in the school setting including both participant-focused and setting-focused interventions. Primary school students with ADHD symptoms were recruited. Two randomized groups (i.e., experimental and control groups) were enrolled with 58 and 56 participants, respectively. Educator and family ratings were adopted to evaluate behavioral, emotional, and social levels of performance at the beginning, during, and after the study. The treatment effect was examined using intention-to-treat multiple responses. Data showed that educators estimated beneficial outcomes on ADHD disorders and adaptive skills. Such effects were not generalized in other settings (i.e., home). As a consequence, the PR program was considered promising to promote and improve adaptive behaviors in children with ADHD, and was assessed as reliable to prevent behavioral problems.

Brunstein-Klomek *et al* [47] addressed the effectiveness and the efficacy of a psychotherapeutic intervention for adolescents with depression who were affected by ADHD and presented learning difficulties. Thus, the treatment combined interpersonal, emotional, and behavioral features. Eighteen adolescents who were aged between 10 and 17 years and presented specific learning disorders, ADHD, and depression or anxiety symptoms. Fifteen completed the intervention. Seven concluded a three-month follow-up. The program included 15 sessions per week and three sessions of follow-up. The skills-based program focused on a specific problematic area and was aimed at improving the participants' capacities of overcoming with their behavioral and emotional problems. Furthermore, their abilities of enhancing both relational and emotional functioning. Data suggested that the treatment was feasible to administrate with high fulfillment. The participants' performances significantly improved. The follow-up evidenced fewer problems and more significant enhancement concerning the depression levels. The three-month follow-up additionally suggested that various of the behavioral modifications for these adolescents could express a delay effect.

Wei *et al* [48] assessed the outcomes of an emotional short-term working memory (EWM) training on cognitive processes. Twenty participants diagnosed with ADHD were randomly included either in an EWM (i.e., experimental group) or a control group. Their chronological mean age was 10.25 and no difference of age was observed between groups. A 1.5 h EWM training was implemented for the treated group. For the non-treated group an occupational program was assessed. Different features of the phases were critically assessed in the control group, notably: at the beginning of the program, with the operant definition of the rehabilitative objectives, the role and knowledge of trainers; during the intervention the use of different methods and structures of the training program; after the intervention the way to facilitate transfer and persistence after the course such as reminders and meetings. Results evidenced the beneficial outcomes of executive functions in the treated group with statistical differences with regard to the non-treated group. Moreover, executive reaction time ability significantly improved in the experimental group and remained unmodified in the non-treated group.

Miranda *et al* [49] evaluated cognitive and social delays in children diagnosed with ADHD, autism spectrum disorders and high functioning (HASD). A systematic comparison with typically developed peers was assessed on different measures of theory of mind (ToM). A second goal concerned the relationship between cognitive processes and social cognition. One hundred and twenty-six children, 52 with HASD, who were aged between 7 and 11 years, 35 diagnosed with ADHD, and 39 with typical development (TD) were recruited and completed the NEPSY II social perception subtests. Adults rated their childrens' ToM skills through the Theory of Mind Inventory (ToMi). Teachers responded to the Behavior Rating Inventory of Executive Functions (BRIEF). Data revealed that ADHD and HASD groups provided worse performance than TD children on the verbal ToM task, and only the scores of the HASD group were worse than the TD group on the contextual ToM task. Additionally, adults evaluated that the HASD group had more problems than ADHD and TD groups on applied ToM. Finally, a relevant difference was observed in the executive functions processes. Specifically, behavioral control such as emotional regulation were closely associated with social and cognitive skills in children with developmental disorders and ADHD. Conversely, meta-cognitive processes such as reasoning and projecting were strictly linked with social cognition in the HASD group.

Smith *et al* [50] carried out a longitudinal study finalized at evaluating the outcomes and correlations between sex, preschool hyperactivity and long-term health risks. Early assessment and strategic approaches were targeted. The primary objective was to clarify the highest long-term negative consequence for mental health. Eighty participants estimated as hyperactive by their parents were compared with 75 non-hyperactive (i.e., control group). They were aged between 14 and 18 years. At aged three, individuals in the hyperactive group presented similar behavioral problems irrespective of being male or female. Once they were adults, these participants evidenced higher levels of ADHD and behavioral disorders, combined with mood problems, anxiety and autism as with intellectual delays. Preschool hyperactivity was a valid predictor of poor adolescent/adult effects for males, across domains with outcomes being specifically driven by impulsivity. Conversely, for females the consequences of preschool hyperactivity were lower and were reduced to non-relevant levels when other preschool difficulties were considered.

Tsai *et al* [51] evaluated the scores of ADHD disorders, behavioral and emotional abnormalities, and physical health among a pediatric population with seizures. Sixty-one participants with epilepsy, who were aged between 6 and 16 years were included and were matched to a control group matched for age, sex, and parent-education. Empirical evidences on demographic, parental reports on the Child Behavior Checklist and Swanson, Nolan, and Pelham, version IV scale (SNAP-IV) and medical treatments were considered. Children with seizures had higher ADHD manifestations, combined with a larger number of behavioral and emotional disorders than the control group. An earlier onset of seizures positively anticipated ADHD outcomes.

8.3.4 Time management

Time management and the awareness of on-task behavior are significantly impaired among students with ADHD and developmental disorders. Thus, individuals affected by ADHD spend a lot of time off-task and are unable to self-manage profitably their time. Academic performance in school and home settings are compromised accordingly. Cognitive-behavioral programs and AT-based interventions within this specific framework are consequently focused on increasing the academic performance, the time of self-management, and the awareness of both. Five contributions were reviewed within this section with 1617 participants enrolled (see table 8.1) [52–56].

Pezzica *et al* [52] verified if students with ADHD could use visual cues similarly to typically developed students. Forty-six participants with ADHD who attended primary school and were aged between 6 and 9 years were systematically compared with 46 peers without ADHD. Participants were requested to perform two specific academic activities within two experimental conditions: (a) on-task versus (b) off-task. The academic activities were examined through the Children's Awareness of Attention via Drawing (CAAD). Results basically evidenced that the performance of both conditions was similar. However, a delay in the awareness of an adequate posture was observed, due to worse development in the management of school tools and higher manifestation of negative feelings over the time. Students with ADHD acquired the awareness of school context but were unable to reach it. Cognitive programs may be useful and helpful, matched to structured learning, for children with ADHD to profitably manage their time.

Geissler *et al* [53] assessed a randomized controlled study which addressed the needs of an intensive cognitive-behavioral intervention with parent-based telephone-assisted self-help for 1160 adolescents with an age ranging between 12 and 17 years, and assessed with ADHD and developmental disorders. The participants underwent an intervention as usual (TAU) observation phase over thirty days. During step 2 those still profoundly affected were randomly assigned to the experimental group with an Individualized Modular Treatment Program (IMTP) or a telephone-assisted self-help program for parents (TASH) as a control group. The experimental group was exposed to a specific treatment with a target to the needs of adolescents with ADHD and developmental disorders. It included 10 trials of individual cognitive-behavioral therapy with the adolescents and/or the parents. The participants selected 3 out of 10 available focus modules (e.g., organizational skills and planning, emotional regulation, problem solving, and stress management, dysfunctional family communication). Primary outcome concerned modification in ADHD symptoms in a clinician-rated diagnostic interview. The data were evaluated at the beginning of the study, after the TAU phase, after the intervention sessions, and following a 12-month follow-up.

Bul *et al* [54] identified which sub-groups of students diagnosed with ADHD highly benefited from playing a Serious Game (SG) program emphasized in a clinical setting to enhance behavioral responses. One hundred and seventy participants were recruited and divided according to pre-test features (i.e., gender, age, intellectual level of functioning, medication use, computer experience, ADHD subtype, severity of inattention problems, severity of impulsivity/hyperactivity problems, oppositional and/or defiant disorder, conduct disorders). Primary outcomes were different collaborative and social skills. Data demonstrated that two groups were recognized such as girls with greater improvements in organization/planning as compared to all the participants included in the sample. Moreover, among boys those with fewer baseline levels of hyperactivity and higher levels of conduct disorders evidenced more enhancements in their projecting capacities when they played Serious Game intervention as compared to the rated treatment effect of the whole sample.

Eyuboglu and Eyuboglu [55] examined sleep problems of 83 children who were aged between 6 and 12 years and had never been exposed any psychiatric intervention and evaluated the effects of such difficulties in functionality. The experimental group was compared to a control group represented by 106 healthy children. A psychiatric diagnostic interview was implemented for all the participants. The parents completed the Conner's Parent Questionnaire to rate the intensity of ADHD in the children, the Children's Sleep Habits Questionnaire (CSHQ) to rate sleep problems and the Weiss Functional Impairment Rating Scale to rate the functionality of the children. Data emphasized that the total scores of subscales and scales of the CSHQ were significantly higher in the experimental group. Participants with ADHD slept one hour later and sleep quantity was 105 h less than the control group. A strong correlation between sleep difficulties, ADHD severity, and functionality of the participants emerged.

Abikoff *et al* [56] compared the effectiveness of two different behavioral programs to enhance organization, time management, and planning problems in third to fifth-grade participants (i.e., age comprising between 8 and 10 years) diagnosed with ADHD. In a dual-site randomized controlled trial, 158 participants were assigned to organizational skills training (i.e., 64 OST participants), a performance-based program that prevented skills training (i.e., 61 children), or a control-list (i.e., 33 children). Interventions were 20 individual clinic-based sessions over 10–12 weeks. The first group (i.e., OST) included skills building delivered primarily to the participant. The second group considered both parents and teachers to reinforce participants contingently for meeting end-point target goals. Primary dependent variables were children's organizational skills scales. Other relevant functions were evaluated. Percentage of participants no longer meeting inclusion criteria for the first group impairments informed on clinical significance. Observations were examined at post-treatment, one-month post-treatment, and twice in the following school year. Data evidenced that significant consolidation outcomes were observed for both interventions. Accordingly, two different targeting organization and time management problems were observed in participants diagnosed with ADHD, which determined relevant functional enhancements. The programs were successful for participants with ADHD and organizational difficulties.

8.3.5 Brain–computer interface (BCI)

Neurofeedback represents a neurophysiological technique aimed at teaching patients and/or users to self-regulate brain activity by themselves. The main objective is to increase cognitive processes functioning and reduce clinical symptoms. Among brain activity patterns, sensorimotor rhythms seem to be highly promising and a crucial target to attempt to improve motor skills. One of the most recent applications is BCI, which represents a specific communication pattern between an improved or a wired brain and an outside technological tool. Usually assistive modules for profoundly impaired persons to foster their control of external equipments or to communicate are usually embedded in a BCI-based intervention. Another issue may concern brain feedback useful to self-control and manage brain activity for the intervention on seizures, ADHD, neurodevelopmental disorders, behavioral problems, or cognitive enhancement among healthy individuals [57, 58]. Four studies were reviewed within this section with 263 participants enrolled (see table 8.1) [59–64].

Park *et al* [59] assessed a game-based program system to examine and improve the reading skills of participants diagnosed with ADHD. A tale-based interactive narrative was implemented as an intervention approach in the behavior, which registered brainwaves and motion-sensing technology. Five participants with ADHD were enrolled (mean age 7.8) for a five-week program on a weekly basis, including a 20-minute long adaptation session and four 40-minute long sessions. The statistical analysis included pre- and post-KNISE-BAAT and general reading questionnaires. Additionally, sensing data were examined. In-depth post-interviews were conducted at the end of the program for qualitative analysis. Paired T-Test on both reading comprehension test demonstrated enhancement in both reading aloud and comprehension. Sensing data suggested an improved attention span and a decreased hyperactivity behavior over the time. The interview analysis corroborated the quantitative test results. Accordingly, data confirmed the efficacy of this approach to ameliorate the reading ability, increase attention span and foster behavior inhibition of children diagnosed with ADHD.

Lim *et al* [60] implemented BCI as a neuro-feedback therapy in a controlled randomized trial to evaluate if an 8-week BCI-based training program fostered inattentive symptoms of participants with ADHD compared to a wait-list-control group, and the effects of a 12-week lower-intensity intervention. One hundred and seventy-two participants, who were aged 6–12 years, and attended an outpatient child psychiatric medical center, diagnosed with inattentive or combined subtypes of ADHD and not exposed either to pharmacological or behavioral intervention, were included in either the experimental group or the waitlist-control group. Intervention included 3 BCI-based programs over 8 weeks, followed by 3 training sessions per month over 12 weeks. Conversely, the control group was exposed to a similar 20-week program after a wait-time of 8 weeks. Results evidenced reduced inattentive symptoms in the experimental group compared to the waitlist-control group. Consequently, data suggested that the BCI-based attention training program can improve ADHD negative outcomes after a minimum of 24 sessions and consolidation may emphasize this improvement.

Qian *et al* [61] evaluated the effects on the topographical alterations of large-scale brain functional network produced by an 8-week BCI based attention program in 66 ADHD males diagnosed with ADHD using resting-state functional magnetic resonance strategy. The boys were aged between 9 and 10 years. Two groups were compared, namely (a) the experimental, and (b) the control group. Results showed a greater reduction of the inattentive symptoms in the experimental group, closely linked with different brain network reorganization observed after the intervention. Specifically, the control group showed an improved functional connectivity within the central attention network and enhanced functional connectivity between task-positive networks and sub-cortical regions. Conversely, the experimental group did not show the aforementioned data. Furthermore, it evidenced decreased degree centrality and clustering coefficient as well as improved closeness in task-positive and the default mode networks after the program. Furthermore, this reduced local functional processing was correlated with fewer inattentive/internalizing difficulties after 8-week BCI-based intervention across ADHD participants. Results corroborated the efficacy of a BCI-based attention program to facilitate cognitive-behavioral improvements in the enrolled boys, by reorganizing brain functional activity from more regular to more random configurations, because it renormalized salience network processing.

Lim *et al* [62] investigated a BCI-based intervention which involved 20 non-medicated ADHD participants, who were aged between 6 and 12 years, with relevant inattentive symptoms (i.e., combined and inattentive ADHD subtypes). The system monitored attention processes through a head band with dry EEG sensors, which was implemented to drive a feed forward game. The system was adopted for each child by measuring the EEG parameters during a Stroop task. The program included 8-week training which consisted of 24 sessions followed by 3 once-monthly booster program sessions. Following the training, both parent-rated inattentive and hyperactive-impulsive symptoms on the ADHD Rating Scale evidenced relevant improvement. Further analysis emphasized that the variations in the EEG based BCI ADHD severity measure were closely associated with the variations in the ADHD Rating Scale scores. Consequently, the BCI-based attention program game system was a suitable intervention for non-mediated children diagnosed with ADHD.

8.4 Discussion

The retained empirical contributions showed the suitability and the effectiveness of cognitive-behavioral interventions and AT-based programs to enhance the independence of children with ADHD. Their constructive engagement and on-task behavior were enhanced and both inattentive, and/or hyperactivity/impulsivity symptoms were reduced. Academic performance and constructive engagement were improved. Results were widely positive, but few and rare failures occurred (i.e., 1.6%). The impact on participants' status, social desirability and image was positive as well as on both parents and caregivers. Data were widely supported by previous findings [63–66] and indicated the following comments.

First, cognitive-behavioral programs and AT-based interventions were successful and effective to profitably increase positive participation, sustained attention, and academic performance. Thus, children with ADHD significantly reduced their inattentive and/or hyperactive/impulsive symptoms and were positively occupied. In fact, they were constructively engaged while dealing with their academic tasks. The executive functions were enhanced, the emotional regulation was fostered, the time management was monitored, and their cerebral activity was controlled [67, 68].

Second, the off-task behavior was significantly prevented. That is, children with ADHD were enabled to complete their academic tasks and their inclusion in both school and home settings was relevantly facilitated. In fact, they were capable of pursuing their academic achievements within the classroom with positive outcomes on their peers and teachers. Specific techniques (e.g., self-monitoring, behavioral interventions, and cognitive training) were helpful for regulating the ADHD children's behaviors. Both cognitive and emotional processes were significantly enhanced with beneficial effects on their immediate environment and/or context (e.g., parents and caregivers) [69, 70].

Third, children with ADHD progressively acquired the awareness of their own behavior and made it purposeful. Thus, the ADHD symptoms were overall controlled and reduced. Because the participants of the reviewed studies were successfully treated, one may argue that the learning process was meaningfully improved. Furthermore, follow-up and maintenance phases demonstrated that ADHD participants confirmed their acquisition and awareness process over the time. Self-management and mastering of the individuals involved were facilitated. The relationship between teachers and students was consolidated. Similarly, parents favorably rated the implemented interventions focused on enhancing attention and reducing inattentive and impulsive symptoms [71, 72].

Fourth, social validation procedures, whenever available, confirmed the interventions' efficacy and suitability in daily contexts. Both social and clinical validity were corroborated accordingly. External raters who had personal or professional experience with developmental disabilities and rehabilitative programs favorably evaluated the use of both AT-based interventions and cognitive-behavioral programs. As a result, even professionals and/or parents of children with learning difficulties who were not included in the interventions could appreciate the implementation of these specific treatments [73–75].

Fifth, the participants' quality of life was relevantly improved. Both direct and indirect measures recorded (e.g., indices of happiness and positive participation or self-report data recorded through questionnaires) suggested that the recruited participants enjoyed the intervention sessions, with positive outcomes on their quality of life. One may argue that the participants' social desirability, image, and status were significantly supported with beneficial consequences on their environment [76–78].

Sixth, although data were largely positive, few failures occurred. One should analyze the failures to examine and identify the plausible causes. For instance, one may argue that the intervention program was not adequately tailored on the targeted users, or the learning process was not sufficiently programmed and considered. Otherwise, the planned time was not adequately prolonged. Each feature should be singly investigated [79, 80].

8.5 Limitations

Although positive, our selective overview should be interpreted with caution. In fact, it was neither a systematic review nor a meta-analysis. Accordingly, further reviews on this specific topic should be carried out. Most of the reviewed studies are groups-based. Few single-case studies have been considered and only rare longitudinal investigations. The generalization process has not been examined. A functional analysis/assessment of the ADHD targeted symptoms should be conducted in future research. The technological devices used in the retained studies were still limited, as well as cognitive-behavioral programs.

8.6 Conclusion

In light of the above, the findings of the current literature overview corroborated the efficacy and the suitability of both cognitive-behavioral programs and AT-based interventions. Thus, inattentive and hyperactive or impulsive symptoms were significantly reduced, and the on-task behavior was increased. Academic tasks were favorably achieved and completed. External raters corroborated such a conclusion. Additionally, beneficial consequences on participants' quality of life were both directly and indirectly evidenced.

Future perspectives on this topic should address the following issues: (a) further extension of the reviewed studies through systematic reviews and meta-analysis, (b) enlargement to further children with ADHD and/or other learning difficulties, (c) functional assessment of the targeted challenging behaviors, (d) new generalization phases, and (e) the use of new and more sophisticated technological devices in order to respond to complex situations caused by the developmental disabilities.

References

[1] Sharma S R, Gonda X and Tarazi F I 2018 Autism spectrum disorder: classification, diagnosis and therapy *Pharmacol. Ther.* **190** 91–104

[2] Goode A P *et al* 2018 Nonpharmacologic treatments for attention-deficit/hyperactivity disorder: a systematic review *Pediatrics* **141** e20180094

[3] Lopez P L, Torrente F M, Ciapponi A, Lischinsky A G, Cetkovich-Bakmas M, Rojas J I, Romano M and Manes F F 2018 Cognitive-behavioural interventions for attention deficit hyperactivity disorder (ADHD) in adults *Cochrane Database Syst. Rev.* **2018**

[4] Chigome A K, Matsangaise M M and Meyer J C 2018 Adult attention deficit hyperactivity disorder and its management *SA Pharm. J.* **85** 31–8

[5] Marraccini M E, Weyandt L L, Gudmundsdottir B G, Oster D R and McCallum A 2017 Attention-deficit hyperactivity disorder: clinical considerations for women *J. Midwifery Women's Health* **62** 684–95

[6] Katzman M A, Bilkey T S, Chokka P R, Fallu A and Klassen L J 2017 Adult ADHD and comorbid disorders: clinical implications of a dimensional approach *BMC Psychiatry* **17** 302
[7] He J A and Antshel K M 2017 Cognitive behavioral therapy for attention-deficit/hyperactivity disorder in college students: a review of the literature *Cogn. Behav. Pract.* **24** 152–73
[8] Hollis C, Falconer C J, Martin J L, Whittington C, Stockton S, Glazebrook C and Davis E B 2017 Annual research review: digital health interventions for children and young people with mental health problems—a systematic and meta-review *J. Child Psychol. Psychiatry Allied Discip.* **58** 474–503
[9] Bikic A, Reichow B, McCauley S A, Ibrahim K and Sukhodolsky D G 2017 Meta-analysis of organizational skills interventions for children and adolescents with attention-deficit/hyperactivity disorder *Clin. Psychol. Rev.* **52** 108–23
[10] Prevatt F 2016 Coaching for college students with ADHD *Curr. Psychiatry Rep.* **18** 110
[11] Asherson P 2016 ADHD across the lifespan *Medicine* **44** 683–86
[12] Satapathy S, Choudhary V, Sharma R and Sagar R 2016 Nonpharmacological interventions for children with attention deficit hyperactivity disorder in India: a comprehensive and comparative research update *Indian J. Psychol. Med.* **38** 376–85
[13] Bluschke A, Roessner V and Beste C 2016 Editorial perspective: how to optimise frequency band neurofeedback for ADHD *J. Child Psychol. Psychiatry Allied Discip.* **57** 457–61
[14] Ng Q X, Ho C Y X, Chan H W, Yong B Z J and Yeo W 2017 Managing childhood and adolescent attention-deficit/hyperactivity disorder (ADHD) with exercise: a systematic review *Complement Ther. Med.* **34** 123–8
[15] Vuori M, Tuulio-Henriksson A, Nissinen H and Autti-Rämö I 2015 Family-based psychosocial interventions for children with attention deficit hyperactivity disorder (ADHD), oppositional defiant disorder, and conduct disorder *Duodecim* **131** 1561–8
[16] Pezzica S and Bigozzi L 2015 A cognitive behavioral parent training and mentalizing for children with ADHD *Psicol Clin Sviluppo* **19** 271–96
[17] Antshel K M and Olszewski A K 2014 Cognitive behavioral therapy for adolescents with ADHD *Child Adolesc. Psychiatr. Clin. N. Am.* **23** 825–42
[18] Philipsen A 2012 Psychotherapy in adult attention deficit hyperactivity disorder: implications for treatment and research *Expert Rev. Neurother.* **12** 1217–25
[19] Rutledge K J, van den Bos W, McClure S M and Schweitzer J B 2012 Training cognition in ADHD: current findings, borrowed concepts, and future directions *Neurotherapeutics* **9** 542–58
[20] Asherson P 2012 ADHD across the lifespan *Medicine* **40** 623–7
[21] Storebø O J, Skoog M, Damm D, Thomsen P H, Simonsen E and Gluud C 2011 Social skills training for attention deficit hyperactivity disorder (ADHD) in children aged 5 to 18 years *Cochrane Database Syst. Rev.* **12** CD008223
[22] Verma R, Balhara Y P S and Mathur S 2011 Management of attention-deficit hyperactivity disorder *J. Pediatr. Neurosci.* **6** 13–8
[23] Newark P E and Stieglitz R-D 2010 Therapy-relevant factors in adult ADHD from a cognitive behavioural perspective *Atten. Deficit. Hyperact. Disord.* **2** 59–72
[24] Knouse L E and Safren S A 2010 Current status of cognitive behavioral therapy for adult attention-deficit hyperactivity disorder *Psychiatr. Clin. N. Am.* **33** 497–509
[25] Melillo R and Leisman G 2009 Autistic spectrum disorders as functional disconnection syndrome *Rev. Neurosci.* **20** 111–31

[26] Knouse L E, Cooper-Vince C, Sprich S and Safren S A 2008 Recent developments in the psychosocial treatment of adult ADHD *Expert Rev. Neurother.* **8** 1537–48
[27] Toplak M E, Connors L, Shuster J, Knezevic B and Parks S 2008 Review of cognitive, cognitive-behavioral, and neural-based interventions for attention-deficit/hyperactivity disorder (ADHD) *Clin. Psychol. Rev.* **28** 801–23
[28] Antshel K M and Barkley R 2008 Psychosocial Interventions in attention deficit hyperactivity disorder *Child Adolesc. Psychiatr. Clin. N. Am.* **17** 421–37
[29] Ramsay J R 2007 Current status of cognitive-behavioral therapy as a psychosocial treatment for adult attention-deficit/hyperactivity disorder *Curr. Psychiatry Rep.* **9** 427–33
[30] Manassis K 2007 When attention-deficit/hyperactivity disorder co-occurs with anxiety disorders: effects on treatment *Expert Rev. Neurother.* **7** 981–8
[31] Safren S A 2006 Cognitive-behavioral approaches to ADHD treatment in adulthood *J. Clin. Psychiatry* **67** 46–50
[32] Barkley R A 2004 Adolescents with attention-deficit/hyperactivity disorder: an overview of empirically based treatments *J. Psychiatr. Pract.* **10** 39–56
[33] Ackermann S, Halfon O, Fornari E, Urben S and Bader M 2018 Cognitive working memory training (CWMT) in adolescents suffering from attention-deficit/hyperactivity disorder (ADHD): a controlled trial taking into account concomitant medication effects *Psychiatry Res.* **269** 79–85
[34] Bikic A, Leckman J F, Christensen T Ø, Bilenberg N and Dalsgaard S 2018 Attention and executive functions computer training for attention-deficit/hyperactivity disorder (ADHD): results from a randomized, controlled trial *Eur. Child Adolesc. Psychiatry* **27** 1563–74
[35] 2015 Initial validation of an assistive technology to enhance executive functioning among children with ADHD *Proc. of IDC 2015: The 14th Int. Conf. on Interaction Design and Children*
[36] Stasolla F, Caffò A O, Perilli V, Boccasini A, Damiani R and Albano V *et al* 2017 Comparing self-monitoring and differential reinforcement of an alternative behavior to promote on-task behavior by three children with cerebral palsy: a pilot study *Life Span Disabil.* **20** 63–92
[37] Fabio R A, Caprì T, Mohammadhasani N, Gangemi A, Gagliano A and Martino G 2018 Frequency bands in seeing and remembering: comparing ADHD and typically developing children *Neuropsychol. Trends* **24** 97–116
[38] Fabio R A and Urso M 2014 The analysis of attention network in ADHD, attention problems and typically developing subjects *Life Span Disabil.* **17** 199–221
[39] Michelini G, Jurgiel J, Bakolis I, Cheung C H M, Asherson P, Loo S K, Kuntsi J and Mohammad-Rezazadeh I 2019 Atypical functional connectivity in adolescents and adults with persistent and remitted ADHD during a cognitive control task *Transl. Psychiatry* **9** 137
[40] Chacko A *et al* 2018 Sequenced neurocognitive and behavioral parent training for the treatment of ADHD in school-age children *Child Neuropsychol.* **24** 427–50
[41] Davis N O, Bower J and Kollins S H 2018 Proof-of-concept study of an at-home, engaging, digital intervention for pediatric ADHD *PLoS One* **13** e0189749
[42] Lynch F A, Moulding R and McGillivray J A 2017 Phenomenology of hoarding in children with comorbid attention-deficit/hyperactivity disorder (ADHD): the perceptions of parents *Compr. Psychiatry* **76** 1–19

[43] Stasolla F, Perilli V, Boccasini A, Caffò A O, Damiani R and Albano V 2016 Enhancing academic performance of three boys with autism spectrum disorders and intellectual disabilities through a computer-based program *Life Span Disabil.* **19** 153–83

[44] Stasolla F, Damiani R, Perilli V, D'Amico F, Caffò A O, Stella A, Albano V, Damato C and Di Leone A 2015 Computer and microswitch-based programs to improve academic activities by six children with cerebral palsy *Res. Dev. Disabil.* **45–46** 1–13

[45] Stasolla F, Caffò A O, Perilli V, Boccasini A, Damiani R and D'Amico F 2018 Assistive technology for promoting adaptive skills of children with cerebral palsy: ten cases evaluation *Disabil. Rehabil. Assistive Technol.* **14** 489–502

[46] Veenman B, Luman M, Hoeksma J, Pieterse K and Oosterlaan J 2019 A randomized effectiveness trial of a behavioral teacher program targeting ADHD symptoms *J. Atten. Disord.* **23** 293–304

[47] Brunstein-Klomek A, Kopelman-Rubin D, Apter A, Argintaru H and Mufson L 2017 A pilot feasibility study of interpersonal psychotherapy in adolescents diagnosed with specific learning disorders, attention deficit hyperactive disorder, or both with depression and/or anxiety symptoms (IPT-ALD) *J. Psychother. Integr.* **27** 526–39

[48] Wei X, Chen X, He L and Liu L 2017 Behavioral inhibition improvement through an emotional working memory (EWM) training intervention in children with attention deficit/hyperactivity disorder *NeuroQuantology* **15** 261–8

[49] Miranda A, Mercader J, Fernández M I and Colomer C 2017 Reading performance of young adults with ADHD diagnosed in childhood: relations with executive functioning *J. Atten. Disord.* **21** 294–304

[50] Smith E, Meyer B J, Koerting J, Laver-Bradbury C, Lee L, Jefferson H, Sayal K, Treglown L, Thompson M and Sonuga-Barke E J S 2017 Preschool hyperactivity specifically elevates long-term mental health risks more strongly in males than females: a prospective longitudinal study through to young adulthood *Eur. Child Adolesc. Psychiatry* **26** 123–36

[51] Tsai F-J, Liu S-T, Lee C-M, Lee W-T, Fan P-C, Lin W-S, Chiu Y-N and Gau S S-F 2013 ADHD-related symptoms, emotional/behavioral problems, and physical conditions in Taiwanese children with epilepsy *J. Formos Med. Assoc.* **112** 396–405

[52] Pezzica S, Vezzani C and Pinto G 2018 Metacognitive knowledge of attention in children with and without ADHD symptoms *Res. Dev. Disabil.* **83** 142–52

[53] Geissler J *et al* 2018 Individualised short-term therapy for adolescents impaired by attention-deficit/hyperactivity disorder despite previous routine care treatment (ESCAadol)-study protocol of a randomised controlled trial within the consortium ESCAlife *Trials* **19** 1469

[54] Bul K C M, Doove L L, Franken I H A, Van Der Oord S, Kato P M and Maras A 2018 A serious game for children with attention deficit hyperactivity disorder: who benefits the most? *PLoS One* **13** e0193681

[55] Eyuboglu M and Eyuboglu D 2018 Behavioural sleep problems in previously untreated children with attention deficit hyperactivity disorder *Psychiatry Clin. Psychopharmacol.* **28** 19–24

[56] Abikoff H, Hechtman L, Klein R G, Gallagher R, Fleiss K, Etcovitch J, Cousins L, Greenfield B, Martin D and Pollack S 2004 Social functioning in children with ADHD treated with long-term methylphenidate and multimodal psychosocial treatment *J. Am. Acad. Child Adolesc. Psychiatry* **43** 820–9

[57] Fabio R A, Gangemi A, Capri T, Budden S and Falzone A 2018 Neurophysiological and cognitive effects of transcranial direct current stimulation in three girls with Rett Syndrome with chronic language impairments *Res. Dev. Disabil.* **76** 76–87

[58] Amin M Z, Zamin N, Rahim H A, Hassan N I and Kamarudin N D 2018 Robo therapist: a sustainable approach to teach basic expressions for special needs children in Malaysia *Int. J. Eng. Technol.* **7** 103–6
[59] Park K, Kihl T, Park S, Kim M-J and Chang J 2016 Narratives and sensor driven cognitive behavior training game platform *2016 IEEE/ACIS 14th Int. Conf. on Software Engineering Research, Management and Applications, SERA 2016*
[60] Lim C G, Poh X W W, Fung S S D, Guan C, Bautista D, Cheung Y B, Zhang H, Yeo S N, Krishnan K and Lee T S 2019 A randomized controlled trial of a brain–computer interface based attention training program for ADHD *PLoS One* **14** e0216225
[61] Qian X *et al* 2018 Brain–computer-interface-based intervention re-normalizes brain functional network topology in children with attention deficit/hyperactivity disorder *Transl. Psychiatry* **8** 149
[62] Lim C G, Lee T S, Guan C, Fung D S S, Zhao Y, Teng S S W, Zhang H and Ranga Rama Krishnan K 2012 A brain-computer interface based attention training program for treating attention deficit hyperactivity disorder *PLoS One* **7** e0046692
[63] Stasolla F, Perilli V and Damiani R 2014 Self monitoring to promote on-task behavior by two high functioning boys with autism spectrum disorders and symptoms of ADHD *Res. Autism Spectr. Disord.* **8** 472–9
[64] Fabio R A and Caprì T 2017 The executive functions in a sample of Italian adults with ADHD: attention, response inhibition and planning/organization *Mediterr. J. Clin. Psychol.* **5**
[65] Fabio R A 2017 The study of automatic and controlled processes in ADHD: a reread and a new proposal *Mediterr. J. Clin. Psychol.* **5** 1–17
[66] Fabio R A and Caprì T 2015 Autobiographical memory in ADHD subtypes *J. Intellect. Dev. Disabil.* **40** 26–36
[67] Fabio R A, Castriciano C and Rondanini A 2015 ADHD: auditory and visual stimuli in automatic and controlled processes *J. Atten. Disord.* **19** 771–8
[68] Fabio R A and Antonietti A 2012 Effects of hypermedia instruction on declarative, conditional and procedural knowledge in ADHD students *Res. Dev. Disabil.* **33** 2028–39
[69] Catherine Joy R, Mercy Prathyusha T, Tejaswini K, Rose Mary K, Mounika M, Thomas George S, Panicker A S and Subathra M S P 2019 Certain analysis on attention-deficit hyperactivity disorder among elementary level school children in Indian scenario *Adv. Intell. Sys. Comput.* **750** 569–76
[70] Jarraya S, Wagnr M, Jarraya M and Engel F A 2019 12 weeks of kindergarten-based yoga practice increases visual attention, visual-motor precision and decreases behavior of inattention and hyperactivity in 5-year-old children *Front Psychol.* **10** 769
[71] Stasolla F, Stella A and Damato C 2014 Verbal prompts to promote on-task behavior by a child with multiple disabilities in classroom *Psicol. Clin. Sviluppo* **18** 211–30
[72] Modesto-Lowe V, Charbonneau V and Farahmand P 2017 Psychotherapy for adolescents with attention-deficit hyperactivity disorder: a pediatrician's guide *Clin. Pediatr.* **56** 667–74
[73] Perilli V, Stasolla F, Caffò A O, Albano V and D'Amico F 2019 Microswitch-cluster technology for promoting occupation and reducing hand biting of six adolescents with fragile X Syndrome: new evidence and social rating *J. Dev. Phys. Disabil.* **31** 115–33
[74] Stasolla F, Caffò A O, Perilli V and Albano V 2019 Supporting locomotion fluency of six children with Cornelia de Lange syndrome: awareness of microswitch responding and social validation *Technol. Disabil.* **30** 209–20

[75] Stasolla F, Perilli V, Caffò A O, Boccasini A, Stella A and Damiani R *et al* 2017 Extending microswitch-cluster programs to promote occupation activities and reduce mouthing by six children with autism spectrum disorders and intellectual disabilities *J. Dev. Phys. Disabil.* **29** 307–24

[76] Lancioni G E, Singh N N, O'Reilly M F, Sigafoos J, Chiapparino C, Stasolla F and Oliva D 2007 Using an optic sensor and a scanning keyboard emulator to facilitate writing by persons with pervasive motor disabilities *J. Dev. Phys. Disabil.* **19** 593–603

[77] Lancioni G E, Singh N N, O'Reilly M F, Sigafoos J, Chiapparino C, Stasolla F, Bosco A, De Pace C and Oliva D 2007 Enabling a young man with minimal motor behavior to manage independently his leisure television engagement *Percept. Mot. Skills* **105** 47–54

[78] Stasolla F, Damiani R, Perilli V, Di Leone A, Albano V, Stella A and Damato C 2014 Technological supports to promote choice opportunities by two children with fragile X syndrome and severe to profound developmental disabilities *Res. Dev. Disabil.* **35** 2993–3000

[79] Stasolla F, Boccasini A, Perilli V, Caffò A O, Damiani R and Albano V 2014 A selective overview of microswitch-based programs for promoting adaptive behaviors of children with developmental disabilities *Int. J. Ambient Comput. Intell.* **6** 56–74

[80] Reale L and Bonati M 2018 ADHD prevalence estimates in Italian children and adolescents: a methodological issue *Ital. J. Pediatr.* **44** 108

Chapter 9

Neuroimaging in attention deficit hyperactivity disorder

Pankhuree Vandana, Shikha Verma and L Eugene Arnold

9.1 Introduction

Attention-deficit/hyperactivity disorder (ADHD) is one of the most common childhood psychiatric disorders. It is chronic: 60%–70% patients have continued symptoms in adolescence and adulthood. According to the National Survey of Children's Health, data gathered from parental report, the prevalence of ADHD diagnosis in ages 4–17 increased by 42% between 2003 and 2011 and was around 11% in 2011 [1, 2]. Based on diagnostic interview data from the National Comorbidity Survey-Adolescent supplement, lifetime prevalence of ADHD among US adolescents ages 13–17 is 8.7%. Males' prevalence is four times as much as females [3, 4]. Adult ADHD prevalence in ages 18–44 was 4.4% according to National Comorbidity Survey Replication (NCS-R) [5]. It is to be noted that these prevalence estimates are based on the *Diagnostic and Statistical Manual IV*.

ADHD is two clusters of symptoms suggesting either predominantly inattentiveness or predominantly increased hyperactivity/impulsivity or combined presentation. Research increasingly looks at ADHD as a dimensional-symptom based disorder rather than as a categorical disorder and as a lifespan disorder rather than a childhood disorder [6–8].

Hyperactivity and poor impulse control decrease with age and, it is mainly inattention and poor organizational skills, which are predominant in late adolescence and adulthood [9, 10]. Untreated ADHD can have adverse psycho-social outcomes [11]. It is possible that the 60%–70% who continue to have symptoms in adulthood constitute a distinct subpopulation having more stable psychopathology and likely different neuroanatomical representation than those whose symptoms subside or decrease significantly with age [12].

Despite the above evidence and the detrimental impact on behavioral, social, psychological and occupational functioning, the authenticity and validity of this

doi:10.1088/978-0-7503-1822-8ch9

diagnosis has been questioned in public and by the media, making it crucial that biological markers for diagnosis be developed for this impairing disorder. Neuroimaging provides an important tool to explore diagnosis, prognosis, and course, and possibly can also guide discovery of novel treatments.

9.2 Gross structural differences in the ADHD brain

Several neuroimaging techniques have been utilized by research groups worldwide to study ADHD structural and functional characteristics and help understand the pathophysiology of this impairing disorder. Anatomically, in children and adolescents who have ADHD, a marked reduction in cerebral volume is reported [13].

Many studies have confirmed that reductions in volumes are even more significant in the prefrontal cortex than overall cerebral volume, particularly in the dorsolateral prefrontal cortex (DLPFC) [13, 14], a region that plays a crucial role in task organization, planning, working memory and attention [12]. Inhibitory controls are through ventrolateral prefrontal regions and emotional control, social behaviors and disinhibitions are mediated by orbitofrontal areas. Results of study done by Hesslinger *et al* in 2002 suggested decreased left orbitofrontal volumes but they were limited by the number of participants in the study [15].

The dorsal anterior cingulate cortex (ACC) not only assists with reward-based learning but also serves an important role in executive functioning, regulating inhibitory control and identifying targets. Overmeyer *et al* reported reduction in right posterior ACC volume in children with ADHD in 2001 [12, 16].

The executive, memory and visuospatial functions are impaired in lesions of cerebellar hemispheres and dentate nucleus. For cognitive functions, lobules VI and VII of the posterior cerebellar lobes are involved [17]. Loss of cerebellar volume is noticed to be more profound than prefrontal volume reduction and, these changes are in parallel with noticed attentional deficits and clinical-rated global scales [18].

Many studies reported a decrease in size of the caudate nucleus in the basal ganglia [13, 14]. A few studies implicated unilateral reduction of the pallidum as well. The basal ganglia are a dopaminergic region supporting motor programs, automatization and procedural learning [12, 13, 16, 19].

Corpus callosum injuries lead to deficits in sustained attention [20], which can contribute further to impaired learning and memory [21]. Posterior corpus callosum volume reductions have been discovered [22–24]. Castallenos *et al* in 2002 indicated that bilateral temporal volume reductions and left occipital volume reductions are likely the result of general volume reduction in children who have ADHD [18]. Effects of sensory processing on cognition and affect or vice versa, due to reduced temporal lobes in children with ADHD, are yet to be determined. Posterior parietal cortex lesions can impair selective attention on the contralateral side and increase attention towards the side of the lesion [25, 26].

9.3 Functional neuroimaging

Research in ADHD has focused on the inattention component of this disorder and so far, three major networks are proposed (figure 9.1) [27–29].

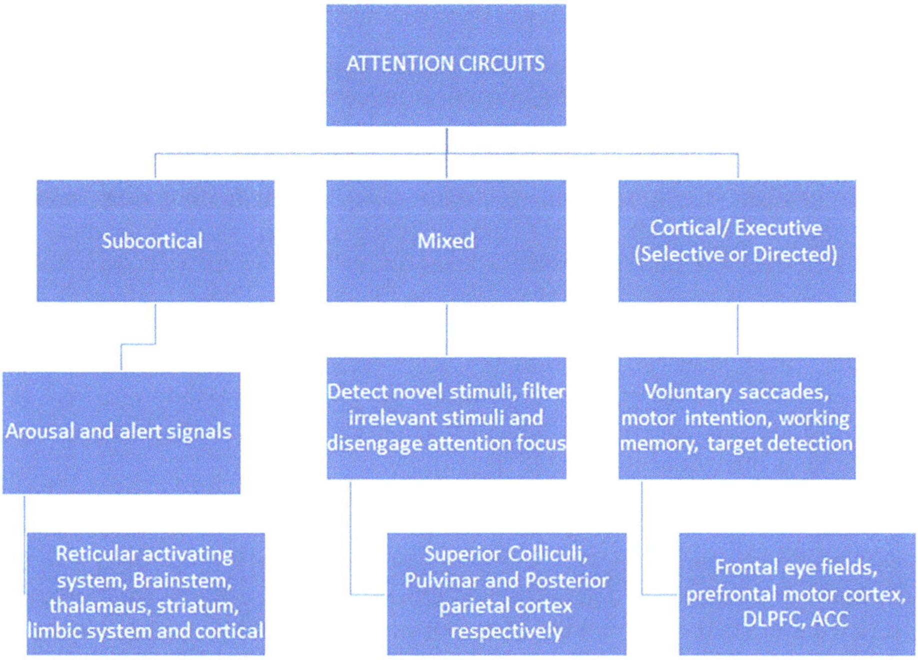

Figure 9.1. Three circuits subserving attention. All three of these circuits were reported to be dysfunctional in children with ADHD in event-related fMRIs by Konrad *et al* [30].

One of the early studies by Zametkin *et al* in 1990 using PET scan for adult ADHD led to an increased interest in utilizing structural and functional neuroimaging in understanding the neurobiology of this disorder [31]. The international ENIGMA-ADHD (enhanced neuroimaging genetics through meta-analysis) working group completed a cross sectional meta-analysis of over 1713 patients with ADHD and 1529 controls supporting the delayed maturation theory of ADHD. Due to the risk of ionizing radiations to developing brain, research has largely restricted techniques to MRI and fMRI in these pediatric studies [32].

9.3.1 ADHD and MRI

Anatomical MRI studies have moved from trying to find clear pathological findings in patients to identifying group level average size differences in different regions of interest in the brain (ROIs). Key findings of recent collaborative and meta-analytic studies have shown smaller basal ganglia, amygdala and hippocampus in children with attention deficit hyperactivity disorder (ADHD). Longitudinal imaging data indicate slower growth of cerebellar white matter in early childhood but faster growth in late childhood [33]. Although the differences and effect size of these differences are modest, they can give powerful insights into the neurobiology of the diagnosis. A comparative meta-analysis done by Normal *et al* showed decreased volume and hypoactivation during inhibitory processing in the putamen and insula in ADHD as compared to reverse findings in obsessive compulsive disorder [34].

9.3.2 ADHD and fMRI

ADHD is a context-based illness and symptom manifestation can vary in severity depending on the task at hand. fMRI studies enable the assessment of regional brain functioning across contexts and cognitive demands [35]. Several studies using fMRI demonstrate hypoactivation in frontal regions and frontal-striatal networks compared to controls during a cognitive control task. Similar findings were noted by Valera *et al* in their adult ADHD study. During a verbal working memory task, adults with ADHD had decreased activation in the left inferior occipital and cerebellar regions as well as a deactivation trend in the right prefrontal cortex pointing towards a possible underactivation in fronto-cerebellar circuitry, similar to the findings in children [36]. Interestingly, Rubia *et al* in 2009 found overall reduced fronto-striato-parietal-cerebellar activation in medication-naive children with ADHD during a cognitive task which 'normalized' with the administration of a single dose of methylphenidate (MPH) [37].

Another circuit of interest in ADHD has been the 'default mode network' (DMN) which includes the medial prefrontal cortex, posterior cingulate, precuneus and medial/lateral/inferior parietal cortices which are believed to be associated with task-irrelevant mental processes and mind wandering [38]. Sonuga-Barke and Castellanos postulated that children with ADHD do not suppress the DMN during task related mental processes, leading to attention deficit. Children with ADHD in a Paterson *et al* study (2009) were unable to suppress DMN activity to the same degree as healthy controls while performing the Stroop Color and Word Test. This underactivity was shown to again 'normalize' with MPH [39].

9.3.3 ADHD and PET studies

An often used functional neuroimaging technique provides a general assessment of functional activity using blood flow and glucose metabolism. Additionally, specific neuroreceptor radiotracers can be used for specific analyses of neurotransmitter binding site density. Keeping in mind the efficacy of stimulant medications in treating ADHD, a few PET studies have focused on dopamine transporter binding, dopamine receptor binding and dopamine metabolism in adolescents and adults with ADHD [40]. These studies have found abnormalities in each of these, supporting the theory of catecholamine deficiency in ADHD. With PET imaging, Volkow *et al* demonstrated lower than normal D2/D3 receptor and DAT availability in the accumbens and midbrain regions in adults with ADHD compared to healthy controls, implicating the dopamine reward pathway which may explain the problem of delayed gratification in ADHD. Additionally, in this study, D2/D3 measures in accumbens were correlated with dimensions of attention, supporting the observation of worsening of attention span during tasks that are boring and not rewarding to the individual [41]. Furthermore, this group utilized a D2 receptor radioligand and PET to assess the effects of oral MPH on extracellular dopamine in the striatum and its association with a rewarding (mathematical problem solving with monetary reinforcement) versus a neutral task. The results showed that MPH when coupled with the mathematical task, significantly increased extracellular dopamine as compared to when it was coupled with the neutral task and increased subjective feelings of motivation. The mathematical task itself did not increase dopamine when coupled with a placebo. This finding supports the increased attention and motivation noted when utilizing MPH in school aged children with ADHD [42].

9.3.4 ADHD and DTI

Diffusion tensor imaging (DTI) has found a novel application in the field of ADHD by allowing study of axonal organization of the brain and white matter structure. DTI studies completed in children and adults with ADHD have pointed towards white matter abnormalities in fronto-striatal and fronto-cerebellar sites. However, these studies have been marred by methodological limitations.

9.4 Clinical application

The extent of literature in neuroimaging and ADHD has rapidly expanded in the last few years with increasing focus on clinical application of this information. Large collaborative studies have been undertaken to delineate the brain structure and function in children and adults due to the heterogeneity in the presentation of this disorder. The functional neuroimaging studies have been helpful in implicating the dopamine reward pathway and its association with important ADHD symptoms of delayed gratification, amotivation when engaged in repetitive and unrewarding tasks as well as deficits in attention.

Supporting the diagnostic specificity and validity of ADHD, meta analytic studies support unique neuroanatomical and neurofunctional differences in individuals with this disorder as compared to others. For example, ADHD is associated with decreased volume and hypoactivation during inhibitory processing in the putamen and insula where obsessive compulsive disorder shows the opposite. With larger multisite collaborative studies trying to find more robust measures of neurological changes, the field hopes to establish neuroimaging as a valid diagnostic tool for clinical use in the future. Limited information is available in regards to neuroimaging data in ADHD patients with co morbid psychiatric disorders, however, fronto-striatal brain regions are most often dysfunctional when comorbid ADHD is present.

In addition to understanding the pathophysiology of this diagnosis and its symptoms, attempts have been made to identify distinct neural changes that may underlie the subtypes of ADHD, namely combined and inattentive presentation. These attempts have faced unique challenges considering the heterogeneous presentations of ADHD symptoms in clinical population. Fair *et al* in their 2013 fMRI study point towards atypical connectivity across multiple systems, particularly, the default network in ADHD-combined versus in ADHD-inattentive, where the functional connectivity differences were more prominent in the b/l DLPF region and cerebellum in children with ADHD-inattentive type versus those with combined type. This study provides a potential pathway for clinical applications of this technique in the future [43].

Several studies have attempted to understand the course and better prognosticate the symptoms of ADHD. Impairment of cerebello-striato-frontal networks have been found in both adult and child ADHD. Several cohort studies have compared neuroimaging data in adults with persistent symptoms of ADHD in adulthood as compared to the remitters. The results of these studies have been mixed, with some studies suggesting a normalization of early microstructural anomalies in the remitters, pointing towards remission being a 'catching up and convergence towards typical dimensions' [44].

The area where neuroimaging studies have been particularly useful is to identify neurological changes that underly the mechanism of action of psychostimulants. The efficacy of psychostimulants to treat the symptoms of ADHD has been supported by extensive high quality clinical research including the NIMH Multimodal Treatment Study of ADHD. Spencer *et al* completed a qualitative review of 29 published MRI studies in an attempt to evaluate the impact of therapeutic dose of stimulants on the brain of patients with ADHD as measured by MRI-based neuroimaging studies. Despite the differences in study design, neuroimaging techniques and, regions of interest studied, as a general finding, brain measures in medicated groups of persons with ADHD are more similar to controls than those in unmediated ADHD groups [45]. This is a very important finding to debunk the controversy around the validity of this very impairing disorder.

9.5 Conclusion

Currently, neuroimaging tools remain primarily valuable for research in the field of ADHD. Creation of large multi-center collaborative study groups will help in providing more robust data of brain structural and functional differences in ADHD [44]. Considering the heterogeneity of this disorder, this would be an important step towards having a large enough sample to pick up on small but diagnosis-specific neurological anomalies that could guide treatment. Despite several methodological limitations in currently available neuroimaging trials in ADHD, it has the potential to become a valuable diagnostic tool as well as guide further research in therapeutic interventions.

References

[1] Visser S N, Danielson M L, Bitsko R H, Holbrook J R, Kogan M D, Ghandour R M, Perou R and Blumberg S J 2014 Trends in the parent-report of health care provider-diagnosed and medicated attention-deficit/hyperactivity disorder: United States, 2003–2011 *J. Am. Acad. Child Adolesc. Psychiatry* **53** 34–46.e2

[2] https://nimh.nih.gov/health/statistics/attention-deficit-hyperactivity-disorder-adhd.shtml

[3] Merikangas K R, He J P, Burstein M, Swanson S A, Avenevoli S, Cui L, Benjet C, Georgiades K and Swendsen J 2010 Lifetime prevalence of mental disorders in U.S. adolescents: results from the National Comorbidity Survey Replication-Adolescent Supplement (NCS-A) *J. Am. Acad. Child Adolesc. Psychiatry* **49** 980–9

[4] NCS-A Lifetime and 12M prevalence estimates 2005 https://hcp.med.harvard.edu/ncs/

[5] Kessler R C *et al* 2006 The prevalence and correlates of adult ADHD in the United States: results from the National Comorbidity Survey Replication *Am. J. Psychiatry* **163** 716–23
[6] Insel T R 2014 The NIMH Research Domain Criteria (RDoC) Project: precision medicine for psychiatry *Am. J. Psychiatry* **171** 395–7
[7] Woo C-W, Chang L J, Lindquist M A and Wager T D 2017 Building better biomarkers: brain models in translational neuroimaging *Nat. Neurosci.* **20** 365–77
[8] Ball G, Malpas C B, Genc S, Efron D, Sciberras E, Anderson V, Nicholson J M and Silk T J 2019 Multimodal structural neuroimaging markers of brain development and ADHD symptoms *Am. J. Psychiatry* **176** 57–66
[9] Biederman J, Faraone S V, Milberger S, Curtis S, Chen L, Marrs A, Ouletter C, Moore P and Spencer T 1996 Predictors of persistence and remission of ADHD: results from a four-year prospective follow-up study of ADHD children *J. Am. Acad. Child Adolesc. Psychiatry* **35** 343–51I/39
[10] Biederman J, Mick E and Faraone S V 2000 Age-dependent decline of symptoms of attention deficit hyperactivity disorder: impact of remission definition and symptom type *Am. J. Psychiatry* **157** 816–8
[11] Biederman J, Faraone S V, Mick E, Spencer T, Wilens T and Kiely K *et al* 1995 High risk for attention deficit hyperactivity disorder among children of parents with childhood onset of the disorder: a pilot study *Am. J. Psychiatry* **152** 431–5
[12] Schneider M, Retz W, Coogan A, Thome J and Rösler M 2006 *Eur. Arch. Psychiatry Clin. Neurosci.* **256** i32
[13] Castellanos F X *et al* 1996 Quantitative brain magnetic resonance imaging in attention deficit hyperactivity disorder *Arch. Gen. Psychiatry* **53** 607–16
[14] Filipek P A, Semrud-Clikeman M, Steingard R, Kennedy D and Biederman J 1997 Volumetric MRI analysis: comparing subjects having attention-deficit hyperactivity disorder with normal controls *Neurology* **48** 589–601
[15] Hesslinger B, Tebartz van Elst L, Thiel T, Haegele K, Hennig J and Ebert D 2002 Fronto-orbital volume reductions in adult patients with attention deficit hyperactivity disorder *Neurosci. Lett.* **328** 319–21
[16] Overmeyer S, Bullmore E T, Suckling J, Simmons A, Williams S C, Santosh P J and Taylor E 2001 Distributed grey and white matter deficits in hyperkinetic disorder: MRI evidence for anatomical abnormality in an attentional network *Psychol. Med.* **31** 1425–35
[17] Schmahmann J D and Sherman J C 1998 The cerebellar cognitive affective syndrome *Brain* **121** 561–79
[18] Castellanos F X *et al* 2002 Developmental trajectories of brain volume abnormalities in children and adolescents with attention deficit/hyperactivity disorder *JAMA* **288** 1740–8
[19] Aylward E H, Reiss A L, Reader M J, Singer H S, Brown J E and Denckla M B 1996 Basal ganglia volumes in children with attention deficit hyperactivity disorder *J. Child Neurol.* **11** 112–5
[20] Ellenberg L and Sperry R W 1979 Capacity for holding sustained attention following commissurotomy *Cortex* **15** 421–38
[21] Zaidel D W 1990 Memory and spatial cognition following commissurotomy ed F Boller and J Grafman *Handbook of Neuropsychology* vol 4 (Amsterdam: Elsevier) pp 151–66
[22] Baumgardner T L, Singer H S, Denckla M B, Rubin M A, Abrams M T, Colli M J and Reiss A L 1996 Corpus callosum morphology in children with Tourette syndrome and attention deficit hyperactivity disorder *Neurology* **47** 1–6

[23] Giedd J N, Castellanos F X, Casey B J, Kozuch P, King A C, Hamburger S D and Rapoport J L 1994 Quantitative morphology of the corpus callosum in attention deficit hyperactivity disorder *Am. J. Psychiatry* **151** 665–9

[24] Hill D E, Yeo R A, Campbell R A, Hart B, Vigil J and Brooks W 2003 Magnetic resonance imaging correlates of attention-deficit/hyperactivity disorder in children *Neuropsychology* **17** 496–506

[25] Posner M I 1995 Attention in cognitive neuroscience: an overview ed M S Gazzaniga *The cognitive neurosciences* (Cambridge MA: MIT Press) pp 615–24

[26] Ro T, Borden C, Driver J and Rafal R 2001 Ipsilesional biases in saccades but not perception after lesions of the human inferior parietal lobule *J. Cogn. Neurosci.* 920–9

[27] Posner M I and Petersen S E 1990 The attention system of the human brain *Ann. Rev. Neurosci.* **13** 25–42

[28] Coull J T, Frith C D, Frackowiak R S and Grasby P M 1996 A frontoparietal network for rapid visual information processing: a PET study of sustained attention and working memory *Neuropsychologia* **34** 1085–95

[29] Fan J, Bruce T, McCandliss D, Fossella J, Flombaum J and Posner M I 2005 The activation of attentional networks *Neuroimage* **26** 471–9

[30] Konrad K, Neufang S, Hanisch C, Fink G R and Herpertz-Dahlmann B 2006 Dysfunctional attentional networks in children with attention deficit/hyperactivity disorder: evidence from an event-related functional magnetic resonance imaging study *Biol. Psychiatry* **59** 643–51

[31] Zametkin A J, Nordahl T E, Gross M, King A C, Semple W E, Rumsey J, Hamburger S and Cohen R M 1990 Cerebral glucose metabolism in adults with hyperactivity of childhood onset *N. Engl. J. Med.* **323** 1361–6 (Seminal large-scale PET study of ADHD adults that showed global and regional hypometabolism in ADHD adults)

[32] Hoogman M *et al* 2017 Sub-cortical brain volume differences in participants with attention-deficit/hyperactivity disorder in children and adults: a cross-sectional mega-analysis *Lancet Psychiatry* **4** 310–9

[33] Shaw P *et al* 2018 A multicohort, longitudinal study of cerebellar development in attention deficit/hyperactivity disorder *J. Clin. Psychol. Psychiatry.* **59** 1114–23

[34] Norman L J, Cartisi C and Lukito S *et al* 2016 Structural and functional brain abnormalities in attention-deficit/ hyperactivity disorder and obsessive compulsive disorder: a comparative meta-analysis *JAMA Psychiatry* **73** 815–25

[35] Lisa W, Swentosky A and Gudmundsdottir B G Neuroimaging and ADHD:fMRI, PET and DTI findings, and methodological limitations *Dev. Neuropsychol.* **38** 211–25

[36] Valera E, Faraone S, Biederman J, Poldrack R and Seidman L 2005 Functional neuroanatomy of working memory in adults with attention-deficit/hyperactivity disorder *Biol. Psychiatry* **57** 439–47

[37] Rubia K, Halari R, Cubillo A, Brammer M and Taylor E 2009 Methylphenidate normalizes activation and functional connectivity deficits in attention and motivation networks in medication-naive children with ADHD during a rewarded continuous performance test *Neuropharmacology* **57** 640–52

[38] Fassbender C A lack of default network suppression is linked to increased distractibility in ADHD *Brain Res.* **1273** 114–28

[39] Peterson B, Potenza M, Wang Z, Zhu H, Martin A, Marsh R and Plessen K J 2009 An fmRI study of the effects of psychostimulants on default-mode processing during stroop task performance in youths with ADHD *Am. J. Psychiatry.* **166** 1286–94

[40] Jucaite A, Fernell E, Hlldin C, Forssberg H and Farde L 2005 Reduced midbrain dopamine transporter binding in male adolescents with attention deficit hyperactivity disorder: association between striatal dopamine markers and motor hyperactivity *Biol. Psychiatry* **57** 229–38

[41] Volkow N *et al* 2009 Evaluating dopamine reward pathway in ADHD *JAMA* **302** 1084–91

[42] Volkow N *et al* 2004 Evidence that methylphenidate enhances the saliency of a mathematical task by increasing dopamine in the human brain *Am. J. Psychiatry* **161** 1173–80

[43] Fair D *et al* 2012 Distinct neural signatures detected for ADHD subtypes after controlling for micro-movements in resting state functional connectivity MRI data *Front. Syst. Neurosci.* **6** 80

[44] Shaw *et al* 2018 ADHD Neuroimaging: What's New? *Psychiatric Times* October https://www.psychiatrictimes.com/view/adhd-neuroimaging-whats-new

[45] Spencer T, Brown A, Seidman L J, Valera E M, Makris N, Lomedico A, Faraone S V and Biederman J 2013 Effect of psychostimulants on brain structure and function in ADHD: qualitative literature review of magnetic resonance imaging-based neuroimaging studies *J. Clin. Psychiatry* **74** 9

IOP Publishing

Neurological Disorders and Imaging Physics, Volume 4
Application to attention deficit hyperactivity disorder
Ayman El-Baz and Jasjit S Suri

Chapter 10

Application of augmented reality in education of attention deficit hyperactive disorder (ADHD) children

Nor Azlina Ab Aziz and Kamarulzaman Ab Aziz

Attention deficit hyperactive disorder (ADHD) children are inattentive, impulsive and often hyperactive. Therefore, providing education for them is challenging. The education plan for these students needs to be stimulating and entertaining in order to capture their attention. It is important to ensure these students receive education so that they are not left behind their peers and to reduce social inequality. Augmented reality (AR) has been adopted in developing lesson plans and proved to improve students' learning experience, and has many benefits. This work focuses on the projects involving application of AR for an ADHD education plan. The advantages and challenges of the approach are presented. The findings show that, like their peers, ADHD students also benefit from an AR learning module but the parties involved need to address the challenges for a more effective educational system for ADHD students.

10.1 Introduction

ADHD is a psychiatric disorder that emerges during childhood and lasts a lifetime. Children with ADHD show symptoms of inattention and/or impulsivity and hyperactivity. According to the *Diagnostic and Statistical Manual* (DSM-V) a person is categorized as ADHD when s/he shows six or more symptoms of inattention and six of more symptoms of hyperactivity and impulsivity for at least half a year [1]. The symptoms of inattention are listed as follows:

- often fails to give close attention to details or makes careless mistakes in schoolwork/chores/other activities;
- often has trouble holding attention on tasks/activities;
- often does not seem to listen when spoken to directly;

- often does not follow through on instructions and fails to finish schoolwork/chores/duties;
- often has trouble organizing tasks/activities;
- often avoids, dislikes, or is reluctant to do tasks that require mental effort over a long period of time;
- often loses things necessary for tasks and activities (e.g. school materials, pencils, books, tools, wallets, keys, paperwork, eyeglasses, mobile telephones);
- often is easily distracted;
- often forgetful in daily activities.

While the symptoms of hyperactivity–impulsivity are:

- often fidgets with or taps hands or feet, or squirms in seat;
- often leaves seat in situations when remaining seated is expected;
- often runs about or climbs in situations where it is not appropriate (adolescents or adults may be limited to feeling restless);
- often unable to play or take part in leisure activities quietly;
- often 'on the go';
- often talks excessively;
- often blurts out an answer before a question has been completed;
- often has trouble waiting his/her turn;
- often interrupts or intrudes on others, for example during conversations or games.

ADHD can be categorized into three categories;

1. combined presentation: where enough symptoms of both inattention and hyperactivity-impulsivity were present for at least six months;
2. predominantly inattention presentation: where enough symptoms of inattention were present but not for hyperactivity-impulsivity; and
3. predominantly hyperactivity–impulsivity presentation: where enough symptoms of hyperactivity–impulsivity were manifested but not the inattention symptoms.

ADHD is also known as hyperkinetic disorder by the World Health Organization (WHO). It is reported that between 5% and 11% children worldwide are affected by ADHD [2–5]. Since DSM-V was published in 1994, the number of ADHD cases reported has shown an increasing trend, as shown in figure 10.1 [2]. Gender-wise, more boys are reported to be affected by ADHD than girls [6].

The causes of ADHD can be categorized as biological and environmental [6]. Biological factors include genetic heredity and brain structure, while environmental factors can be problems during and after birth, like premature birth, exposure to toxins like lead, high artificial food additive diet, usage of mobile phone by young children and parenting.

The disorder impacts the individual's performance, behaviour and social skills. ADHD children are known to be impulsive, day dreamers, inattentive, forgetful,

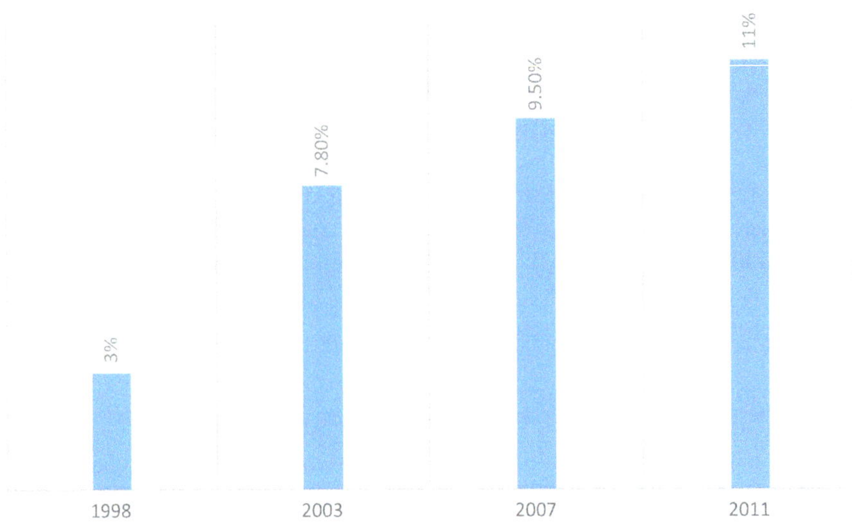

Figure 10.1. Reported ADHD cases.

sensitive, aggressive and overly active. Therefore, an education system for ADHD students needs to be tailored to better suits these students. One technology with great potential to benefit ADHD students is augmented reality (AR). AR is a variation of virtual reality (VR). However, unlike VR, where users are brought into a virtual/synthetic environment, AR merges virtual objects with the real world. Hence, AR is supporting the real world rather than replacing it with a synthetic environment. The usage of AR in education for ADHD students is able to capture the students' attention and interest [7]. In the following section, the application of AR in education specifically for ADHD students is reviewed and the challenges are presented.

10.2 ADHD and education

Studies show that students with ADHD tend to persistently perform poorly in school and frequently are among the group of underachieving students [8]. School and teachers play an important role in recognizing possible ADHD cases. The time children spend in school allows teachers to observe any possible symptoms of ADHD and alert the guardian and healthcare provider. On the other hand, one of the contributing factors to low performance of ADHD students is caused by the negative impact of the ADHD diagnosis, where it causes the parents and teachers of ADHD students not to place emphasis on the education of these children due to fear of overburdening the students [9]. The diagnosis is also found to lower the self-esteem of the students, which also leads to their poor performance.

Education plans for ADHD students need to simulate and capture the students' interest and attention to overcome their inattentiveness and easy distraction. An up-to-date teaching method which is more fun and engaging will be able to improve the learning ability of ADHD students. A stimulating approach with some physical activities is good to capture their attention. Computer aided education naturally allows interaction between a student and the subject taught and also involves multi-sensory modality. Among the technology available is AR.

10.3 Augmented reality, education and ADHD

The AR technology emerged in the 1990s and started to accelerate from 2010 due to advancement in computing power [10]. The AR technology had also been integrated to mobile applications. The most famous commercial application of AR is the Pokemon Go. The Pokemon Go is a mobile game where the players need to hunt for Pokemons in their surroundings. The Pokemons are superimposed on the surroundings and can be seen via the handphone camera.

Other than gaming, AR had been applied in many other fields, such as tourism [11–13], retail [14, 15], health [16] and military [17, 18]. Education had also taken interest in AR. Many projects involving AR for education had been proposed. Mobile AR games like the Pokemon Go are popular among children and teenagers and had been shown to be able to provide positive impact to many aspects of players including education [19]. Among the advantages of an AR based module for education are [20, 21]:

- its ability to excite and motivate learners to stay interested and engage in the subject taught;
- abstract and complex concepts can be better represented and visualized using AR;
- the sensory engagement of AR promotes better remembering among learners by experiencing the content;
- its ability to encourage students' creativity by allowing them to be bold and adventurous within a safe virtual environment; and
- the fluid support of collaboration among learners.

In [22, 23], the researchers focussed on the role of AR towards collaborative learning where students needed to communicate among themselves while using an AR module. The students in [22] worked in pairs for an AR based electricity system experiment (figure 10.2). The relation between resistance and current are experimented on using AR, where the students were able to observe how brightness of a bulb changes according to resistance value. AR provided a safe environment and a low risk experiment. The collaboration among the students was studied and it was found that AR gives positive impact to collaborative learning. Students are motivated and engaged during the process, and, more importantly, they interact and communicate with each other throughout the experiment. The communication and interaction are the main objective of collaborative learning. AR is also observed to provide positive impact to collaborative learning in younger school children and subsequently helps in their social skills development [24].

A two-year study was conducted in [25] to look into the application of AR in higher learning institutions. The study focussed on a free application, the HP Reveal, which is a repository of mobile AR with educational content. HP Reveal

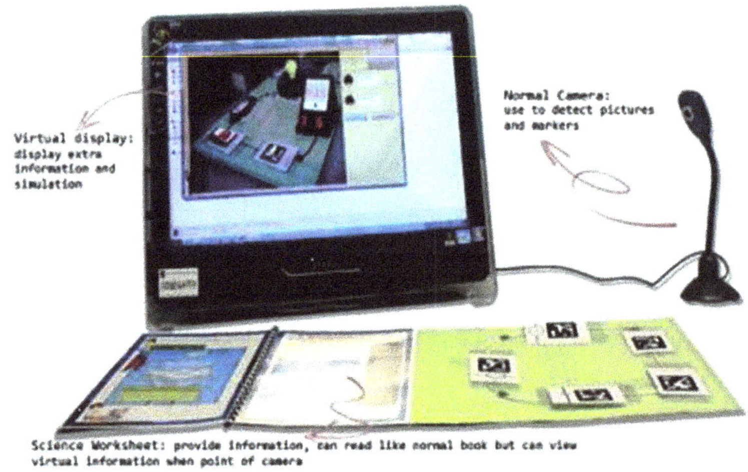

Figure 10.2. AR circuit system. Reproduced from [22] with permission of Universiti Teknologi Malaysia.

supports collaboration, interaction and engagement among its users through the social media-like follow, like and share features. The study revealed that educators are motivated to adopt mobile AR in their lesson plan due to its ability to support interaction, collaboration, digital storytelling and cultural exploration.

An AR biology module based on the Malaysian secondary school syllabus is developed in [26]. The module allows better visualization of complex concepts such as meiosis, mitosis and respiration. Virtual teacher and 3D storytelling are used in the module developed. The module objective is to improve the students' understanding and remembering of the selected complex biological processes. It also allows personalized learning while at the same time supporting the learning collaborative aspect.

Application of AR in history education is able to provide students with immersive learning experience which gives them sense of empathy to the historical events [27]. This cannot be achieved through traditional classroom and textbook. Students who are exposed to an AR based history class are reported to have better perspective on the history by experiencing the event virtually. They scored highly in tests. The immersive learning also promotes long-term memory of the subject.

Application of AR for educational purposes among ADHD students can be seen as suitable due to gamification. Numerous studies had recognised the potential of gamification and AR [28–30]. According to [31], gamification is the application of games mechanics, design and thinking or approach in order to engage users, motivate certain actions or reactions including for learning and solving problems. In [32], it was proven that there is a clear relationship between gamification on learners' motivation and engagement. Furthermore, [33] highlighted that specific games design elements have niche psychological effects. There are three main categories of how gamification is used in education [34]: (1) cognitive, where students get rules of play that promote experimentation and exploration; (2) emotional, where with gamification creates engaging emotional experiences; and

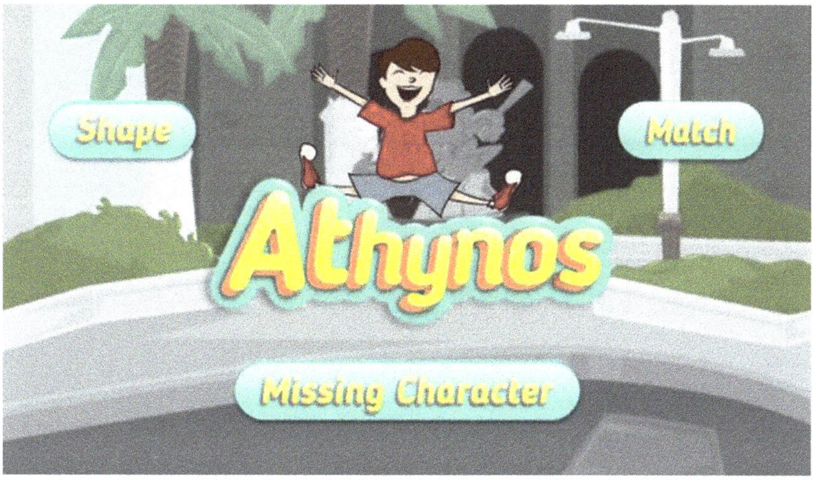

Figure 10.3. Screenshot of ATHYNOS [35]. Copyright 2019 with permission of Springer.

(3) social, where the students get to role play and take decisions as they navigate from the role's point of view. Thus, arguably education products using AR with gamification will be able to engage ADHD students better and overcome challenges pose by the ADHD symptoms, namely hyperactivity–impulsivity and inattention.

The following section will review further AR for ADHD education by highlighting some of the existing examples of AR for ADHD education products.

10.3.1 Augmented reality for ADHD education

AR is a suitable tool for inclusive education which makes it a good choice for enhancing the education plan for ADHD and special need students [21]. ATHYNOS (figure 10.3) is a prototype of an AR based serious game for ADHD therapy; it is proposed in [36, 37]. A serious game is a game design for 'serious' purpose instead of entertainment. A serious game is often used for teaching and training. It could provide hands-on experience in a safe environment. ATHYNOS is developed to improve the concentration of ADHD children. It was tested on eleven 7–10 years old children under the supervision of two specialized therapists over the period of two weeks. The findings show that ATHYNOS improved the concentration of the children. The serious game and AR approach are proven to be successful in capturing their interest, which in turn increases their participation rate. ATHYNOS also received a good response from the therapists.

An AR based project called ADHD-Edu (figure 10.4) was reported in [38], where a prototype was developed based on the pre-school English curriculum. ADHD-Edu provides an interactive and exciting education module for pre-school ADHD children so that they can learn effectively and not be left behind by other children of their age. The project focuses on pre-school, as this age is when the symptoms of ADHD start to manifest.

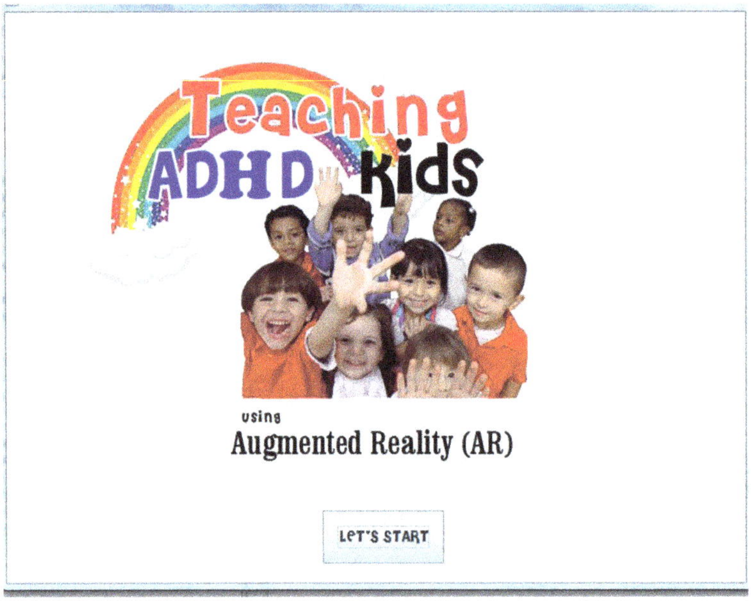

Figure 10.4. Start screen of ADHD-Edu. Reprinted from [38] with permission of UTPedia.

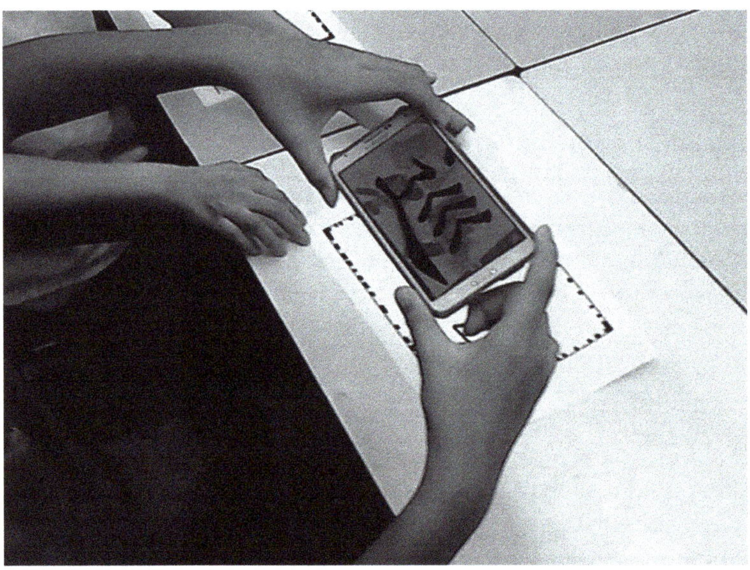

Figure 10.5. Application of MAR in Chinese word learning for ADHD [39]. Reprinted by permission of Taylor & Francis Ltd.

Application of a Chinese words learning module using mobile AR (MAR) towards education of ADHD children is studied in [39]. The study involved two 11-year-old ADHD students with two experienced special education teachers. The study was conducted over the period of three months. Figure 10.5 shows the application of MAR by a student. MAR was found to motivate and increase students' participation during the lesson, which improved their literacy. The teachers also noted that MAR is easy to use and has a positive impact on the students' confidence.

The application of Empowered Brain®, which combines smartglasses with educational modules for coaching of social communication and cognitive skills in reducing the ADHD related symptoms, is studied in [40, 41]. The research involved eight participants with age ranging from 7 to 20 years old. The participants were asked to wear smartglasses, which provide a private augmented reality experience to the wearer (figure 10.6). The augmented reality aims to enhance attention through a gamification approach. The user's attention is tested by providing augmented reality distraction. The findings show the reduction of hyperactivity, inattention and impulsivity symptoms among the participants. A study on the effect of application of the smartglass in socio-emotion coaching for a 13-year-old autism male by the same group of researchers is presented in [42]. The findings show that the technology helps in improving the student's social communication, motivation, cognition, interest and repetitive behaviour. The Face2Face module used encourages the user to maintain face-to-face communication

In [43], a study is conducted focusing on the effect of AR to increase frustration tolerance among ADHD children. Frustration is a negative feeling due to inability of achieving a certain goal. ADHD children are reported to have low frustration tolerance level. The study involved 11 participants using an AR based mathematic module. The findings show that AR positively improves the frustration tolerance of the children and makes the learning session more exciting and enjoyable.

A study conducted in [44] involving four autism students from the age of 5 to 9 years old and four teachers showed positive response from the teachers towards the usage of edutainment in the classroom. The proposed edutainment mechanism includes the usage of AR together with a virtual game, online game and animation. The teachers noted the edutainment potential in improving students' coordination and concentration.

Sinaptiks which is a developer of healthcare mobile application developed mSinaptiks, an eHealth platform [45]. The platform contains various medical and health apps which can be used by a medical practitioner in a face-to-face or remote session with patients. Among the apps on the platform is a VR ADHD assessment

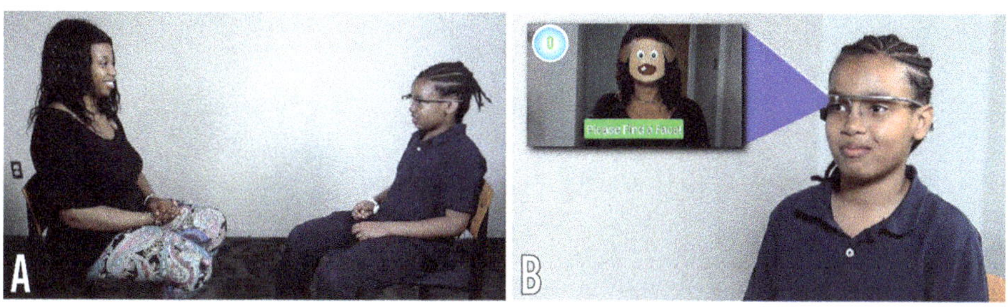

Figure 10.6. Participant wearing smartglass for Empowered Brain® [41]. Reproduced with permission.

tool. The ADHD assessment app has a virtual classroom with a series of distractors to evaluate the attention of the patient (figure 10.7). Similarly, a virtual classroom project for ADHD assessment is proposed at the Virtual Environment Laboratory, University of Southern California [46]. The virtual classroom is designed with three scenarios with different level of distraction. In [47], pre-research on the potential of VR for ADHD therapy is investigated. Two children are involved in the study and it is found that the VR therapy has potential to reduce their inattention, hyperactivity and opposition behaviour.

These projects reviewed here improve the learning process of ADHD students through exciting game-like features which motivate the learner to stay engaged. The sensory element of AR also helps to tackle the inattentiveness of ADHD children and improve their coordination. The collaborative element of AR, on the other hand, assists in enhancing the social skills of the students.

10.4 Challenges

The projects reviewed in section 10.3.1 involve a small number of participants from different ages, therefore, the observation reported could be biased. Despite the many advantages of AR reported by the projects, there are several issues to be taken into consideration for successful adoption of the technology [10, 20, 21, 48, 49]. Among the issues are:

- stable and good internet connection to ensure an uninterrupted session;
- the complexity of the module needs to suit the leaners' capability;
- the teachers need to be trained to use the AR modules so that the learning session can be handled efficiently;

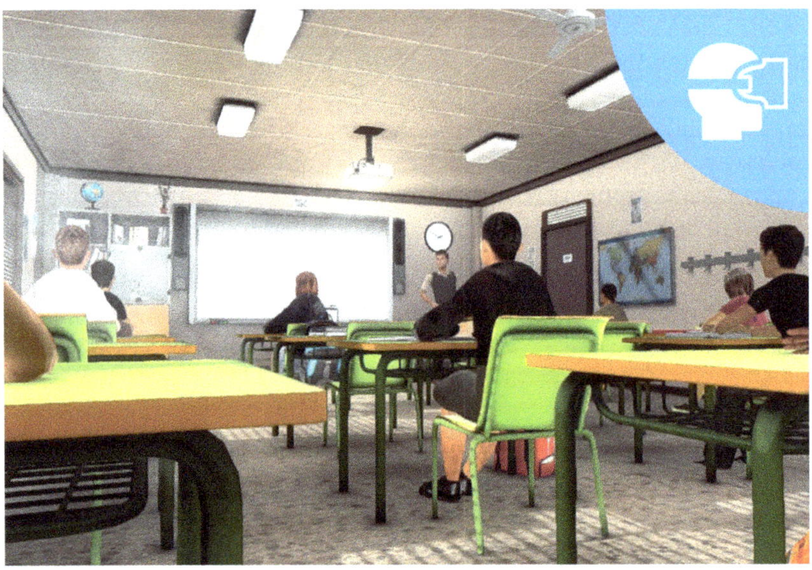

Figure 10.7. mSinaptiks virtual classroom for ADHD assessment [45]. Reproduced with permission.

- a good technical support system is required to address technical problems such as faulty devices;
- balance between the entertainment feature of AR with the content;
- over gamification may lead to binging behaviour that is common among gamers [50];
- to ensure inclusiveness of the solution and readiness of the intended users [51].

Most of the challenges listed above are on ensuring an uninterrupted learning session, as ADHD learners tend to have low attention and frustration levels. An interrupted session, whether due to technical or individual issues, will hamper the benefits of application of AR towards education of ADHD students. Although the entertainment feature of AR is the contributing factor that makes it engaging, as highlighted by [27], fun does not mean that a student is learning effectively. Too much of the fun element could be the cause that distracts a student from the learning content.

Furthermore, caution is needed in terms of ensuring inclusiveness of the solutions for all ADHD students from all economic strata. It cannot be assumed that all of the young generations nowadays are familiar with gadgets, apps, etc. Those that do not have prior access to technology will struggle to use the products, which will only increase the risk of frustration and bringing out their ADHD symptoms.

Digital divide is still a real societal problem around the globe. Assuming equal access and familiarity to technology may only compound further the disadvantages ADHD students from lower income groups have to overcome.

10.5 Conclusion

Multiple works involving the adoption of AR in education specifically for ADHD students have been studied here. Among the benefits of AR are that they are exciting and engaging, and that they promote collaborative, stimulating and immersive learning. The literature reviewed shows that ADHD students are able to learn better, and improve their coordination and social skills through an AR learning module. This work also highlights several issues to be tackled to ensure the benefit of AR based education can be fully gained.

References

[1] American Psychiatric Association 2000 *Diagnostic and Statistical Manual of Mental Disorders* 4th edn (Arlington, VA: American Psychiatric Association) Text Revision

[2] te Meerman S, Batstra L, Grietens H and Frances A 2017 ADHD: a critical update for educational professionals *Int. J. Qual. Stud. Health Well-being* **12** 1298267

[3] Rubia K 2018 Cognitive neuroscience of attention deficit hyperactivity disorder (ADHD) and its clinical translation *Front. Hum. Neurosci.* **12** 1–23

[4] Banaschewski T, Becker K, Döpfner M, Holtmann M, Rösler M and Romanos M 2017 Attention-deficit/hyperactivity disorder *Dtsch. Arztebl. Int.* **114** 149–59

[5] Matthews M, Nigg J T and Fair D A 2013 Attention deficit hyperactivity disorder *Curr. Top. Behav. Neurosci.* **16** 235–66

[6] Singh A, Yeh C J, Verma N and Das A K 2015 Overview of attention deficit hyperactivity disorder in young children *Heal. Psychol. Res.* **3**
[7] Ab Aziz N A, Ab Aziz K, Paul A, Yusof A M and Mohamed Noor N S 2014 Providing augmented reality based education for students with attention deficit hyperactive disorder via cloud computing: its advantages *Int. Conf. on Advanced Communication Technology (ICACT 2012)* pp 577–81
[8] Loe I M and Feldman H M 2007 Academic and educational outcomes of children with ADHD *J. Pediatr. Psychol.* **32** 643–54
[9] Owens J and Jackson H 2017 Attention-deficit/hyperactivity disorder severity, diagnosis, & later academic achievement in a national sample *Soc. Sci. Res.* **61** 251–65
[10] Garzón J, Pavón J and Baldiris S 2019 Systematic review and meta-analysis of augmented reality in educational settings *Virtual Real.* **23** 447–59
[11] Marimon D, Sarasua C, Carrasco P, Álvarez R, Montesa J, Adamek T, Romero I, Ortega M and Gascó P 2010 *MobiAR: Tourist Experiences Through Augmented Reality* (Barcelona: Telefonica Research & Development)
[12] Han D-I, Jung T and Gibson A 2013 Dublin AR: implementing augmented reality in tourism *Information and Communication Technologies in Tourism 2014* ed Z Xiang and I Tussyadiah (Cham: Springer) pp 511–23
[13] Jung T and Han D 2014 Augmented reality (AR) in urban heritage tourism *e-Review Tour. Res.* **5** https://e-space.mmu.ac.uk/id/eprint/608512
[14] Boletsis C and Karahasanovic A 2018 Augmented reality and virtual reality for retail innovation *Magma Tidsskr. økonomi og ledelse.* **7** 49–59
[15] Poushneh A 2018 Augmented reality in retail: a trade-off between user's control of access to personal information and augmentation quality *J. Retail. Consum. Serv.* **41** 169–76
[16] Zhu E, Hadadgar A, Masiello I and Zary N 2014 Augmented reality in healthcare education: an integrative review *PeerJ* **2** e469
[17] Livingston M A, Rosenblum L J, Julier S J, Brown D, Baillot Y, Swan J E II, Gabbard J L and Hix D 2002 An augmented reality system for military operations in urban terrain *Interservice/Industry Training, Simulation, & Education Conf. (I/ITSEC'02)* pp 1–8
[18] Livingston M, Rosenblum L, Brown D, Schmidt G, Julier S, Baillot Y, Swan J E II, Ai Z and Maassel P 2011 Military applications of augmented reality *Handbook of Augmented Reality* ed Borko Furht (Cham: Springer) pp 671–706
[19] Arriaga P, Esteves F and Fernandes S 2013 Playing for better or for worse?: Health and social outcomes with electronic gaming *Handbook of Research on ICTs for Human-Centered Healthcare and Social Care Services* (IGI Global) pp 48–69
[20] Saidin N F, Abd Halim M D and Yahaya N 2015 A review of research on augmented reality in education: advantages and applications *Int. Educ. Stud.* **8** 1–8
[21] Quintero J, Baldiris S, Rubira R, Cerón J and Velez G 2019 Augmented reality in educational inclusion. A systematic review on the last decade *Front. Psychol.* **10** 1–14
[22] Matcha W and Awang Rambli D R 2016 Time on task for collaborative augmented reality in science experiment *J. Teknol.* **78** 137–44
[23] Eh Phon D N, Ali M B and Abd Halim M D 2014 Collaborative augmented reality in education: a review *Proc., 2014 Int. Conf. Teach. Learn. Comput. Eng. LATICE 2014* pp 78–83
[24] Bistaman I N M, Idrus S Z S and Rashid S A 2018 The use of augmented reality technology for primary school education in Perlis, Malaysia *J. Phys. Conf. Ser.* **1019** 012064

[25] Marcel F 2019 Mobile augmented reality learning objects in higher education *Res. Learn. Technol.* **27** 1–10

[26] Weng N, Bee O, Yew L and Hsia T 2016 An augmented reality system for biology science education in Malaysia *Int. J. Innov. Comput.* **6** 8–13

[27] Challenor J and Ma M 2019 A review of augmented reality applications for history education and heritage visualisation *Multimodal Technol. Interact.* **3** 39

[28] Mohamed Noor N, Yusoff F H, Yussof R L and Ismail M 2015 The potential use of augmented reality in gamification *Proc. of the 5th Int. Conf. on Computing and Informatics, ICOCI 2015 (Istanbul, August 2015)* 048

[29] Eleftheria C A, Charikleia P, Iason C G, Athanasios T and Dimitrios T 2013 An innovative augmented reality educational platform using Gamification to enhance lifelong learning and cultural education *Int. Conf. on Information, Intelligence, Systems and Applications (IISA) (Piraeus)* 1–5

[30] Schroeter R, Oxtoby J and Johnson D M 2014 AR and gamification concepts to reduce driver boredom and risk taking behaviours *Proc. of the 6th Int. Conf. on Automotive User Interfaces and Interactive Vehicular Applications. Association for Computing Machinery* pp 244–51

[31] Kapp K M 2012 Games, gamification, and the quest for learner engagement *Train. Dev.* **66** 64–8

[32] Alsawaier R S 2018 The effect of gamification on motivation and engagement International *J. Info. Learning Technol.* **35** 56–79

[33] Sailer M, Hense J U, Mayr S K and Mandl H 2017 How gamification motivates: An experimental study of the effects of specific game design elements on psychological need satisfaction *Comput. Human Behav.* **69** 371–80

[34] Lee J J and Hammer J 2011 Gamification in education: what, how, why bother? *Acad. Exchange Quart.* **15** 2

[35] Avila-Pesantez D, Vaca-Cardenas L, Delgadillo Avila R, Padilla Padilla N and Rivera L 2019 Design of an augmented reality serious game for children with dyscalculia: a case study *Technology Trends CITT 2018* ed M Botto-Tobar, G Pizarro, M Zúñiga-Prieto, M D'Armas and M Zúñiga Sánchez (Communications in Computer and Information Science vol 895) (Cham: Springer)

[36] Avila-pesantez D, Rivera L A, Vaca-cardenas L, Aguayo S and Zuñiga L 2018 Towards the improvement of ADHD children through augmented reality serious games: preliminary results *2018 IEEE Glob. Eng. Educ. Conf.* pp 843–8

[37] Avila-Pesantez D F and Rivera L A 2016 Augmented reality serious games design to improve attention of children with ADHD *IEEE 11th Colombian Computing Conf.* pp 1–3

[38] Abdullah M A and Rambli D R A 2013 *Teaching ADHD Kids Using Augmented Reality* (Petronas: Universiti Teknologi)

[39] Lin C-Y, Yu W J, Chen W-J, Huang C W and Lin C-C 2016 The effect of literacy learning via mobile augmented reality for the students with ADHD and reading disabilities *Universal Access in Human–Computer Interaction. Users and Context Diversity UAHCI 2016* ed M Antona and C Stephanidis (Lecture Notes in Computer Science vol 9739) (Cham: Springer) pp 103–11

[40] Vahabzadeh A, Keshav N U, Abdus-Sabur R, Huey K, Liu R and Sahin N T 2018 Improved socio-emotional and behavioral functioning in students with autism following

school-based smartglasses intervention: multi-stage feasibility and controlled efficacy study *Behav. Sci.* **8** 85

[41] Vahabzadeh A, Keshav N U, Salisbury J P and Sahin N T 2018 Improvement of attention-deficit/hyperactivity disorder symptoms in school-aged children, adolescents, and young adults with autism via a digital smartglasses-based socioemotional coaching aid: Short-term, uncontrolled pilot study *J. Med. Internet Res. Ment. Heal.* **5** 1–13

[42] Sahin N T, Abdus-Sabur R, Keshav N U, Liu R, Salisbury J P and Vahabzadeh A 2018 Augmented reality intervention for social communication in autism in a school classroom: rated by teachers and parents as effective and usable in a controlled, longitudinal pilot study *PsyArXiv* 1–10

[43] Ocay A B, Rustia R A and Palaoag T D 2018 Utilizing augmented reality in improving the frustration tolerance of ADHD learners: an experimental study *Proceedings of the 2nd International Conference on Digital Technology in Education (ICDTE 2018)* (New York: Association for Computing Machinery) pp 58–63

[44] Mohd Yusof A, Daniel E G S, Low W Y, Ab Aziz K and Yingprayoone J 2013 Perception on adapting the edutainment technologies in private special school: Malaysian case study *5th Int. Sci. Soc. Sci. Eng. dan Energy Conf.* pp 1–6

[45] Alsina-Jurnet I, Del Águila F, Peris J and Moreno P 2015 MSinaptiks: an eHealth platform for virtual and augmented reality mobile applications *CEUR Workshop Proc.* 1547 pp 40–6

[46] Rizzo A A, Buckwalter J G, Bowerly T, Van Der Zaag C, Humphrey L, Neumann U, Chua C, Kyriakakis C, Van Rooyen A and Sisemore D 2000 The virtual classroom: a virtual reality environment for the assessment and rehabilitation of attention deficits *Cyberpsychology Behav.* **3** 483–99

[47] Musalek M, Kovar I and Sysala T 2019 Use of virtual reality for the therapy of children with attention deficit hyperactivity disorder *MATEC Web Conf.* **292** 01042

[48] Elmqaddem N 2019 Augmented reality and virtual reality in education. Myth or reality? *Int. J. Emerg. Technol. Learn.* **14** 234–42

[49] Khan T, Johnston K and Ophoff J 2019 The impact of an augmented reality application on learning motivation of students *Adv. Human–Computer Interact.* **2019** 7208494

[50] Welbers K, Konijn E A, Burgers C, de Vaate A B, Eden A and Brugman B C 2019 Gamification as a tool for engaging student learning: A field experiment with a gamified app *E-Learning and Digital Media* **16** 92–109

[51] Ab Aziz K 2016 Convergence and inclusive innovation in the communications sector *18th Int. Conf. on Advanced Communication Technology (ICACT) (Pyeongchang)* pp 218–22

Lightning Source UK Ltd.
Milton Keynes UK
UKHW050747050121
376410UK00004B/100

9 780750 317993